Meditation

To my colleagues

Joan Emerson, Ellen McGrath, Gerald Piaget,
Johanna Shapiro, and Roger Walsh,
who have offered support, firmness,
therapy, and friendship

as we, alone and together,
struggle to

"blend," "time-share," "synthesize,"
"integrate," and/or "transcend"

power and intimacy,
spirituality and the ways of the world. . .

and

to my "babies"

Shauna and Jena, who already know how

Meditation

Self-regulation strategy and altered state of consciousness

Deane H. Shapiro Jr.

AldineTransaction
A Division of Transaction Publishers
New Brunswick (U.S.A.) and London (U.K.)

First paperback printing 2008
Copyright © 1980 Deane H. Shapiro, Jr.

All rights reserved under International and Pan-American Copyright Conven-
tions. No part of this book may be reproduced or transmitted in any form or by
any means, electronic or mechanical, including photocopy, recording, or any
information storage and retrieval system, without prior permission in writing from
the publisher. All inquiries should be addressed to AldineTransaction, A Division
of Transaction Publishers, Rutgers—The State University of New Jersey, 35
Berrue Circle, Piscataway, New Jersey 08854-8042. www.transactionpub.com

This book is printed on acid-free paper that meets the American National Standard for Permanence of Paper for Printed Library Materials.

Library of Congress Catalog Number: 2008016638
ISBN: 978-0-202-36240-3
Printed in the United States of America

Library of Congress Cataloging-in-Publication Data

Shapiro, Deane H.
   Meditation : self-regulation strategy and altered state of consciousness / Deane
   H. Shapiro.
          p. cm.
   Includes bibliographical references and index.
   ISBN 978-0-202-36240-3 (alk. paper)
      1. Meditation. I. Title.

BF637.M4S5 2008
158.1'2--dc22

                                                              2008016638

Table of Contents

Overview   xiii

Preface   xviii

1. Perspectives on Meditation: 1
    Clinical and Psychotherapeutic Applications

2. Meditation and Psychotherapy: 55
    Case Study—James S.

3. A Content Analysis of the Meditation Experience   85

4. Practical Instructions   119

5. Meditation as a Self-Regulation Strategy: 133
    The Empirical Literature

6. A Model for Comparing Self-Regulation Strategies: 163
    Zen Meditation and Behavioral Self-Management,
    A case in point.

7. Meditation as an Altered State of Consciousness   187

8. Components of Meditation   209

9. Mediating Mechanisms   229

10. Methodological Issues in Meditation Research: 253
    An Applied Clinical Model

11. Epilogue: A Personal Essay   265

Appendices   273

A. Motivation, Expectation, Adherence Questionnaire   274

B. Notes   279

C. References   281

Author Index   309

Table and Figures

Chapter One:

Table 1.1   What Effect Does the Teaching of   10-11
Meditation Have on an
Individual Who Practices, and Why?

Table 1.2   Examples of Concentrative Meditation   17

Figure 1.1   A Five-Step Model of Zen Breath Meditation   21

Chapter Two:

Figure 2.1   Sleep: Baseline Data Weeks One and Two   61

Figure 2.2   Weekly Mean of Sleep and Non-Sleep (Hours)   74

Figure 2.3   Nights Per Week Without Valium   75

Table 2.1   Weekly Mean of Sleep, Non-Sleep (in hours),   76
and Number of Times Awoke Total, With Valium
and Without Valium

Figure 2.4   Mean Hours of Sleep and Non-Sleep: 77
With and Without Valium

Chapter Three:

Table 3.1   Coding Instrument   96

Table 3.2   Percent of Breath Blocks: Thought   98
and Non-Thought (By Session)

Figure 3.1   Percent of Breath Blocks: Thought and Non-Thought   98

Figure 3.2   Mean Time of Breaths in Thought and Non-Thought   99
Blocks/Session

Table 3.3   Mean Time of Breaths in Thought and Non-Thought   100
Blocks/Session

Figure 3.3   Mean Time of Breaths, In Seconds: 101
Comparison of Cycles Within Session

Table 3.4	Mean Time of Breaths, In Seconds: Comparison of Cycles, Within Session	102
Figure 3.4	Percentage of Thought and Non-Thought Blocks/Cycle: Mean Across All Ten Sessions	103
Table 3.5	Thought and Non-Thought Blocks per Cycle	104-105
Figure 3.5	Percent of Breath Blocks/Session of Positive, Negative, and Neutral Thoughts	107
Table 3.6	Percent of Breath Blocks/Session of Positive, Negative, and Neutral Thoughts	108
Table 3.7	Number of Thoughts (and Percentage) Across Ten Sessions, Per Coding Category	108
Table 3.8	More Detailed Breakdown of Category II: "Thoughts Related to Task at Hand"	110
Figure 3.6	Percent of Positive, Negative, and Neutral Thoughts in Each Cycle	111
Table 3.9	Percent of Positive, Negative, and Neutral Thoughts in Each Cycle	111

Chapter Five:

Table 5.1	Studies on Fears and Phobias, Stress and Tension Management	136-138
Table 5.2	Studies on Addictions: Drugs/Cigarettes/Alcohol	143
Table 5.3	Studies on Hypertension	145
Table 5.4	Summary of Indian Yogic Tradition Based Partially on Woolfolk (1975)	147
Table 5.5	Summary of Studies of Transcendental Meditation Based Partially on Woolfolk (1975)	148-149
Table 5.6	Summary of Studies of Zen Meditation Based Partially on Woolfolk (1975)	150
Table 5.7	Summary of Studies Comparing Meditation with Other Self-Regulation Strategies: Physiological Measures	155-156
Table 5.8	Summary of Studies Comparing Meditation with Other Self-Regulation Strategies: Clinical Measures	158

Chapter Six:

| Table 6.1 | Meditation and Behavioral Self-Control: Comparison and Contrast | 178-181 |

Chapter Seven:
Table 7.1   Subjective Changes Following Meditation   200-201
Table 7.2   Studies on Attention and Perception   203

Chapter Eight:
Figure 8.1   An Omni-Determinism Model of Mediating   211
               Mechanisms of Meditation
Table 8.1   Meditation: An Omni-Determinism Analysis   213

Chapter Ten:
Figure 10.1   An Interactive Systems Theory Model for   255
               Utilizing Meditation as a Self-Control
               Technique in the Management of a Clinical Problem

Acknowledgements

I wish to thank the following:

—Those journals, where my articles have previously appeared, for permission to reprint portions.

—Ann Reeder, for her perseverance, care, and thoroughness in typing the numerous drafts of this manuscript as it evolved over the past several years, and to Susan Fontana for her extra help and effort in the final months of the book.

—David Giber, for his work on the tables in Chapters Five and Seven; Roger Walsh for his work on tables in Chapter Five; Don Hansen and David Bezanson for their help in the data analysis of the article in Chapter Three; and David Bezanson for his technical assistance on the bibliography and text.

—Ted Barber, David Bezanson, Albert Ellis, Robert Kantor, Ellen McGrath, Gerald Piaget, Gary Schwartz and his student William Pelonsky, Johanna Shapiro, John Smolowe, Miles Vich, and Roger Walsh for their generosity of time in offering comments on previous drafts of this book.

—John Wander, at Aldine, who encouraged me to take the risk, and produce this volume as an accompaniment to the volume of edited readings.

—Two Laguna Beach Bakeries:
Renaissance Bakery, for whole wheat croissants.
Scandia Bakery for poppyseed cake; and both for table space to work on this manuscript!

Portions of this book have appeared in previous articles in the following journals:

New England Journal of Medicine
Archives of General Psychiatry
American Psychologist
Behavior Therapy
Journal of Humanistic Psychology
Journal of Transpersonal Psychology
*Psychologia: An International Journal of Psychology
   in the Orient*

and in presentations made at state, regional, and/or national meetings of the following organizations:

American Association for the Advancement of Science
American Psychological Association
Association for the Advancement of Behavior Therapy
American Education Research Association
Association of Humanistic Psychology
Association of Transpersonal Psychology

Partial support for the writing has come from funds through the National Institute of Mental Health under contract No. 278-77-0040LSM, *Holistic Medicine;* and funds through the National Institute of Education under contract No. NE-C-00-30061.

Although every effort has been made to review all the experimental literature on meditation published in the major English language journals, because of the ever-present problem of time lag while a book is in press (and as a temper to obsessive-compulsive tendencies), a cut-off date was needed, and some studies may have been missed. I apologize to those whose recent efforts are not included, and, while promising their inclusion in future revisions, I can only hope that the main themes discussed in this volume are based upon a body of evidence sufficient to provide a comprehensive overview of the current state of the art.

Overview

Preface

THE PREFACE cites the four goals for the book: 1) Providing a comprehensive scientific approach to meditation; 2) Showing its clinical applications — indications and contraindications (bridging research literature and clinical practice); 3) Pointing out potential blinders to scientific study of meditation; and 4) Combining the scientific approach with a personal one.

CHAPTER ONE: *Perspectives on Meditation:*
Clinical and Psychotherapeutic Applications.

Chapter One poses the question which provides the structure for the book: What *Effect* does the *Teaching* of *Meditation* have on the *Individuals* who *Practice* it. After exploring potential areas of paradigm clash and overviewing the book, I examined each of the key words in this sentence. *Effects:* Positive and adverse effects are mentioned. *Teaching:* The therapist's orientation is discussed from a psychoanalytic, humanistic, behavioral, and transpersonal perspective. Further topics include the role of relationship; resistance and (counter) transference; the qualities of the "good" therapist; and whether meditation might be useful for the therapist; adverse effects, and how the therapist deals with them. *Meditation:* A working definition is offered; different types of meditation are reviewed and comments made on the difference between meditation as a self-regulation strategy and as an altered state of consciousness. *Individuals:* A discussion of the literature bearing on who seeks out meditation and why? What is their motivation? Are they a particular, definable subpopulation? Of those who begin to meditate, who drop out, who continue? Of those who continue, who have a "successful" experience; who have "adverse" experiences? *Practice:* Issues of adherence and compliance are explored, including the importance of practice to the outcome of treatment.

CHAPTER TWO: *Meditation as a Self-Regulation Strategy: Case Study—James Sidney.*

This case explores in practical terms issues raised in Chapter One. The therapist's orientation, and belief in the efficacy of the strategy are noted; and the client's background, presenting problem, expectation and motivations are explored. Baseline information is gathered on client concerns—insomnia, assertiveness, social skills, general stress, and job—and both meditative and non-meditative interventions utilized. Specific indications and contraindications of meditation for this client are cited, and the role of relationship issues, selection of a meditation technique, and use of a tape are discussed. Results are presented as well as a discussion of whether meditation and therapy worked effectively for this client, and if so, why.

CHAPTER THREE: *Meditation as an Altered State of Consciousness: Case Study— A Content Analysis of the Meditation Experience.*

This chapter explores the importance of phenomenologically based research and cites previous research on the phenomenology of meditation. Four hypotheses are generated regarding thoughts (images, sensations) and non-thoughts during meditation, and the affect associated with them—positive, negative, neutral. Subject background, including type and length of meditation; adherence and compliance; initial motivation and commitment (maintenance of the practice) are cited. The setting, procedures, coding instrument are presented, followed by results, discussion and implications of the case-study experiment.

CHAPTER FOUR: *Practical Instructions.*

Practical instructions for a breath meditation technique are presented. Topics include how to present meditation to the client; cultic versus non-cultic meditation; specific instructions; issues of generalization and adherence; more advanced meditative techniques; ways to combine informal meditation with behavioral self-control skills; and a note to therapists on evaluation.

CHAPTER FIVE: *Meditation as a Self-Regulation Strategy: The Empirical Literature.*

This chapter contains a brief definition of a self-regulation strategy and a description of "round one" literature showing meditation's effect on stress and stress disorders, psychotherapy, the addictions, hypertension, and physiological changes. The second section of the chapter describes the "round two" literature comparing meditation with other self-regulation strategies, both physiologically and clinically.

CHAPTER SIX: *A Model for Comparing Self-Regulation Strategies: Meditation and Behavioral Self-Control— A Case in Point.*

A rationale for comparing self-regulation strategies is offered, followed by a discussion of different behavioral self-management techniques and a comparison with meditation: behavioral self-observation, self-evaluation, goal setting, environmental planning (stimulus control) and behavioral programming. Ways for clinically combining behavioral self-control strategies with formal and informal meditation are discussed and a therapeutic rationale offered.

CHAPTER SEVEN: *Meditation as an Altered State of Consciousness: The Empirical Literature.*

A working definition of altered state of consciousness is offered, followed by a discussion of problems in studying altered states, as well as approaches available. Research bearing on the following topics is then presented: subjective experiences during meditation, concurrent validity for subjective experiences, subjective reports of changes in attitude and perceptions after meditation, and non-self-reported indications of attitude and perceptual change. Implications of these findings are discussed.

CHAPTER EIGHT: *Components of Meditation.*

A contextual model of omni-determinism—mutual causality among multiple parts, in which behavior (meditation), environment, and the person all interact with each other—is presented. Then, the components of meditation are reviewed, including the following: antecedent variables of preparation and environmental planning and components of the behavior itself; physical posture (or movement)—lotus versus half-lotus versus sitting—; attentional focus and style; and breathing. The following questions are explored. Which posture is most stable for whom? What is the relationship between practice and attention, between the ability to attend, and clinical improvement? How important is the object of attention? mantra versus non-mantra? What is the most suitable style of attention—e.g., active or passive?

CHAPTER NINE: *Mediating Mechanisms.*

A summary overview of the mechanisms posited to mediate meditation effects is cited. Then this chapter looks at *physiological mechanisms:* general constellations of change, specific variables (e.g., oxygen consumption; skeletal relaxation), ergotropic/trophetropic states. Also considered is the role of *cognitive mechanisms* including expectation effects and demand characteristics; and finally *attentional mechanisms;* active versus passive attention; deautomization; the role of discrimination; the information-processing literature; global desensitization. The chapter concludes with a discussion of the technique-specific and state-specific nature of mechanisms.

CHAPTER TEN: *Methodological Issues in Meditation Research: An Applied Clinical Model.*

This chapter outlines an interactive model for applied clinical research on meditation. Issues include the need for a precise theoretical rationale between the independent and dependent variables; care in matching treatment strategy to the clinical concern of a particular individual; care in noting indications and contraindications for treatment; more precise specification of both the independent and the dependent variables; relevance of data-gathering strategies (group design or N = 1); and comments about the philosophy of science in relation to meditation research.

CHAPTER ELEVEN: *Epilogue: A Personal Essay.*

A personal offering of unanswered questions with regard to meditation in general and this book in particular. Issues focused on include the struggle of how to integrate a scientific approach with a personal one without doing a disservice to both; the role of ego; the difficulty of "practicing what you preach"; and a discussion of the tasks that are left, the challenges that remain.

APPENDIX

The Appendices consist of a Motivation, Expectation, Adherence Questionnaire—(Appendix A); and the references for the book—(Appendix B), including 424 references.

A NOTE ON FURTHER READING

For individuals who wish more in-depth reading, there is a list of suggested readings at the end of all chapters (except the two case studies, Chapters Two and Three, and the methodological and personal summaries, Chapters Ten and Eleven).

Many of these suggested readings—both reprints and original articles—may be found in the forthcoming volume, D.H. Shapiro and R.N. Walsh (Eds.), *The Science of Meditation*, New York: Aldine, 1980.

Preface

I BEGAN THIS BOOK with three goals. First, I wanted to provide a book which offered the most comprehensive, up-to-date, scientific approach available to the study of meditation. That book became the product of over three and one-half years preparation and involved reading every scientific article on meditation published in any major English language journal.

Second, based on my research, training, and experience as a clinical psychologist and behavioral scientist, I wanted the book to show the potential health-care, medical, and therapeutic uses of meditation: both indications and contraindications. As more and more people begin to meditate in our culture, sensitive clinicians and therapists are faced with the need to know about the nature of meditation, both its positive and adverse effects.

Although there has been a dramatic increase in the number of meditation studies, the quality remains variable; many of them are trivial, and most remain unreplicated. In addition, meditation research has been plagued by insubstantial theorizing, global claims, and the substitution of belief systems for grounded hypotheses. With this in mind, I hope this book can puncture some of the myths.

For example, some hold meditation to be a global panacea, though it is unlikely that any unimodal technique will ever be the treatment of choice for all clinical problems. Not only does meditation not serve all populations equally well, but its varying components may not all be equally effective. How is the clinician to know which of the plethora of different meditative techniques to use? Or, how to choose between meditation and an alternative form of self-regulation such as biofeedback, hypnosis, autogenic training, behavioral self-control? Clinicians need to know *when* meditation will be useful for themselves, for *which* of their clients, for *which* clinical problems. They need to know how meditation compares in terms of effectiveness with other self-regulation strategies. Further, they must know when their patients misuse it.

By attempting to provide a well-reasoned, objective critique of the literature, this book tries to answer the above questions as completely as currently possible while attempting to support and provide impetus for a thorough follow-through where more information is needed, as suggested by the American Psychiatric Association, (1977):

> "the Association strongly recommends that research be undertaken in the form of well controlled studies to evaluate the specific usefulness, indications and contraindications of various meditation techniques. The research should compare the various forms of meditation with one another and with psychotherapeutic and psychopharmacological modalities" (p. 720).

To facilitate this effort, in each of the chapters there is a discussion of the major questions to be addressed, followed by a detailing and critique of important theoretical, clinical, and research issues. In several instances the reader will find to his or her chagrin as well as, I can assure you, mine, that questions seem to beget questions: research bearing upon certain issues may be contradictory, or not yet of sufficient thoroughness. In these cases, I have tried to suggest the specific kinds of future research necessary to resolve the current issues. In this way we can determine which claims about meditation are justified, and which are not.

I hope this approach can help provide a bridge between research and clinical practice. Currently the profession of psychology itself is, and has been, in a polarized debate between the "practitioners" and the "experimentalists." The latter accuse the former of being "soft, non-empirical, non-scientific," while the practitioners accuse the experimentalists of conducting research which is essentially irrelevant to human concerns. On the one hand, this book attempts to look at issues in a refined "reductionistic" way; however, at the same time, it attempts to show the practical applications of the research and not lose sight of the human perspective.

The third goal I have for this book is to shed light upon potential biases we as Western scientists might have in approaching meditation as an area of study and to help to prevent what I might call a meditation backlash. In other words, once it is seen that meditation is not a panacea, I am concerned that it might be totally dismissed by the scientific community as a useless curiosity at best, or as a harmful, illusory artifact of morbid psychological processes at worst. In light of these biases, it is well to remember that biases against altered-state phenomena are not new, that during most of the last century hypnosis was regarded by the scientific establishment as illusory, that those physicians who practiced it were considered suspect and were unable to have their papers accepted by any reputable scientific or medical journal. The power of this bias was such that some patients were accused of maliciously colluding with surgeons in pretending to feel no pain while major amputations were performed on them. Biases against meditation are likely to prove just as harmful to science and psychotherapy as uncritical enthusiasm.

Therefore, as we look at these claims and counterclaims, I believe we must be aware that caution is needed "on both sides." We the scientists need to critically examine the data to temper others' uncritical enthusiasm and evangelic fervor. Yet we must also be cautious of our own cultural blinders and the resultant potential paradigm clashes when we try to place meditation within our scientific clinical perspective. Meditation is a technique developed within a religious/philosophical framework to give individuals a new sense of self-understanding and meaning, a harmony within themselves, and with the world around them. It should be noted that this book deals only briefly with the theoretical values and goals of meditation, and the background of Eastern psychology and philosophy which provided the context and *raison d'etre* of meditation (see Shapiro, 1978b for a more detailed discussion). Some of the issues of potential paradigm clash are raised in Part I, and one subtitle of the book—Self-Regulation Strategy and Altered State of Consciousness—is my attempt to make this potential clash explicit. The West primarily views meditation as a possible self-regulation strategy for use in clinical problems. The East sees meditation as a vehicle for altered states of consciousness and enlightenment, be it called *Nirvana, Satori, Kensho,* or *Samadhi.* We must become aware of and acknowledge these differences and their potential hindrance in our efforts to study meditation.

Finally, in the course of writing the book a fourth goal has evolved. About two years ago, having already spent nearly a year and a half on the book, I became aware of it, a goal somewhat difficult for me to articulate. I realized that the first two, and to a certain extent the third, goals of this book remain firmly within the orthodox scientific tradition. I have great respect for the utility and necessity of that approach. But I became conscious of certain general, and for a book of this nature particular limitations. For example, how could I presume to be able to *objectively* and scientifically read and report on the meditation literature? Call it authorship bias if you will, but clearly the fact that I lived for fifteen months in the Orient studying Zen and Eastern thought and that I have now meditated on a regular basis for nearly ten years would surely influence my reading and interpretation of the data. Further, my personal background and experience was one of the critical motivations in my interest to write a book of this nature in the first place. Finally, I became aware that a complete understanding of meditation was *not* going to come from keeping my own personal meditation experiences separate from my scientific study through research and writing. Though this insight may seem trivial to some, for me it was a difficult one, one which caused me much fear. During my meditation training I had been admonished repeatedly as to the danger of analysis and intellectual endeavors, and I feared that I would be in danger of placing my personal meditation experience in the service of science, thus sabotaging that experience. I decided to take that risk, and, therefore, the fourth goal involves having the book provide a model for what I have termed a "scientific/personal" exploration. I do not mean to imply by this term that the book will involve a review of my "personal" meditation journals. I do not yet feel ready for that intimacy with an audience. However, I did want to become more a part of the book (or acknowledge where I already had, but was not aware of it). The clearest examples of this occur in Chapters Two (where I am the therapist); Chapter Three (where I am the subject) and in the "Epilogue: A Personal Essay" where I try to share some of the implications of this new model. I realize this is only a beginning effort, and ask the readers to be gentle in their critiques, as it still feels a somewhat vulnerable experiment.

From a personal standpoint, as I noted earlier, I am just as concerned about exaggerating meditation's benefits as I am about uncritical dismissal. The book strives for an accurate appraisal between these two extremes—what might be called Buddha's Middle Way and what I have called a scientific and personal exploration. I am trying, in the best tradition of the philosophy of science, to tread a middle ground: acknowledging where we do not have the conceptual, methodological, and research tools to ferret out the experiential subtleties and delicacies of meditation, and where meditation does or does not meet its purported claims. It is my contention that it is only this middle way which will prevent us from doing a disservice to both the spiritual disciplines of the East and the scientific research of the West.

At this point I need to acknowledge, in light of the scientific/ personal exploration, a certain hubris in deciding to write a book on the state of the art of meditation. On the one hand, since meditation is purported to have a pronounced effect on human attitudes and behavior, it is certainly a subject worth close scientific examination. On the other, one wonders, for example, what relevance this book might have for yogins or Zen masters.

At times, during the writing, I empathized with the sentiments expressed by e.e. cummings in his poem, "oh sweet spontaneous," in which the probing fingers of researchers and philosophers analyze and dissect the meaning and significance of the seasons, and the earth responds with a flower. There often seemed a contradiction in analyzing and dissecting a technique which was developed in the Eastern philosophical and religious tradition as a means for learning sensitive, non-analytical, non-verbal living in the here and now. I believe that all of us who study and practice meditation need to be careful that the research and methodological analysis do not obscure and distort the very essence of the technique which we are attempting to study.

I believe that a balance between these two poles—scientific analysis and experiential (personal) knowledge—is not only possible but also necessary. To this balance, this middle way, this book is dedicated.

                              D.H.S.
                              Palo Alto and Laguna Beach

Perspectives
on Meditation:
Clinical and
Psychotherapeutic Applications

What effect does the teaching of meditation have on an
individual who practices?

1.1 Effects

AT FIRST GLANCE, the answer to this question would be an overwhelming "several!" A brief review of the literature reveals that meditation has been found to influence an impressive number of different outcome criteria in a positive direction. For example, meditation has been shown to be effective for clinical concerns such as stress, substance abuse, fears and phobias (Shapiro & Giber, 1978), psychosomatic complaints (Udupa, 1973, Vahia et al., 1973), reduction of neuroticism and

1

depression (Ferguson & Gowan, 1976; Vahia et al., 1973), increasing congruence between a person's real and ideal self (Bono, 1980 in press), fostering self-actualization (Seeman, Nidich & Banta, 1972; Nidich, Seeman & Dreskin, 1973), helping an individual develop a sense of personal meaning in the world (Osis et al., 1973; Kohr, 1977; Goleman, 1971), a sense of personal responsibility (Shapiro, 1978a, 1980 in press), increased internal locus of control (Hjelle, 1974), and an increase of positive self-statements, feelings of creativity, and a concomittant decrease of negative self-statements (Shapiro, 1978a).

In addition to the literature on positive effects, there has recently been a small, though growing literature suggesting some of the adverse effects which might occur with meditation (e.g., French et al., 1975; Lazarus, 1976; Otis, 1980 in press).

1.2 Clinician's/Trainer's Orientation

BECAUSE OF THE broad range of positive effects meditation seems to produce with different dependent variables, clinicians and therapists from several orientations have been attracted to it. Some have conceptualized it as a self-regulation strategy useful in behavioral medicine (Stroebel & Glueck, 1977; Schwartz & Weiss, 1977), or as a clinical tool for anxiety and the addictions within the behavioral framework (Shapiro & Zifferblatt, 1976a; Shapiro, 1978b, Berwick & Oziel, 1973; Woolfolk & Franks, 1980 in press). Some have conceptualized it as a useful means of becoming aware of one's own self-actualizing nature, of developing increased congruence between one's real and ideal self, as a way of taking more responsibility for one's life and therefore useful in humanistic psychotherapy for clients and therapists (e.g., Keefe, 1975; Schuster, 1979; Lesh, 1970); as an integral part of holistic medicine (e.g., Hastings & Fadiman, 1980 in press). Others have conceptualized meditation as an "evocative" strategy which allows repressed material to come forth from the unconscious (e.g., Carrington & Ephron, 1975) and allows for controlled regression in the service of the ego (e.g., Shafii, 1973); and as therefore useful from a psychoanalytic viewpoint. From another viewpoint, meditation has been conceptualized as a technique that helps individuals let go of thoughts, become relatively egoless, yielding, present centered; and is therefore useful in transpersonal psychotherapy (e.g., Weide, 1973; Goleman, 1971; Clark, 1977; Shapiro, 1978b; Walsh & Vaughan, 1980).

From a historical perspective, this interest in meditation and Eastern thought by Western scientists and health-care professionals is relatively recent. For example, a little over thirty years ago Carl Jung (1947) wrote a foreword to D.T. Suzuki's *Introduction to Zen*. This represented one of the first attempts by a psychologically trained Westerner to interact with and write about Eastern thought and philosophy. And as recently as the late sixties, Charles Tart (1969) noted in his book on altered states that by including two articles on meditation, he was including two thirds of the published English-language experimental work. Since Tart's book, and a related book edited by Robert Ornstein (1972), the scientific literature on meditation has increased exponentially. Further, there have been increased attempts to look for theoretical insights, combinations, and blendings between Eastern thought and Western psychology, ranging across many theoretical orientations from Sullivanian interpersonal theory (e.g., Stunkard, 1951) through psychoanalysis (e.g., Fromm, 1960) and existentialism (e.g., Boss, 1965) to behavior therapy (e.g., Shapiro, 1978b).

Why this sudden interest? It appears that Western scientists and health care professionals have begun to look seriously at Eastern techniques such as meditation for four primary reasons. First, the interest of the Western scientific community was catalyzed in the mid 1960's by reports from India and the Orient detailing extraordinary feats of bodily control and altered states of consciousness by meditation masters (Wenger & Bagchi, 1961; Gundu Rao et al., 1958; Kasamatsu et al., 1957; Anand, Chinna & Singh, 1961b). These reports from the East were not summarily dismissed because they paralleled a rather major shift in Western scientific *zeitgeist* and models. For example, Miller and DiCara, among others, were showing that voluntary control of the autonomic nervous system was possible (Miller, 1969; Di Cara, 1970; Shapiro, Tursky & Schwartz, 1970; DiCara & Weiss, 1969); and Tart (1971) was pointing out how a variety of arcane, seemingly incomprehensible phenomena of non-Western psychologies could be rendered understandable within the framework of state-dependent technologies. Further, increased sophistication in scientific instrumentation gave rise to the possibility of replicating and substantiating these anecdotal reports.

Second, there is a growing dissatisfaction among health-care professionals in our culture who find themselves treating stress-related disorders with pharmacological solutions (cf. Glueck & Stroebel, 1975, Benson, 1975). This has resulted in attempts to find non-drug-related self-regulation strategies by which individuals may learn to better manage their own internal and external behaviors. Meditation is viewed as one such potential self-regulation strategy.

Although Western psychology and psychiatry were born out of a concern with pathology (e.g., Freud's index contains four-hundred references to neurosis and none to health; *all* the psychiatric diagnostic categories of the DSM [Diagnostical and Statistical Manual] are pathological), recently there has been a shift in interest toward exploring positive mental health (e.g., Maslow, 1968; Walsh & Shapiro, 1980). There is a recognition of the self-fulfilling power of scientific models in general (Kuhn, 1971) and of models of the person in particular (Bandura, 1974). This interest in models of positive health has led to a turning to other traditions, such as the Eastern, in which years of effort have already been expended toward developing and seeking to implement an expanded vision of our human potential.

Fourth, many individuals in this society are looking for values and meaning alternative to those of our competitive, fast-paced technological culture, and the Eastern tradition offers them one such alternative. A Gallup Poll in November, 1976 noted that nearly eight percent of the American population—sixteen million people—were involved with Eastern disciplines and Eastern techniques such as meditation and yoga. Further, according to the Transcendental Meditation organization, as of December, 1978 more than one million Westerners had been instructed in the specific TM practice. This large number of individuals provides Western science with a potential subject pool of meditators instructed in a standardized practice, thereby facilitating opportunities for research. Finally, more and more researchers, clinicians, and health-care professionals either meditate themselves or come into contact with clients or patients who do, and therefore need to be at least conversant with the meditation literature.

1.3 Areas of Potential Paradigm Clash: Science, Religion, Experience and Analysis

WHEN WE, as Western scientists and clinicians, attempt to understand, study, and/or utilize, either personally or professionally, a technique which originated in a different philosophical and cultural framework, some problems may occur. Although we may not be able to totally avoid them, a certain sensitivity to their potential existence becomes important.

First, it is critical to acknowledge that both science and religion are based upon belief systems. Acknowledging that religion is based on quite a strong belief system—i.e. faith—scientists are often less willing to acknowledge their own preconceptions—"paradigms"—of the world (Kuhn, 1971, Tart, 1972; Polanyi, 1958). These "scientific" belief systems (concepts, models, paradigms) not only may affect the *content* of what is observed, but also the *process* by which it is observed and interpreted. They may act as self-fulfilling prophetic filters for experimental and experiential knowledge, acquisitions, and interpretations.

Infrequently recognized by Western science, two basic types of knowledge exist—1) experiential (non-symbolic, direct) and 2) map knowledge (cartographic, conceptual, symbolic, inferential) —and three modes of knowledge acquisition: 1) physical (science), 2) conceptual (philosophy), and 3) contemplative (religion, spiritualism). Failure to recognize these fundamental distinctions results in a variety of errors (called category errors) which result in miscommunication and misunderstanding between Eastern and Western approaches (Wilbur, 1977).

For example, scientists attempt to gain conceptual knowledge of phenomena. This involves setting up hypotheses, hypothetico-deductive reasoning, empirical testing, and evaluation of results. From this process, we gain a map, primarily in linguistic or symbolic form. The meditation traditions point out the critical difference between conceptual and experiential knowledge and the danger of confusing them (category error) or of obliterating the experiential by the conceptual. They state that only through direct experience can "true" reality be understood. As D.T. Suzuki noted (1956, p. 9), true understanding involves, "a special transmission outside the scriptures: no dependence on words or letters." Lao-tsu observed (1972, p. 56):

> Those who know do not talk.
> Those who talk do not know.

The type of approach represented by Lao-tsu, Suzuki and the meditation traditions in general is a scientist's nightmare. How can we form testable hypotheses about experiences which cannot be conceptualized or talked about, and in which the practitioners themselves say that any attempt to analyze will cause one to completely lose the experience itself? This is a real dilemma. Unfortunately, scientists have often reacted by dismissing mystical experiences as "epiphenomena" not worthy of consideration, or by trying to place those experiences within their own Western paradigm, and calling them delusional, psychotic, catatonia-like (e.g., Alexander, 1931; Group for Advancement of Psychiatry Report, 1977).

The mystical traditions, on the other hand, have for the most part ignored scientific analysis and therefore have no scientific frame of reference for evaluating the efficacy of their hypotheses and practices. Scientists are expected to use the data from their research to evaluate the veracity of their hypotheses, and where data do not accord with belief, change their beliefs. Those who believe only on faith, use data (whether confirming or negating their beliefs) as a means of strengthening what they already believe.

Can these two models complement each other? Although my belief is that they should, the task is not easy. First and foremost, the very act of translating "holistic" (direct, non-symbolic knowledge) experiences into verbalizations about these experiences (symbolic, cartographic, knowledge by inference) is fraught with difficulty (Franks, 1977), perhaps analogous to the difficulties encountered in quantum physics in measuring the properties of a subatomic particle (e.g., Heisenberg, 1963). As soon as one begins to analyze one's "altered state," it changes. Therefore, the Eastern tradition is correct in admonishing us not to equate conceptual knowledge with subjective experience.

Nevertheless, it is true that the two modes may complement each other. For example, we may use pinpointed analysis to learn more precisely about the subjective experience of meditation

(Osis et al., 1973) and how these experiences are influenced by a subject's anxiety level, prior meditative experience, and adherence to meditation (e.g., Kohr, 1977). This can help us better teach and transmit the technique of meditation. Conversely, the experiential knowledge gained from practicing meditation can help us develop more sophisticated and sensitive research hypotheses and methodologies for scientific study.

What seems critical at this point is a complementary science which combines the experience of the practitioner with the experimental rigor of the researcher. Especially in studying meditation research and its clinical applications, we need to be careful not to make two errors: a) scientific and conceptual study without experiential knowledge; or b) experiential practice without scientific evaluation.

As scientists, we need to honestly and openly look with precision at the variables involved in the phenomena we are studying. In the case of meditation, this analysis does not need to negate the poetic, transcendent qualities and the visionary experiences that can occur. Although reading and writing about meditation are not meditation, I believe it is possible to feel and live the experiential and poetic *and* also be willing to honestly assess and evaluate the nature and causes of those effects. The scientific tradition requires this level of openness and intellectual honesty in its practitioners.

1.4 Overview of the book

WITH THE ABOVE context in mind, let us return to the question with which we opened this chapter: What *effect* does the *teaching* of *meditation* have on an *individual* who *practices?* What is the best way to answer this question? The approach utilized in this book is to look in a very precise, fine-tuned way at the key words of the sentence: 1. effect; 2. teaching; 3. meditation; 4. individual; and 5. practices. A useful analogy is to look at this sentence and these words under a microscope. We begin the inspection at a low power and then subject it to increasingly higher and more detailed examination.

For example, we have already looked briefly at the first key word in our sentence *effects* (Chapter One, 1.1). We then need to review in more detail the question does meditation work? For what types of concern? In Chapter Five we attempt to define self-regulation and then look at meditation as a self-regulation strategy to see its clinical effects for stress management, psychotherapy, dealing with the addictions, decreasing hypertension, and its general physiological effects. We then ask the next level of questions: How do the effects of meditation compare with other self-regulation strategies on these clinical and physiological parameters? Is meditation unique? How different is it from other self-regulation techniques? In Chapter Six we offer a model for comparing self-regulation strategies. We then attempt to define "altered states" and look at meditation as an altered state of consciousness to determine subjective experiences during meditation, concurrent validity for these changes, and subjective changes following meditation (Chapter Seven).

The next key word is *teaching*. Here we need to explore two issues. First, we need to look at the teacher's (psychotherapist's, clinician's, guru's) orientation. What are the teacher's hopes, expectations (demand characteristics) in teaching the strategy? What is the teacher's experience and style of teaching? A related issue is the *relationship*. Here we need to look at issues of trust and confidentiality, the establishment of rapport, the length of the therapeutic contact, how issues of resistance* and transference*/counter-transference are dealt with. We briefly mentioned the issue of therapist orientation in Chapter One (1.2) and will explore issues related to teaching in more detail at the end of this chapter (1.11-1.13).

The third key word is *meditation*. We initially (Chapter One, 1.3) ask the basic question of what is meditation and attempt to develop a working definition. We explore different types of formal meditation and the difference between formal and informal meditation. Finally, still at a basic level, we offer a model to describe the different levels or depths of the meditation experience. Later (Chapter Eight) we refine our analysis even more and discuss the different components of meditation. For example,

---

*I do not use these terms in their classical Freudian sense (1912). They refer here to patient/client resistance to learning the technique; and student/ teacher, client/clinician issues of a *general* interpersonal nature that might effect treatment outcome.

we look at the antecedent or preparatory variables, and at the components of the behavior itself: attentional focus and style, posture, breathing. We do this in order to further our understanding of which components of the descriptive label "meditation" may be active in determining treatment effects and which inert.

The fourth key word is *individual*. What is the psychological profile of the person who wants to learn meditation? What are his/her expectations, initial motivations? What is the profile of the person who drops out of meditation, the person who continues, the person who continues and has "successful" outcome (Chapter One 1.8-1.9)?

The fifth word we look at is *practice*. This involves questions of prior experience, adherence and compliance, nature and length of practice, and intensity of effort directed toward the training (Chapter One, 1.10).

The above five issues, though presented separately, obviously interact. For example, the orientation of the psychotherapist/ spiritual teacher who is presenting the technique determines what effects are being sought. The motivation of the individual effects the length of practice and adherence to the technique, etc.

In Chapter Eight, we present a general systems model of reciprocal interaction and omni-determinism to help give a context to our discussion and to show the way these different topics interact. Finally, in Chapter Nine, *Mediating Mechanisms,* we look at the question of "why" the practice of meditation does (or does not) have an effect on an individual. We look in particular at physiological, cognitive, and attentional mediating mechanisms.

The above material provides an overview for the issues we are going to deal with throughout the book. Table 1.1, summarizing the issues embodied in the sentence, *What effect does the teaching of meditation have on an individual who practices, and why?* may be useful for the reader to refer to in order to maintain an overview of the structure of the book.

The first part of this chapter (1.1, 1.2) looked briefly at the effects of meditation and the therapist's orientation. The rest of the chapter provides a brief overview for the remaining parts of the sentence; therefore, let us now turn to the question of "What is meditation?"

What *Effect*[1] does the *Teaching*[2] of *Meditation*[3] have on an *Individual*[4] who *Practices*[5], and *Why*[6]?

1. *Effects*

1.1. Self-Regulation
  1.1a. Toward a working definition
  1.1b. Stress
  1.1c. Addictions
  1.1d. Hypertension
1.2. Comparison with other self-regulation strategies

1.3. Altered State
  3a. Toward a working definition
  3b. Subjective Experiences
  3c. Concurrent validity

1.4. Comments on Adverse Effects

2. *Teaching*

2.1 Clinician/Psychotherapist/Teacher
  2.1a. Orientation
  2.1b. Demand Characteristics: beliefs, hopes
  2.1c. Experience
  2.1d. How it is taught

2.2 Relationship
  2.2a Trust, confidentiality
  2.2b Resistance
  2.2c Non-technical transference/ counter-transference
  2.2d Length of contact

2.3 Other "Teaching" Factors
  2.3a Modeling
  2.3b Style-e.g., successive approximation, reinforcement, etc.

3. *Meditation*

3.1 What is Meditation?
  3.1a. Toward a working definition
  3.1b. Types of Meditation
  3.1c. Levels of Meditation
  3.1d. Cultic vs. non-cultic

3.2 What are the components of meditation?
  3.2a Antecedent/Preparatory
  3.2b The Behavior
    Posture
    Attention
    Cognitions
  3.2c Post Meditation Components

4. *Individual*

4.1 Individual Profile
4.1a. Initial expectation/motivation/
      beliefs
4.1b. Commitment

4.2 Who is attracted to it

4.3 Who drops out

4.4 Who continues

4.5 Who continues and has positive
    experience

5. *Practice*

5.1 Adherence/compliance

5.2 Depth of experience

5.3 Length of practice

6. *Why*

6. Mediating Mechanisms

6.1 Physiological
    6.1a General: Trophotropic
         response,Hypometabolic state
    6.1b Specific: muscular; oxygen

6.2 Attentional

6.3 Cognitions

6.4 Non-specific
    Discussion of uni, reciprocal, and
    omni-determinism models

1.5 *What is Meditation:*
Toward a Working Definition

ONE OF THE problems in studying meditation is the lack of a clear definition. Because of its effects, some have tried to define it as a relaxation technique (e.g., Benson, 1975). This raises problems similar to those encountered in the relaxation literature (Davidson & Schwartz, 1976) where a relaxation technique is defined as one producing certain effects—decreased skeletal-muscular tension, decreased sympathetic arousal, etc. Defining a technique by its effects, however, is tautological and not very useful, as we shall see in subsequent sections on meditation's effects, components, and mediating mechanisms. For example, one might describe one type of meditation as a "technique in which one focuses on one's breathing in a calm way." Therefore, a definition of the independent variable would be "calm, attentional focus on breathing." The effect of this focus (dependent variable), interestingly enough, has been shown to be decreased respiration (Hirai, 1974)! Further, some have argued that decreased oxygen consumption—an anaerobic state—is the primary mediating mechanism accounting for meditation's effect (Watanabe, Shapiro & Schwartz, 1972)!

Others have defined meditation by its goal: a state of complete concentration with no extraneous thoughts (i.e. concentrative meditation), a state of complete mindfulness, living in the here and now, a choiceless awareness, without analysis and intellectual constructs (opening-up awareness). These definitions are useful in that they provide an end state. However, they are not really a definition of the process of meditation, and therefore may blind us to what may actually occur during meditation—e.g., discrimination training, covert self-instructions, etc. Further, many of the insights that individuals gain from meditation are a result of *learning about* what happens to them while meditating.

A third definition of meditation often used comes directly from the *Random House Dictionary of the English Language (1973):* To meditate is to "engage in thought or contemplation, reflect. Synonym 1. contemplate, plan, devise, contrive. Synonym 2. ponder, muse, ruminate, cogitate, study, think." This definition equates meditation with thinking or planning as in, "I want to meditate about my future direction in life." Although this type of rumination may take place during meditation, as noted in definition two above, it is not its goal or central characteristic. Therefore, to equate meditation with cognition does not give us a complete definition either.

Another problem is that there are many different types of meditation. Some involve sitting quietly and produce a state of quiescence and restfulness (e.g., Wallace, Benson, & Wilson, 1971); some involve sitting quietly and produce a state of excitement and arousal (e.g., Das & Gastaut, 1955; Corby et al., 1978). Some, such as the Sufi whirling dervish, Tai Chi, Hatha Yoga, Ishiguro Zen involve physical movement to a greater or lesser degree (e.g., Hirai, 1974; Naranjo & Ornstein, 1971). Sometimes these "movement meditations" result in a state of excitement, sometimes a state of relaxation (e.g., Davidson, 1976; Fisher, 1971).

Accordingly depending on the type of meditation, the body may be active and moving, or relatively motionless and passive. Attention may be actively focused on one object of concentration to the exclusion of other objects (e.g., Anand, Chinna, & Singh, 1961). Attention may be focused on one object, but as other objects, thoughts, or feelings occur, they too are noticed, and then attention is returned to the original focal object (e.g., Vipassana, TM). Attention may not be focused exclusively on any particular object (e.g., Zen's Shikan-taza, Kasamatsu & Hirai, 1966; Krishnamurti's choiceless awareness, 1979).

From this plethora of different types of meditation techniques, to find one, all-encompassing definition becomes quite difficult. The definition should take into account the limitations of the other definitions discussed above, and encompass the variety of techniques—specific, attention-focusing strategies—which are subsumed under the label meditation. We may be helped to formulate our definition by a brief digression into the neurophysiology of attentional processing mechanisms. According to Pribram (1971), brain attentional mechanisms are similar to a camera and of two types: 1) when the focus is similar to a wide-angle lens: a broad sweeping awareness, taking in the entire field; and 2) when the focus is similar to a zoom lens—a specific focusing on a particular restricted segment of the field. The attentional strategies in meditation seem to involve either one or the other of the above types of awareness; or a shifting between them: i.e. a focus on the field, a focus on an object within the field, or a shifting back and forth between the two.

Therefore, as a working definition, let me suggest the following:

Meditation refers to a family of techniques which have in common a conscious attempt to focus attention in a non-analytical way, and an attempt not to dwell on discursive, ruminating thought.

If we look closely at the above definition, we notice several important things. First, the word conscious is used. Meditation involves intention: the intention to focus attention either on a particular object in the "field," or on "whatever arises." Second, the definition is non-cultic. It does not depend on any religious framework or orientation to understand it. This statement does not intend to imply that meditation does not or cannot occur within a religious framework. It does suggest however, that what meditation is, and the framework within which it is practiced, though interactive, are two separate issues and need to be viewed as such. Therefore, although there may be overlap in terms of the concentration on a particular object, or repetition of a sound or phrase, we should not *a priori* equate meditation with prayer. This is particularly true when the intent of the prayer has a goal-directed focus outside oneself (e.g., asking a higher power to absolve one of one's sins).

Third, the word attempt is used throughout. This allows us to deal with the process of meditation. Since meditation is an effort to focus attention, it also involves how we respond when our attention wanders; or how we respond when a thought arises. There is a continuum of instructions, from quite strong to quite mild, in terms of how to deal with thoughts (Carrington, 1978). For example, Benson (1975) instructs students to "ignore" the thoughts; Deikman (1966) to exclude them; a fifth century Buddhist treatise to "...with teeth clenched and tongue pressed against the gums, he should by means of sheer mental effort hold back, crush and burn out the thought..." (Conze, 1969, p. 83); the Vipassana tradition instructs one to merely notice and label the thought (e.g., thinking thinking); or, in Zen, to merely notice, observe with equanimity, and when weary of watching, let go (Herrigel, 1953).

Fourth, there is an important "meta-message" implicit in the definition: namely, the *content* of thoughts is not so important: They should be allowed to come and go. Consciousness, or awareness of the *process* of thoughts coming and going, is more important. The context—conscious attention—is stated to be the most important variable. Although cognitions and images may arise, they are not the end goal of meditation. Thus, although there may be overlap in content, we should not *a priori* equate meditation with techniques of guided imagery (Kretschmer, 1969); daydreaming (Singer, 1975); covert self-instructional training (Meichenbaum & Cameron, 1974); hetero-hypnosis (Paul, 1969); self-hypnosis (Fromm, 1975); or other cognitive strategies (cf. Tart, 1969).

1.6 Types of Meditation

THE "FAMILY" of meditation techniques may conveniently be divided into three groupings: concentrative meditation, opening-up (mindfulness meditation), (Naranjo & Ornstein, 1971; Goleman, 1972), and a combination of the above (Washburn, 1978). Let us turn to a brief discussion of opening-up and concentrative meditation techniques and illustrate the differences by the results of two now classic research studies, one by Anand, Chinna, and Singh (1961a) studying Rāja Yogins practicing concentrative meditation; and one by Kasamatsu and Hirai (1966) studying Zen masters practicing opening-up meditation.

CONCENTRATIVE MEDITATION

There are almost as many different types of concentrative meditations as there are spiritual disciplines. For example, the Taoist focus is on the abdomen; the Zen practitioner focuses on a *koan*—a "nonsense" question such as, what is the sound of one hand clapping?—or on breathing; the Christian focuses on a phrase or the cross; the Yogin focuses on a *chakra*—areas near major endocrine glands—or symbol. However, all types of concentrative meditations have certain elements in common. In all types of concentrative meditation, *an attempt is made to restrict awareness by the focusing of attention on a single object.* Other stimuli in the environment are usually ignored, and complete attention is focused on the stimulus labelled the "object of meditation." During the act of meditation an attempt is made to be directly aware of the object in a non-analytical way rather than indirectly, via thought. For example, in his instructions to people focusing on a blue vase, Deikman (1966) stated:

> "By concentration I do not mean analyzing the different parts of the vase, or thinking a series of thoughts about the vase, or associating ideas to the vase, but rather, trying to see the vase as it exists in itself, without any connections to other things. Exclude all other feelings or sounds or body sensations. Do not let them distract you, but keep them out so that you can concentrate all your attention, all your awareness, on the vase itself. Let the perception of the vase fill your entire mind" (p. 103).*

The "object of meditation" can be located in either the external or internal environment. Examples of objects in the external environment include a kasina—a plain disc (Theravada Buddhism), abdomen (Taoism), the cross (Christianity) or a vase. The meditator can also focus on internal stimuli, such as visual images, the third eye, the vault of the skull (e.g., as done by Rāja Yogins); or internally generated sounds such as a mantra, sutra; a prayer; a sentence (e.g., a Zen koan).

The element in common in all these types of concentrative meditation is the attempt to restrict awareness to a single object and to the focus on that object over a long period of time.

The now classic study of Rāja Yogins practicing concentrative meditation was carried out by Anand, Chinna and Singh (1961) in

---

*I would slightly change these instructions, to minimize the law of reverse effects (formulated by Allport 1955; discussed by Shapiro, 1978b, with reference to cognitive focusing strategies). Simply stated, it argues that sometimes our instructions to ourselves seem to have the opposite effect: e.g., an injunction, "Do not eat that thick, lovely, gooey pastry" may cause us to eat it; or an injunction, "For the next five seconds *Don't Think of Pink Elephants*"...1...2...3 ...4...5, may cause you to. Therefore instead of *exclude* I would instruct: "If other feelings, sounds, or bodily sensations arise, notice them, and then return your focus to the vase. Try to concentrate all your attention, all your awareness on the vase itself. Let the perception of the vase fill your entire mind." For a further discussion of techniques, see Chapter Four.

India. These Rāja Yogins practiced concentrative meditation by pinpointing consciousness on the back of their skulls, a third eye, or the tip of their nose. During meditation their eyes were closed. In this experiment, a variety of external stimuli were administered to the Yogins: photic (strong light), auditory (loud banging noise); thermal (touching with a hot glass tube); and vibration (tuning fork). According to the authors:

> None of these stimuli produced any blockage of alpha rhythm when the yogis were in meditation. When the yogis' hands were immersed in cold water (four degrees centigrade) for forty-five to fifty-five minutes, there was persistent alpha activity both before and during the period which their hands were immersed. In other words, the yogis did not see, hear, or feel the stimuli presented to them (p. 453).

TABLE 1.2 *Examples of Concentrative Meditation*

	Auditory	Visual	Tactile
overt, external environment	verbal—Sufi dervish call mantra	kasina mandala cross vase abdomen	touching thumb to each finger
internal environment	verbal—mantra koan	third eye vault of skull symbol of guru (image)	heart beat breathing

(After Shapiro, 1978b, p. 39)

These results are consistent with the stated purpose *during concentrative meditation* of reducing reactivity to stimuli in the environment. As we shall see in the next paragraph, they present a marked contrast to the EEG responses of experienced meditators practicing opening-up, or mindfulness meditation.

OPENING-UP MEDITATION

In opening-up, or mindfulness meditation, an attempt is made to be responsive to all stimuli in the internal and external environment, but not to dwell on any particular stimulus. In the Kasamatsu and Hirai study (1966), Zen subjects meditated with their eyes open. As with the Rāja Yogins, soon after the onset of meditation (fifty seconds) alpha waves were recorded in all brain regions. The longer the monk had been in training, the more pronounced the changes in his alpha activity. However, when a click sound was made, there was alpha blockage for two or three seconds. The click sound was repeated twenty times, and each time there was alpha blockage for two or three seconds followed by a resumption of alpha waves. As noted above, this presents a marked contrast to the results of the experiments with the Rāja Yogins, whose alpha waves were not blocked even though very strong stimuli were presented.

COMBINATION

Some meditation techniques integrate elements of both concentrative and opening-up types. For example, a person may focus on breathing (Zen and Vipassana meditation) or a mantra (e.g., Transcendental Meditation) but be willing to allow attention to focus on other stimuli if they become predominant, and then return to the breathing (or mantra). In other words, they remain open to other stimuli, but have an "anchor" to which to return their attention. Also, in the classic texts, a distinction is made between fixed concentration, i.e. focus on a single object continuously; and momentary concentration in which, during opening-up meditation, attention shifts from object to object as one object becomes salient and another loses salience.

FORMAL VERSUS INFORMAL MEDITATION

Formal meditation refers to the practice of meditation at certain times during the day, usually in a consistent, specified place and generally in a specific posture (classically the lotus or half-lotus position). Informal meditation is practiced throughout the day, in no specified posture or specified place. It involves an attempt to be conscious of everything that one does, to attend very closely to one's everyday actions, without judging or evaluating.

As Walpole Rahula (1959) noted,

> "Be aware and mindful of whatever you do, physically or verbally, during the daily routine of your work and your life. Whether you walk, stand, sit, lie down, or sleep, whether you stretch or bend your legs, whether you look around, whether you put your clothes on, whether you talk or keep silent, whether you eat or drink, whether you answer the calls of nature—in these and other activities you should be fully aware and mindful of the act performed at the moment, that is to say, that you should live in the present moment, the present action" (p. 71).

In informal meditation, conscious attention becomes a way of life. I mention informal meditation here because most Western researchers focus primarily on formal practice. However, the end goal of meditation is not simply to be able to "make an effort to consciously focus attention" twice a day during formal sittings but to maintain and generalize that "conscious attention" to all parts of the day.

1.7 Comments on Meditation as a Self-Regulation Strategy and Altered State of Consciousness

IN PREVIOUS EFFORTS (Shapiro & Zifferblatt, 1976a; Shapiro & Giber, 1978; Shapiro, 1978b), I have, for heuristic purposes, conceptualized meditation both as a self-regulation strategy and as a means for inducing altered states of consciousness. Because that division forms one of the primary bases for the organization of this book, I review it here, presenting also a critique of that distinction.

The distinction grew out of a need to clarify meditation as an independent variable. Western research has primarily conceptualized meditation as a self-regulation strategy and looked for its effects on dependent variables such as stress (Glueck & Stroebel, 1975), addictive behaviors (Marlatt et al., in press 1980),

and hypertension (Benson et al, 1974a, 1974b). The primary rationale for meditation as a treatment for these dependent variables
has been its relaxation effects (Wallace, Benson, Wilson, 1971).

Meditation, however, was originally conceived within the
religious philosophical context of Eastern spiritual disciplines. It
was a technique utilized in those traditions primarily as a means
for developing insight (wisdom), purification (lack of anger, greed
and selfishness), concentration, as well as inducing altered states
of consciousness. In these ways, meditation was a means for
changing an individual's perception of the world and for developing a more veridical, unified, and accepting view of one's self, of
nature, and of other people. The research literature on meditation
as an altered state of consciousness suggests that subjective
phenomenological changes occur during meditation, ranging from
relatively strong alterations of perception in short-term
meditators (Deikman, 1966; Maupin, 1965) to more pronounced
feelings of "self-transcendence," "felt meaning in the world," "a
heightened sense of connectedness with the world and with others,
a sense of purpose and meaningfulness, deep positive emotion"
(Osis et al., 1973; Kohr, 1977).

One way of visually representing this distinction is by looking
at meditation as involving different levels of depth of experience.
On the opposite page is a simple, 5-step model of Zen breath
meditation that offers such a distinction. I use the word simple
because each level may be refined several-fold more, both within
this meditation technique, as well as across different techniques,
for example, a discussion of the Jhānas in the Abhidamna
(Goleman, 1972) or the classical texts of the Mahāmudra tradition
(Brown, 1977). However, for the purposes of illustrating this
distinction, it seems a useful and sufficient model.

The division of meditation into different steps is used here
only as a heuristic device to help understand the "process" of
meditation, not to give the impression that meditation consists
of discrete, nonoverlapping steps. Further, the different steps
discussed should be considered only as plausible hypotheses until
verified by additional research.

STEPS ONE AND TWO:
MEDITATION AND ORDINARY AWARENESS

These two beginning steps involve similarities to ordinary

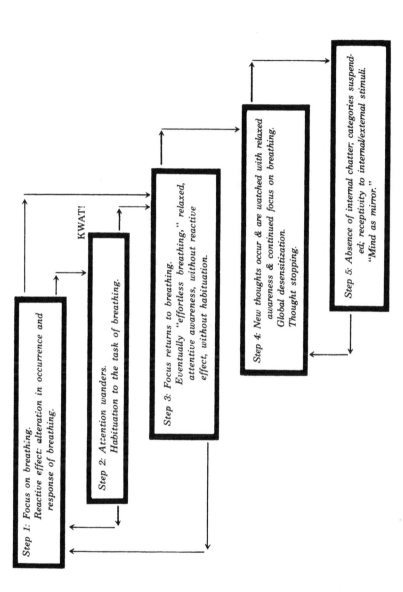

FIGURE 1.1 *A Five-Step Model of the Zen Breath Meditation*

awareness: a reactive effect (step one) and habituation to task (step two). Anecdotal data suggest that when the person is first asked to observe his or her breathing, there is often an alteration in this behavior. The person has difficulty letting the air "come," catches his/her breath, and breathes more quickly and shallowly than normal. Often the person complains about not getting enough air and of "drowning" (step one, Shapiro and Zifferblatt [1976]).

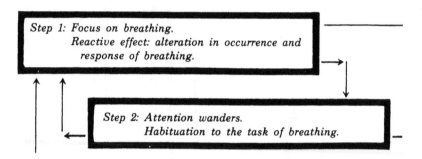

Soon, however, the meditating person forgets the task at hand, stops focusing on his/her breath, and unrelated thoughts and images occur (step two). When this nonattentive dialogue occurs and the individual becomes aware of it, s/he is asked to bring attention back to the act of breathing. In Japan, the meditator is aided in this task by the Zen Master, who walks around the meditation hall, carrying a big stick. The Master watches each of the meditators to make sure they are alert and receptive. Since sleepiness *(kanchin)* is not desirable in Zen training, when the Master sees one of the students sagging, or not concentrating, he approaches that person and bows. (The meditator, if aware of a wandering mind, can also initiate the bow.) The Master then raises the stick and gives a blow (called a *kwat,* after the Zen Master Rinzai), intended to return the individual to conscious alertness immediately.

When no Master is present, the beginning meditator is told to be his or her own master: to learn to identify when attention wanders from the task of breathing and to bring it back to that task.

STEPS THREE AND FOUR:
MEDITATION AS A SELF-REGULATION STRATEGY

With practice the individual learns to focus on breathing without altering the behavior of breathing (the reactive effect of step one)

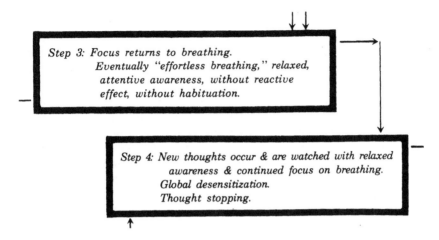

Step 3: *Focus returns to breathing.*
Eventually "effortless breathing," relaxed,
attentive awareness, without reactive
effect, without habituation.

Step 4: *New thoughts occur & are watched with relaxed*
awareness & continued focus on breathing.
Global desensitization.
Thought stopping.

and without habituating to the task (as in step two). Step three, described as "effortless breathing," is what Benson (1975) refers to when he discusses the relaxation response; it may be the critical one in the reduction of blood pressure, stress and tension, and insomnia.

In the fourth step of meditation the individual maintains the effortless breathing of the third step, yet new thoughts occur. However, when new thoughts occur, the meditator is able to "just observe them...and let them flow down the river."

That is, in the fourth step an individual does not enter into dialogue with a thought, but merely watches it, and lets it go, while maintaining the effortless breathing of the third step. This step seems to have an important effect in helping an individual overcome anxieties, phobias, and other concerns. We assume this effect occurs because whatever is important to a person comes into awareness; and, the relaxed, physically comfortable posture prevents what does come into awareness from becoming threatening.

An illustration from some of my research with heroin addicts vividly illustrates this fourth step (Shapiro & Zifferblatt, 1976a). One of the subjects noted that while meditating he saw a movie screen, on which flashed pictures of his life and questions such as, "Hey man, what are you doing with your life? You're really blowing it. What are you going to do with yourself?" He said that normally these questions would cause him a great deal of anxiety and turmoil and lead him to use heroin again. However, becoming aware of these questions while meditating, he felt none of the anxiety, none of the guilt: "I could merely be an observer of my own life." In other words, the fourth step of meditation serves to present whatever is of concern to the person at that time in a calming, non-emotional manner. As new thoughts are self-observed, the meditator is able to take note of them and to continue focusing on breathing. Because the person is in a relaxed, comfortable, and physically stable posture, he is able to self-observe with equanimity everything that comes into awareness: fears, thoughts, fantasies, guilts, decisions, and other covert events. No attempt is made to systematically structure the covert stimuli; rather, there occurs what may be referred to as a "global hierarchy" consisting of things currently "on a person's mind" (Goleman, 1971). In this way, the individual learns to discriminate and observe all covert stimuli that come into awareness, without making any judgment, thereby desensitizing him/herself (unstressing) to those covert images and statements (step four).

As Eugene Herrigel (1953) noted in *Zen and the Art of Archery*,

> As though sprung from nowhere, moods, feelings, desires, worries, and even thoughts incontinently rise up in a meaningless jumble...the only successful way of rendering the disturbances inoperative is to...enter into friendly relations with whatever appears on the scene, to accustom oneself to it, to look at it equitably, and at last grow weary of looking (pp. 57-58).

Meditation as an Altered State: Step Five

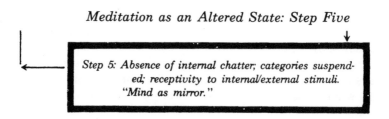

Step 5: *Absence of internal chatter; categories suspended; receptivity to internal/external stimuli.* "Mind as mirror."

The fifth step of meditation is the step that has been referred to in various Eastern literatures as *satori, nirvana, kensho, samadhi.* In the West it has been referred to as an altered state or higher state of consciousness. It involves an ability to observe with equanimity and mindfulness, and eventually to reduce the "internal chatter" of covert thoughts and images; a sense of timelessness (Kairos), as opposed to chronological time (Chronos), goallessness and non-striving: an openness and receptivity to what is occurring in the moment. Davidson (1976) has suggested the term "mystical states" for those experiences which occur during meditation and involve an alteration in consciousness. Stace (1960), after reviewing the literature, described certain qualities associated with this state, such as "deeply felt positive mood"; "unity" or "union"; "a oneness with all things"; "a sense of ineffability"; "an enhanced sense of reality"; "an alteration of time and space." Davidson (1976) points out that these mystical experiences do not occur in most meditation experiences.

Altered state, as I am using the term, needs to be seen along a continuum. On one end of the continuum are "full blown" mystical and spiritual experiences (e.g., nirvana, satori, kensho, samadhi), at the other, profound, intense, but more common alterations of perception.

COMMENTS ON UTILITY
AND LIMIT OF THIS DISTINCTION

This distinction between meditation as self-regulation strategy and as altered state of consciousness has proved to be a useful one. First, it allows more precision in viewing meditation as an independent variable, thereby influencing the dependent variable selected for study, and in turn helping researchers to develop a stronger theoretical rationale between independent and dependent variables. Second, different research strategies may be appropriate depending on how meditation is conceptualized. For example, if seen, as suggested by Shapiro and Giber (1978), as a self-regulation strategy, it needs to be compared with other self-regulation strategies in controlled group designs to evaluate its clinical utility. If conceptualized as an altered state, at this stage of our knowledge, well-designed $N = 1$ studies may be more appropriate. Finally, as we will see in Chapters Eight and Nine, different components and mediating mechanisms may be operating, depending upon how meditation is being conceptualized as an independent variable (e.g., altered state or self-regulation strategy) and the nature of the dependent variable being investigated.

However, as with any distinction, there may also be limitations and areas of imprecision; for example, the Shapiro and

Giber (1978) article leaves several questions unanswered about
this distinction. First, no real definition of a clinical self-
regulation strategy is given. Rather effects of the strategy serve
to define the strategy: i.e. meditation helps reduce stress,
therefore, it is a self-regulation strategy. A similar problem
occurs with meditation as an altered state of consciousness; i.e.
viewing meditation as a vehicle for altered states of consciousness does not define meditation, but merely illustrates one
of its results. A further compounding problem with this distinction is that its division between self-regulation and altered state
may be at times arbitrary. For example, literature on meditation
as altered state suggests that meditation may provide individuals with a new sense of meaning and purpose, a new perspective on personal reality. This would obviously have a pronounced
influence on levels of stress and tension. Conversely, the relaxation effect of meditation may be important in calming an individual, helping him or her feel more peaceful and tranquil,
thereby influencing attentional focusing, "clearing the mind,"
and having some resultant altered state effects. Accordingly, in
Chapters Five and Seven, additional attempts at refining and
clarifying this distinction will be made.

1.8 The Individual:
Initial Motivation and Expectations

IT IS QUITE likely that many individuals in our culture
want to learn meditation for its self-regulation
qualities: as a strategy for stress management, relaxation, reducing blood pressure, etc., based on the "demand characteristics"
of the data in our scientific journals. Others may be attracted to
it for "spiritual reasons," i.e. meditation as an altered state of
consciousness, based on the "demand characteristics" of reports
in meditation texts. For those who want self-regulation, perhaps
the mystical garb (e.g., Katz, Note Two) and even the label itself
(e.g., Barber & Calverley, 1964) may be a hindrance. For those
looking for a "new meaning," perhaps the mysticism is important to successful outcome.

Although several studies have attempted to control for expectation effects (e.g., Smith, 1976; Malec & Sipprelle, 1977), to my
knowledge no article has been published which *assesses* subjects'

expectations prior to meditation* (cf. Chapters Two and Three for examples). It may be critical to determine why people meditate: what they perceive this "technique" as being able to do for them. For example, if they meditate for "relaxation," do they ever have an altered state experience? If they meditate for "spiritual meaning," do they relax as well as those who are meditating just for relaxation?

An issue related to expectation effects is motivation. How much does a person want to "learn to relax" to find "new meaning"? For example, Maupin (1965) noted that those who entered his study had a strong "therapy-seeking motivation." Are individuals who begin to meditate looking for "personal growth," self-actualization, relief from painful stress and tension, or seeking a cognitive avoidance strategy with which to escape from problems? How much do they want to change or grow? How intensely committed do they perceive themselves as being to working for this change? Additional issues involve the relationship between motivation, tension, arousal, and outcome. These are as yet unanswered questions, but empirically testable ones.

Two studies offer some clues to the relationship between initial motivation and treatment outcome. Kubose's (1976) study gave indirect support for the importance of motivation and suggested the potential importance of attitudes toward expectations in determining a treatment's effectiveness. Studies prior to Kubose had noted that changes on the POI (Personal Orientation Inventory) occurred in those who practiced meditation for eight weeks (Seeman et al., 1972). This finding was later replicated by the same group of experimenters in 1973 (Nidich et al.). However, in Kubose (1976) these findings failed to replicate. Kubose (1976, p. 9) noted that "although subjects were curious about meditation, the major motivating factor was probably the fact that participation was one of the ways to satisfy their introductory psychology course experimental participation requirement." Therefore, they might not have been as highly motivated as those who had paid money or who were desirous of being initiated into TM training.

Goldman, Domitor, and Murray (1979) performed the first study which actually looked at the relationship between motiva-

*To facilitate further research in this area, a brief expectation, motivation, assessment questionnaire is provided in the appendix.

tion and treatment outcome. Half their subjects were fulfilling an introductory psychology research requirement (subject-pool subjects) and half were recruited through a college newspaper advertisement (volunteer subjects). The authors noted that volunteer subjects had significantly more altered states of consciousness, and improved their Zen meditation practice over time whereas the subject-pool individuals responded worse over time.

Thus, the subject's initial desire to learn the technique may be an important additional variable in determining treatment outcome. It would be useful to administer a brief subjective questionnaire to measure subject's expectations and motivation level prior to beginning meditation practice. It would then have to be determined, however, how well initial motivation translates into long-term commitment, as evidenced by adherence and compliance.

A final issue, before discussion of subject profile, is initial skills: e.g., the ability to sit for a certain period of time, the ability to focus attention. As Stroebel and Glueck (1977) noted, "quite seriously ill, hospitalized psychiatric patients can learn the meditation techniques *if* they are able to comprehend the instructions."

1.9 Subject Profile

FOUR MAIN ISSUES need to be addressed regarding subject profile: 1) Are there differences between those interested in learning meditation versus those who are not? 2) For those interested, how do those subjects who drop out compare with those who continue? 3) What are the qualities of those who continue to a successful outcome? 4) Information on those who continue and experience adverse effects*.

---

*It should be noted that these studies on expectation and motivation as well as subject variables all pertain to Western meditators. Another interesting question, and one which has not yet received attention, is what is the psychological profile of "Eastern" people who meditate? Of those in the East who really commit themselves? Of those who drop out? And of those who have positive outcome? We are just beginning to investigate these cross-cultural issues (Shapiro, Note Four).

QUESTION ONE: DIFFERENCES BETWEEN THOSE
INTERESTED IN LEARNING MEDITATION
AND THOSE WHO ARE NOT

Stek and Bass (1973) looked at the differences between those interested in meditation and those less interested. They took four groups of students with different interest levels. Group One was self-selected and had attended two free introductory lectures and paid an enrollment fee in a four day course; Group Two was self-selected and had attended one of the two free introductory lectures; Group Three participated in the study for partial fulfillment of the requirements of a course—they were aware of meditation but not interested in attending; and Group Four was an unselected control group who participated in this study for course requirements. The lack of significant differences among the groups on either the Rotter Internal/External Locus of Control Scale or Shostrom's POI suggest that those interested in the practice of meditation and those who are not do not differ at least in terms of these dimensions. Though it intuitively seems that there would be differences in populations, this issue awaits further research.

QUESTION TWO: DROPOUT PROFILE;
CONTINUATION PROFILE

In one of the first studies to look at meditation "dropouts," Otis (1974) noted that those subjects who dropped out stated that they had fewer problems before they began Transcendental Meditation and noted that they felt less change after learning the technique than a comparable group who continued. In addition, dropout subjects were more likely to describe themselves as "withdrawn, irritable and anxiety ridden" than a control group. In the second experiment conducted by Otis (1974), the dropouts at pretest felt "less positive about themselves" or "had serious problems." Otis suggested that individuals who stopped meditating are more disturbed and yet are less likely to admit their problems. Those who do continue may be less disturbed but are willing to admit their problems.

Smith (1978), in a systematic follow-up of personality correlates of continuation, noted that out of thirty possible pre-test predictors, continuation (defined as having practiced TM at least once in the last month of the project), correlated most highly with low scores on the Tennessee Self Concept Scale (TSCS) Psychosis Scale and high scores on the TSCS Self-Criticism Scale. Further, those that did drop out scored lower on the TSCS Self-Criticism Scale and considerably higher on the TSCS Psychosis Scale. Smith noted that dropouts may defensively need to see or present themselves in unrealistically healthy or favorable terms. Conversely, those who continued are more likely to admit to a wide range of possibly unfavorable statements. Continuation with TM correlated significantly with a low degree of psychosis, a high degree of self-criticism, as well as with having considered psychotherapy prior to the onset of the project. These findings are interesting in light of Maupin's (1965) comment that those who entered his study had a "therapy-seeking motivation" and Bono's study (1980, in press) which suggested that meditators, prior to meditation, had a significantly lower self-concept than non-meditators.

QUESTION THREE:
QUALITIES OF THOSE WHO CONTINUE
AND HAVE SUCCESSFUL OUTCOME

Smith's study (1978) and a related study by Beiman et al., (1980, in press) also cast light on the nature of individuals who not only continue to meditate but seem to benefit from meditation. In both studies, outcome was assessed by anxiety measures. The two predictors Smith found to correlate most highly with outcome were Cattell's 16 PF factor M "autia" and Factor A, "schizothymia." Cattell (1957; Cattell et al., 1970) suggested that core features of autia can be variously described as a strong inner life, a preoccupation with inner ideas and emotions, good contact with the inner world. At the opposite pole from autia is praxernia. As might be expected, this trait is characterized by a tendency to be practical, conventional, guided by objective realities, and concerned with immediate interests and issues. As Smith noted, praxernic subjects were less likely to benefit from meditation. The second quality, schizothymia, reflects, according to Cattell, a low variability in behavioral and emotional expression, "steadiness of purpose," and a tendency of a habit not to disappear with a lack of reward. The schizothymic finds it easy to turn inward. Behaviors correlated with schizothymia reflect behavioral and emotional invariability as well as withdrawal. Emotionally they are "cool," "flat," and display relatively few fluctuations in mood. The opposite of schizothymia is affectothymia. Smith (1978) noted that "individuals possessing this trait are outgoing, warm, emotional, likely to work with people, and as we found, less likely to benefit from meditation." In order of significance, successful outcome on anxiety measures correlated significantly with a) not having considered psychotherapy prior to the onset of the project; b) schizothymia; c) autia; d) high anxiety State Trait Anxiety Inventory (STAI-A trait).

Beiman et al., (1980, in press) noted that the more internal locus of control that participants reported prior to treatment (cf. Rotter, 1966), the more they benefited from TM, as measured by the Fear Survey Schedule and two electrodermal measures of autonomic arousal. The Internal-External Locus of Control Scale predicted thirty-four percent to sixty-two percent of the variance in three of the five dependent variables analyzed. Higher internal locus prior to training was consistently associated with more improvement in the dependent variables after training in meditation. Conversely, those with a higher external locus benefited less from meditation.

There are a few other studies which provide additional information about subject profile. Anand, Chinna and Singh (1961a) noted anecdotally that less experienced Rāja Yoga meditators whom they studied were found to a) be quite enthusiastic and b) have high alpha in the resting state. Some of the earlier studies tried to determine the relationship between personality factors (independent variable) and response to meditation (dependent variable). Maupin (1965) looked at "capacity for adaptive regression in the service of the ego and tolerance for unrealistic experiences" as personality characteristics which might predict responses to meditation. He found meditators who had "deeper levels" of experience also had a higher incidence of primary process responses to the Rorschach and a greater tolerance for "unrealistic experiences." Lesh (1970), using the Fitzgerald Experience Inquiry (a test of openness to and tolerance of regressive, altered state, and peak experiences) also found that the more openness and tolerance, the greater the correlation with depth of experience. And Akers et al., (1977) found these meditators with a higher score on the hypochondriasis scale of the

Minnesota Multiple Personality Inventory, MMPI, (i.e. individuals who endorse items which indicate more concern with their physical or psychological well-being) evidenced greater psychophysiological response to meditation (measured by increase in EEG alpha) than individuals who endorse items which indicate less concern.

Kanas and Horowitz (1977) in their study of individuals' reactions to a stress film, noted that pre-meditators emerged significantly different from the other three groups (control group, non-teaching meditators, and meditation teachers). The pre-meditating group was "significantly more stressed, angry, and disgusted in response to the stress films and they perceived themselves as more nervous, sad, and fearful both before and after seeing the films" (Kanas & Horowitz, 1977, p. 435). After viewing the films there was a meditation or sitting period. Then subjects were given an intrusive thoughts and film reference questionnaire. On the questionnaire the pre-meditators were more preoccupied with life issues and fantasies than with the films and experimental tasks. Kanas and Horowitz suggested that one cannot assume that these "stressed" pre-meditators become relatively less stressed after learning to meditate. They noted that this would only be true if all the meditators came from the same population as the pre-meditators. However, they noted that this may not be so because of the large dropout rate dependent upon motivation. After a four month telephone follow-up, three of the eight pre-meditators contacted (thirty-eight percent) had already stopped meditating. This then led them to the conclusion that, "with dropout rates this high, it is possible the successful meditators (those who continue meditating regularly) seem to come from a reasonably healthy sub-population of meditators, while those who drop out seem to represent more emotionally distressed persons" (Kanas & Horowitz, 1977, p. 435).

QUESTION FOUR: THOSE WHO CONTINUE
AND REPORT ADVERSE EFFECTS

One final subject population, on which there has been almost no research, is comprised of those who *continue* meditation, but report *adverse* experiences (Otis, 1980, in press). Why do they continue? Are these "pain-dependent" people? Do they believe the "adverse" effects are a stage (necessary and sufficient; necessary but not sufficient) after which more learning will come;

is it a stage necessary for learning, i.e. a higher sensitivity to formerly defended material? The only report to date on subject profile (Walsh & Rauche, 1979) reported case reports of psychotic breaks during intensive meditation in individuals with a prior history of schizophrenia. Clearly this seems an important area for further investigation.

SUMMARY OF THE INDIVIDUAL

The profiles that emerge from the above studies are based on small numbers with a wide range of variability between subjects. However, some interesting trends seem to emerge. First, there may be a certain type of individual who will be most successful at meditation. This person already has a high "internal locus of control" (Beiman et al., 1980, in press), is enthusiastic (Anand, Chinna & Singh, 1961a), has high baseline alpha to begin with (Anand, Chinna & Singh, 1961a), is more interested in internal, subjective experiences, has flatter, less labile affect (Smith, 1978), may already be a better attender (that is, has better ability to maintain attentional focus, Vahia et al., 1972), and is more able to be open to and tolerant of "unrealistic" altered state experiences (Maupin, 1965; Lesh, 1970). Another subject variable which is worth noting is what Pelletier and Peper (1977) describe as the "chutzpah factor"—the importance of believing in the possibility of one's success (cf. Bandura, 1977).

This discussion gives us a frame of reference from which to begin to understand subject variables involved in meditation. Even seemingly contradictory findings may be understandable within the context of the above profile. For example, Smith (1978) noted that high anxiety was correlated with positive outcome, and Bono (1980, in press) showed that prior to TM, subjects had a lower real-ideal correlation. However, high anxiety, willingness to be self-critical, *and* the belief in one's own internal locus of control may all be part of the profile of the successful meditator.*

---

*An interesting question raised by Robert Kantor involves the issue of whether socio-economic status has been controlled for in any of these studies. To my knowledge, it has not, and that would offer a profitable line of inquiry.

The profile of those who drop out of meditation is a rather negative one. Drop-outs were highly defensive (Otis, 1974; Smith, 1978), scored higher on the Psychosis Scale of TSCS (Smith, 1978), had serious problems (Otis, 1974), and were emotionally disturbed (Kanas & Horowitz, 1977).

Why might this "negative" profile be occurring? First, there is a slick meditation "hype," a Madison Avenue sales pitch given by some organizations. This sales pitch may attract individuals to meditation, as if it were "sugar-coated tofu"—i.e. a simple, fun, relaxing technique to solve all problems*. And it is not. Meditation involves work, often a willingness to sit quietly and "face oneself," which can be frightening. Unless one is truly motivated to change or work on oneself, it is easy to drop out. Meditation may be attracting a group of individuals who are not willing to make the effort.

On the other hand, there may be at least two other sub-sets of populations which drop out—a fact not accounted for by the above data. Some may wish to learn meditation to reduce anxiety. After several weeks of faithful practice, this occurs. Then, subsequent meditation may not seem to be having as pronounced an effect—they may feel they have reaped all the benefits they can from it (Glueck & Stroebel, 1975). Also, it is possible some of these subjects are achieving similar effects to those gained from meditation from other idiosyncratic sources: listening to music, running. Another group may be those who have "somatic anxiety" and who meditate. Somatic anxiety refers to feelings of anxiety which occur in the body, e.g., butterflies in the stomach, sweaty palms, tight jaw, etc. Cognitive anxiety involves what a person says: I feel out of control, helpless, tense, a "whirring" mind. If the views of Davidson and Schwartz (1976) are borne

---

*There is an interesting philosophical question regarding "sales pitch." One the one hand, some researchers have said that we need subjects who are not long-term meditators enmeshed in belief systems (e.g., Woolfolk, 1975). In this way, we can determine the variance in successfulness of treatment due to the technique itself. Therefore, what are needed, Woolfolk concluded, are naive subjects, people without belief systems. Yet, from a clinical standpoint, we are aware of the power of belief systems (e.g., Frank, 1963); Pelletier & Peper, 1977). Therefore, from a clinical perspective, we would want to *maximize* expectations and beliefs, *but* only within the limitations of honesty and integrity.

out (Schwartz, Davidson & Goleman, 1978), then meditation, a cognitive focusing strategy, may not be as beneficial for those with somatic (as opposed to cognitive) anxiety. These individuals may realize this, and if their reasons for beginning to meditate were anxiety reduction, and instead somatic anxiety intensifies, they may drop out. Therefore, a further refinement of the subject "drop-out population," seems necessary.

My own clinical experience disinclines me to believe that all meditators who drop out have such a negative profile. As in any self-regulation procedure, continued practice requires enormous discipline. I should think there would be healthy students who drop out of meditation just as in any other self-regulation strategy (including medical adherence, dental floss adherence! etc.). The profile up until now does not seem specific enough, and will require further research and refinement.

Finally, it should be noted that most of the "predictors" of meditation success have involved "trait" personality descriptions. Given the rather convincing review of the situational specificity of behavior (Mischel, 1968), it might be important to try to define non-trait skills (attentional skills, ability to sit quietly) and/or cognitive beliefs, and their abilities to predict successful outcome (Shapiro, Note Five). Further, successful outcome has most often been measured by variables relating to anxiety. However, it is quite possible that some introverted, "shy" individuals may turn to meditation because it fits their temperament. They may show a reduction of anxiety, and therefore be "successful meditators." However, from a therapeutic standpoint, meditation may not be a sufficient intervention for them. They may need, for example, assertiveness training, social skills, training in risk-taking behavior (See Chapter Two; & Shapiro, Note Five).

1.10 Practice.

THE PRIMARY ISSUES in this section involve the length of practice, and subject's willingness to continue the practice. Adherence to treatment is an important variable in any self-regulation strategy. In meditation research, it presents a particular dilemma in evaluating meditation's effectiveness against reported claims. Specifically, much of the research which has been done in the West has been done with relatively short-term meditators as subjects, whereas claims from the Orient are based on experiences of subjects who were skilled masters and have spent decades perfecting the discipline through intense practice. Past studies have shown that a large percentage of meditators, ranging from twenty-five to fifty percent and sometimes higher, do not continue to practice the technique. For example, Kanas and Horowitz (1977) note that within four months of beginning, three out of eight subjects had already dropped out of the meditation group. Similarly, Stroebel and Glueck (1975) noted that the greatest difficulty was in getting patients with significant depression or younger teenage patients to meditate regularly.

Since many of the effects of meditation may be cumulative and a result of practice (e.g., Kasamatsu & Hirai, 1966), adherence seems an important variable. For example, Davidson, Goleman and Schwartz (1976) suggest that the longer the practice, the greater the increase in concentration. Further, Ikegami (1973) showed that the more experienced the meditator, the more physically stable the posture.*

There are three critical issues here: a) whether subjects *say* they practiced, b) whether they in fact practiced, and c) how to maintain adherence. Goldman, Domitor and Murray (1979), to ensure practice, had subjects meditate in a laboratory setting, and debriefed them after each session to determine the nature of their experience to see if they were meditating "correctly." This certainly ensures practice during the intervention phase, a point about which experimenters cannot always be sure. However, it is cumbersome and expensive, and thereby usually results in a short experiment, e.g., Goldman, Domitor and Murray's (1979) lasted only five days. Further, the issue of adherence also involves the question of what happens once the intervention is

---

*Physiologically, however, there are some contradictory findings about the effects of long-term practice. For example, in the Morse et al. study (1977) and in the study by Cauthen and Prymak (1977) the length of experience of the meditator did not seem to have any effect on the physiological outcome variables. As Morse noted, subjects trained in hypnosis (one month to four years) or TM (two months to five years) did not have significantly better results than subjects untrained in either modality.

completed. Marlatt et al. (in press, 1980) monitored adherence to different relaxation strategies and noted that after the invention phase, when given a choice, individuals, almost without exception chose to discontinue all types of treatment, ranging from pleasurable reading, to meditation (Benson's method) and Progressive Relaxation. Glueck and Stroebel (1975), noted that all subjects in their biofeedback and Autogenic Training groups dropped out, as well as, at a later time, a sizable number of their meditation group.

What steps might be taken to increase adherence? First, we need a common definition of adherence. For example, Smith (1976) defined adherence as having practiced meditation once within the last month of the intervention. This seems a rather broad definition. In another study (Note One) Smith defined adherence as practicing one time per day for twenty minutes. Whatever the definition, researchers should specify it clearly, and monitor adherence closely as an important outcome variable.

One study has looked primarily at the role of adherence and its relationship to preparation (Note One). Smith took two groups of students and taught one Benson's relaxation procedure and the second group a series of five gradated, successive approximations to meditation with each one more difficult and "meditation-like," i.e. more passive, effortless, internal, and subtle.* The results show that there was no difference in anxiety scores on the Spielberger STAI trait scale, but that the comprehensive meditation program subjects displayed a significantly greater decrease in physiological symptoms as measured by a personalized stress and anxiety questionnaire that Smith devised. In addition, those in the comprehensive meditation training program practiced ninety percent of the total possible seventy practice sessions whereas the treatment group subjects practiced fifty-two percent. Counting full participation as regular meditation at least once a day during the last four weeks of the project, sixteen out of the twenty-two in the comprehensive meditation program continued to meditate while five of the seventeen in the Benson treatment continued. The major problem with this study, however, is that we are comparing Benson's relaxation treatment to a treatment

*It is not clear whether those in the comprehensive meditation training actually received meditation instructions.

which actually changed every week or ten days, thereby providing novel stimuli and a new additional component. This may
not be a justifiable comparison for adherence qualities because
the novelty effect may account for continued adherence (Berlyne,
1960). Although not a convincing study, it is cited here to encourage others to share their experiences and ideas about ways
to improve adherence.

In addition to preparation, Smith (Note One) and Glueck and
Stroebel (1975) stressed the importance of follow-up checking to
ensure adherence. Other ideas include developing self-contracting
at least in the initial stages with the client, deciding on time and
place in advance, building in initial reinforcements, providing for
successive approximations to the desired time limit, carefully
understanding the client's initial motivation and desire to learn
meditation, and using positive images of desired consequences as
ways of facilitating and of increasing motivation to continue the
practice.

1.11 The Role of the Teacher: The Therapist's (Clinician's/Teacher's) Orientation

CLINICIANS, psychotherapists and/or health-care professionals need to know certain things about meditation to help determine whether it will be the treatment of choice.
For which clients/patients, with what types of problems will
meditation be effective? To answer this question, they must be
as aware as possible of personal preconceptions, values, and
biases toward therapeutic treatment. For at least one part of the
question of whether meditation is effective will depend upon the
therapist's (or researcher's) theoretical orientation and what s/he
decides to measure as criteria for "successful outcome."

In Chapter One (1.2) brief mention was made of how
therapists from several different orientations were utilizing
meditation in their practice. As a way of elaborating on this
issue, four viewpoints will be briefly presented, including a
discussion of how meditation, when viewed as a positive
therapeutic tool, is utilized within the context of each: classical
(id) Freudian psychoanalysis; ego (humanistic) psychology—

holistic medicine; behavioral therapy—behavioral medicine; and transpersonal psychology.

PSYCHOANALYTIC THEORY AND MEDITATION

For psychoanalytically oriented therapists, the task of therapy is to uncover and understand the initial traumatic event, "to make the unconscious conscious, recover warded off memories, and overcome infantile amnesia" (Greenson, 1968, p. 4). As Freud noted in a preliminary communication to Breuer (1893, cited in Greenson, 1968, p. 11), "each individual hysterical symptom immediately and permanently disappeared when we had succeeded in bringing clearly to light the memory of the event by which it was provoked and in arousing its accompanying affect, and when the patient had described that event in the greatest possible detail and had put the affect into words." This statement illustrates two important aspects of classical psychoanalytic theory which remained unchanged throughout Freud's writing: 1) hysteria is merely a symptom that has its etiology at some point in the past (normally in the child's psychosexual stages of development) and 2) insight into the etiology is necessary and sufficient for curing the symptom.

The analytically oriented have attempted to use meditation as one means of evoking or uncovering repressed material; of breaking down defenses, the "protection of the ego against instinctual demands" (Freud, 1936, p. 146). Those individuals when utilizing meditation with their patients see it as a positive vehicle for inducing primary-process thinking, for avoiding or bypassing rational defense mechanisms and for recollecting memories of traumatic events. They feel however, that in-depth discussion, "i.e. putting the affect into words," is also necessary. The use of meditation is considered "successful," therefore, if it helps "uncover" repressed material. However, it is considered only as an adjunct to psychotherapy. Further, in-depth discussion of the issue is necessary to "describe the event in the greatest possible detail and to put the affect into words."

EGO (HUMANISTIC) PSYCHOLOGY— HOLISTIC MEDICINE

Freud stated in *Civilization and Its Discontents* (Freud, 1961, pp.

57-58) that "men are not gentle creatures who want to be loved; they are, on the contrary, creatures among whose instinctual endowments is to be reckoned a powerful share of aggression."

Rogers, on the other hand, a representative of ego (humanistic) psychology, noted, "The organism has one basic tendency and striving—to actualize, maintain, and enhance the experiencing organism" (Rogers, 1951, p. 491). Therefore, the goal of therapy, according to Rogers, was to get the client to move away from facades, oughts, meeting expectations, pleasing others, and to move towards self-direction—being more autonomous, increasingly trusting and valuing the process which is him/herself (Rogers, 1961, Chapter 8). Ego psychologists believe there is a basic innate self-actualizing quality within each individual. Therefore, the task of the therapist is to provide a warm, supportive trusting environment, to allow this self to be seen and accepted, so that the client can see that s/he "is a person who is competent to direct himself and who can experience all of himself without guilt" (Rogers, 1957, p. 41).

Humanistically oriented psychologists who use meditation in their practice view it as a technique for helping a person become sensitive to his/her innate, self-actualizing nature, for turning from an external to an internal orientation. From the perspective of holistic medicine, meditation is viewed as a way of enhancing individual client responsibility and a way of teaching the client to develop non-pharmacological approaches to taking care of oneself. Meditation is considered to be a successful strategy if the client is able to become more in touch with his/her "true" self; more inner-directed; to take more self-responsibility; and to be more psychologically and physically "centered."

BEHAVIORAL APPROACH

Behavior modification uses principles derived from the experimental analysis of behavior (cf. Skinner, 1953) and Social Learning Theory (Bandura, 1969, 1977) to modify maladaptive behaviors and/or to inculcate more adaptive habits. Behavior therapy consists of activities implying a contractual agreement between therapist and patient (or client) to modify a designated problem behavior—with particular application to neurosis and affective disorders (Wolpe, 1969, Lazarus, 1971).

Behavioral medicine is the application of these principles to physical disease. As Schwartz and Weiss (1977, p. 379) note, "Behavioral medicine is the field concerned with the development of behavioral science knowledge and techniques relevant to the understanding of physical health and illness and applications of this knowledge and these techniques to diagnosis, prevention, treatment and rehabilitation." Pomerleau (1979, p. 655) defines behavioral medicine as "a) the clinical use of techniques derived from the experimental analysis of behavior—behavior therapy and behavior modification—for the evaluation, prevention, management or treatment of physical disease or physiological dysfunction; and b) the conduct of research contributing to the functional analysis and understanding of behavior associated with medical disorders and problems in health care."

Behaviorally oriented individuals who use meditation in their practice view it primarily as a self-regulation strategy for dealing with clinical, health-related, and stress-related concerns. Meditation is considered to be a successful treatment if it proves effective in significantly reducing the target behavior concerns.

TRANSPERSONAL

The transpersonal approach is probably most clearly aligned with the original spiritual intent of meditation practices of the East. It includes many of the qualities associated with the humanistic tradition (i.e. developing inner directedness, a strong sense of oneself) but also goes beyond them. Maslow (1969) referred to the goal of therapy as learning how not only to build a strong sense of ego, but learning how to surrender the ego. The individual is taught how not to identify with his/her thoughts. As Goleman noted (1971, p. 19), "the phenomena contemplated are distinct from the mind contemplating them." The goal of therapy is to develop a high degree of perceptual clarity about one's thought patterns, habits, behaviors, but without the accompanying affect; a mindfulness of each moment.

According to this viewpoint, the definition of successful meditation becomes quite elusive, and rather all-encompassing. Pleasant and unpleasant experiences, even wandering mind all occur in "correct" meditation. The goal is to keep as sensitively mindful as possible to these experiences; to cultivate an attitude of compassionate acceptance; to utilize each experience as "grist for the mill," new learning to be observed, new objects of awareness.

Effective, or successful meditation becomes, therefore, a misnomer. It is not an end state, but a path, a vehicle for "transcending" the personal ego boundaries of the self, and for feeling a sense of spiritual harmony.

THE ORIENTATION AS "DEMAND"

The therapist's orientation (or the religious training organization's belief system,) creates a certain "demand" on the client/patient/student. This "demand" postulates implicitly or explicitly the following: a) I (we) believe in this technique, b) if you believe as we do and practice as we do, this technique will help you achieve a desired effect. The demand characteristics of the therapeutic orientations as noted above are readily apparent.

Further, most religious traditions set forth a certain vision for the student, stating that if these meditation disciplines are correctly practiced, certain positive consequences will follow (Orne, 1962). This demand, as we see in Chapter Eight, has an effect on treatment outcome, moving it, as we would suspect, toward the effect postulated by the therapist/teacher (cf. Smith, 1976).

These demand characteristics have both positive and negative aspects. On the one hand, belief in the efficacy of one's treatment strategy or orientation appears to be an important factor in therapeutic success (e.g., McReynold et al., 1973). Further, the transmission of this belief to the client, and the client's belief in its credibility are also important factors. The only possible adverse effect of these "demands" is when the therapist or organization holds them so strongly as to be unwilling to question them, and/or have them altered by invalidating evidence. Then the orientation, rather than being a useful method for organizing information and hypotheses about the world, becomes a blinder to new information and may cause a type of evangelical fervor to convince others of the rightness of one's view.

1.12 Relationship.

DEPENDING UPON the orientation, the relative emphasis on relationship ranges from unimportant (e.g., taped instructions of meditation) to the critical variable (e.g., Rogers, client-centered therapy). As Rogers noted (1957), the necessary and sufficient variables for therapeutic personality change to occur must be two people in close interpersonal contact, the therapist's empathetic understanding of the client's frame of reference and unconditional positive regard for the client (both of which the client perceives). Truax and Carkhuff developed scales for measuring congruence and genuineness; non-possessive warmth; and non-judgmental accurate empathy; and concluded from their research that these three variables are characteristics of human encounters that change people for the better (Truax & Carkhuff, 1967, p. 41).

The analytic perspective also views the relationship as an important variable particularly around the issues of transference and counter-transference. Technically, transference is defined as the experiencing of feelings, drives, attitudes, fantasies and defenses toward a person in the present which do not benefit that person but are a repetition of reactions originating in regard to significant persons of early childhood, unconsciously displaced onto figures in the present (cf. Freud, 1912). The problem with transference, as Greenson (1968, p. 155) noted, is that it is repetitious and inappropriate. As I use the terms here, they refer (non-technically) to the relationship between the client and therapist: how the client perceives the therapist (transference), e.g., does the client want an authority figure, male or female therapist, warm individual, etc.? And how the therapist perceives the client (counter-transference) e.g., can s/he work with this client? Does s/he dislike the client? These are variables which might effect the therapist's ability to work with the client, or to teach the client a self-regulation technique.

The transpersonal, or spiritual perspective, has two different views with regard to the role of the teacher/therapist, and relationship. Initially it is seen as critical to have someone as a guide. Much as in classical psychoanalysis, this person should be someone who has gone through the practice, the spiritual discipline. The idea behind this is that one can only teach (guide) another as far as the teacher him/herself has gone: i.e. you can only teach what you know. However, ultimately, in many traditions, although the role of the teacher is acknowledged, eventually the individual must leave the teacher and experience for him/herself. As Watts noted (1961), the basic position of the Zen master is that s/he has nothing to teach. Or, in Hesse's *Sidd-*

hartha, Siddhartha met Buddha but left him, "for Siddhartha had...become distrustful of teachings and learning...I have little faith in words that come to us from teachers" (Hesse, 1951, p. 28).

The role of the therapist and therapeutic relationship is emphasized much less in the behavioral tradition. The emphasis is on the utility of the strategy, and therefore tape-recorded or other semi-automated methods of disseminating techniques to individuals are considered appropriate and useful.

Implicit in the above discussion of relationships is the issue of trust. Is the client willing to trust the therapist? How important is this as a variable in positive therapeutic actions?

RESISTANCE

Resistance is a technical term first used by Freud and refers to the two aspects of the person waiting between life (eros) and death (thanatos). Freud saw this as a battle the person under treatment must fight every step of the way, between that part striving toward recovery and the opposing forces, urging destruction and chaos. Therefore, Freud, as therapist, felt he had to fight against the patient's resistance. He did this by representing himself as infallible, as in the case of Frau Elizabeth Von R. in which he said, (e.g., "Tell me what's happening, I know there is more,") and with Lucy R. in which he pitted his will and efforts against her contrary insistence and desires (Freud, 1959).

In teaching an individual meditation, the therapist needs to be sensitive to several potential resistances, as well as how s/he will deal with resistance to the chosen therapeutic orientation.

Why do some people resist meditating? Carrington and Ephron (1975) made useful comments on why there is refusal to learn or continue to meditate: 1) incompatibility with the individual's lifestyle or belief system, 2) a fear of loss of control, 3) difficulty in giving up the parent/child roles of transference, 4) misconceived "shoulds" about how they should meditate, 5) reluctance to give up of symptoms useful to the patient. In addition, a person may feel "pressured" to learn the technique by a spouse or intimate who recently learned meditation. Often, there can be an evangelic fervor with which a person who practices meditation encourages a spouse to "seek the higher truth." One client told me, "My wife now feels I must begin to meditate. She says if I don't I'll never get out of my rut. I do feel I want to learn it, to try it, but I don't like being forced. In fact, I feel she is beginning to live in a more and more sterile world, afraid to relate to me. My wife is a meticulous person who has always tried to control everything in her life; and when she can't she now retreats into her meditation." So, we need to look at the general family (significant-other) system of a person who wishes to begin, or thinks s/he might want to begin learning meditation. Also, learning an essentially non-analytical technique may be frightening to individuals who have been brought up in a culture which places such a high value on the analytical skills.

How the therapist responds to therapeutic "resistance" in general, and to meditation in particular depends upon the particular orientation. Some specific suggestions from my own orientations are discussed in the case study in Chapter Two.

QUALITIES OF THE THERAPIST: CAN MEDITATION HELP THE THERAPIST?

Implicit in the above discussion is the issue of what therapist qualities facilitate positive therapeutic outcome. The transpersonal approach emphasizes that the therapist be someone who "practices" what s/he preaches; i.e. be on the same path. The humanistic approach as noted emphasizes therapeutic qualities of congruence, empathy, warmth. Freud (1912a), in his recommendations to physicians practicing psychoanalysis, insisted that to be successful, the therapist must shift from participant to observer, from problem-solving to intuition, from a more involved to a more detached position; to have empathy, s/he must "renounce for a time part of his own identity, and for this he must have a loose or flexible self-image" (Greenson, 1968, p. 382).

WOULD MEDITATION BE USEFUL FOR THE THERAPIST?

Complementing discussion of the use of meditation for the client, there has been some writing about the use of meditation for the therapist (Carrington & Ephron, 1975; Schuster, 1979; Keefe, 1975). On a theoretical and anecdotal case-report level, the following have been suggested as benefits for the therapist: greater stamina when patient hours follow in continuous succession, ability to maintain a focus of attention and awareness on present events (Keefe, 1975), increased empathy (Schuster, 1979), enhanced awareness of one's feelings, less tendency toward drowsiness resulting from work stress, and less discomfiture from patients' negative transference reactions (Carrington & Ephron, 1975).

Two studies have looked at the potential effects of meditation on the therapist. Lesh (1970) found that counselors in training who meditated were more empathic—as measured by response to an affective sensitivity videotape—than those who did not. Leung (1973) did a similar study comparing both internal and external concentration and used as his dependent variable two counseling behaviors—empathic understanding of the client, as measured by an analytical empathy measurement, and ability to perceive specific "notice-authority statements" from the client. Leung found that with fourteen hours of training (seven hours internal concentration, seven hours external concentration) the undergraduate subjects significantly increased their ability in the two counseling behaviors described above.

These findings with undergraduates or with counselor trainees in addition to the anecdotal reports of clinicians who meditate, though tentative, suggest a potential utility of meditation for the therapist. They also raise an interesting question for the therapist—*should the nonmeditating therapist offer a meditation technique to a client?*

In the absence of empirical literature directed to this question let me make some suggestions. On the one hand, I think we can carry the argument of matching therapist to client to treatment to an absurd conclusion: i.e. women must counsel only women; black men with stress must counsel only black men with stress; etc. On the other hand, it seems that in teaching a self-regulation skill, the therapist can serve as a useful model. Further, the literature suggests the importance of the therapist's believing in the rationale of the technique (McReynolds et al., 1973). Seemingly, in addition to knowledge of the research literature, one must at least have some first-hand experience to have "faith" in the efficacy of a particular treatment as well as competency and skill in transmitting the technique. The skill at teaching involves being able to be sensitive to problems in learning adherence, as well as the ability to be sensitive to client concerns about certain kinds of experiences that may be quite novel, i.e. altered state experiences. How these experiences are viewed by the therapist—e.g., dismissed, seen as delusional, hallucinatory, viewed as positive, transcendent—would depend in part on the therapist's own personal knowledge of such experiences.

ADVERSE EFFECTS AND CONTRAINDICATIONS:
WHAT SOME MIGHT BE,
HOW A THERAPIST DEALS WITH THEM.

Carrington and Ephron as well as Stroebel and Glueck point out the importance, with psychiatric patients, of having the therapist available to aid with any material that comes into the patient's awareness. Therefore, Carrington (1978) noted that borderline psychotics or psychotic patients should not be prescribed meditation unless their practice of it can be supervised by a psychotherapist familiar with meditation. In this regard almost all meditation researchers and those who use it in their clinical practice are cautious in stating that there should be careful instruction, training, and follow-up observation by the therapist. This is especially true as we become more sensitive to unpleasant and sometimes negative experiences that patients sometimes have during meditation (cf. VanNuys, 1973; Kohr, 1977; Otis et al., 1973; Otis, 1980, in press). For example, Stroebel and Glueck and also Carrington and Ephron note that some of the unpleasant feelings which may occur with meditators include occasional feelings of dizziness, feelings of disassociation, and other adverse feelings produced by the release of images, thoughts, and other material that they had not been sensitive to. In addition to anecdotal reports, there have been three case reports in the literature suggesting the negative effects of meditation (Lazarus, 1976; French, Schmid & Ingalls, 1975; and Walsh & Rauche, 1979). There is also one study (Otis, 1980, in press) with a large N which discusses potential adverse effects of meditation.

Otis reanalyzed data which he had collected previously and examined in particular subjects who had reported a considerable increase (fifty-one percent or over) of feelings in a negative or adverse direction. He found that the longer an individual meditated, the more likely it was that adverse effects would occur. These adverse effects included increased anxiety, boredom, confusion, depression, restlessness, and withdrawal. He also noted that teacher trainees who were long-term meditators reported more adverse effects than long-term meditators who had not made a commitment to become teachers. Although there are many ways to analyze the data, it seems that there is a percentage of people for whom meditation will have negative effects.

For example, certain individuals are attracted to meditation for inappropriate reasons, seeing it as a powerful cognitive avoidance strategy, or attracted to the technique of concentrative meditation as a way of blocking out unpleasant areas of their lives. Similarly, many individuals lacking basic social skills (i.e. those shy or withdrawn) may be attracted to meditation. For these individuals meditation may not be a useful therapeutic intervention (certainly not as a sole intervention strategy). Rather, it may be more appropriate for them to have some kind of social skill or assertiveness training, either in place of or in addition to the meditation treatment (Shapiro, 1980). Further, meditation may not be a useful therapeutic intervention for chronically depressed individuals, who may need to have their arousal level activated (cf. also hypotensives, hyperactive children). Also, many therapists consider arousal one of the prime conditions facilitating therapeutic change (cf. Yalom et al., 1977) and therefore meditation would not be considered a treatment of choice if used as a strategy to calm or relax a person. In addition, it may not be a useful strategy for individuals with somatic but low cognitive anxiety (Davidson & Schwartz, 1976). Meditation may not be the treatment of choice for individuals with high external locus of control, or with clinical problems such as migraine headaches or Raynaud's Disease, which, as Stroebel and Glueck (1977) note, are not as amenable to amelioration by meditation as to temperature and EMG biofeedback for eliciting vasodilation and muscle relaxation.

Additional issues to be considered regarding negative effects are the following: Is the individual meditating for too long a time, thereby impairing reality testing (cf. French et al., 1975; Lazarus, 1976). Is the person spending too much time letting go of thoughts (not analyzing them) and therefore not gaining pinpointed cause and effect awareness. Thus, even though affect may be lessened, has the person learned the antecedent conditions which cause reflex inappropriate, maladaptive behaviors? Have they learned, in addition to skills of letting go of thoughts and goals, the skill of setting goals: existentially choosing who they want to be and how they want to act.

There is also the important issue of preparation. Negative effects may occur if the individual has not been given sufficient preparation. For example, a self-critical, perfectionistic, Western goal-oriented individual who learns meditation will probably bring that same cognitive orientation to the task of meditation. S/he may, therefore, be highly critical: e.g., I am not doing it right, each thought may be seen as a defeat, an internal fight may ensue to "stop" thoughts. As James S. noted in the case to follow, "I became distracted by thoughts, then worried about being distracted; but I couldn't stop the flood of thoughts; I started crying; it was almost impossible for me to then return to breathing."

HOW MAY THESE ADVERSE EFFECTS BE DEALT WITH?

A distinction needs to be made between negative (harmful) effects and unpleasant experiences. As Roger Walsh notes, "Equating unpleasant with negative comes out of an unacknowledged pleasure = good, pain = bad world view, which is the very content which all meditation disciplines say must be transcended" (Personal communication). Therefore it is important to hold the context in mind when we discuss these experiences. Difficulties along the road do not necessarily mean we are on the wrong path. On the other hand, we need to be careful not to dismiss "harmful" experiences too readily. Eastern philosophy, with a world view espousing acceptance, says all things, good and bad, should be accepted with equanimity. Philosophically and theoretically, once a person can do that, life becomes free from suffering, as Buddha noted in his Fourfold Truth.

The transpersonal, or spiritual perspective therefore gives an answer elegant in its simplicity for dealing with adverse effects. Namely: watch that process; don't get caught up in it; let it be a learning experience for yourself, a new awareness of your resistance and defenses; keep the context. The answer to every dilemma becomes: adverse effects are only part of the path. Stay centered. It takes years of practice. On the one hand, I subscribe to this advice. On the other, I find it too absolute; it strikes me as similar to the classical psychoanalytic diction: insight causes cure. If you are not cured, by definition more insight is needed. Similarly, if you are not keeping the context, practice keeping it more. This is similar to the behavioral approach of cognitive restructuring: change your thoughts and you'll feel better. But what about the *process* of how this occurs? Here the therapeutic relationship is critical, as well as non-attachment to verifying the effectiveness of any particular technique.

Further, in the personal growth movement, there is a danger of equating "if it hurts, it must be good for me," or "if it isn't working, try the same thing, only harder: i.e. meditate more." As I note in the epilogue and in the case study, (Chapter Two), if used inappropriately, meditation can become just another vehicle for self-criticism.

Also, even though each "negative" effect may be the fault of incorrect training or attitude, it is important to take these negative effects seriously, become precise about why they are occurring, and see if there are ways to correct them.

Personally, I have learned over the past few years that my preferred attentional style is an overview wide-angle lens approach. I like to take in the field, to get an overview. On Rorschach blots, I see a complete picture, encompassing all the parts in one whole. I do not like concentrative meditation. I fear "tuning out." Therefore, in order for me to concentrate on a task, I need a relatively stimulus-free environment, so that there are no other distractions in the field, and the field becomes the task.

Thus, it is difficult for me to begin concentrating in a noisy stimulus-demanding environment. When I meditate, I like a quiet, peaceful environment so that *my* thoughts can come up. The positive side of this "opening-up style" is that I can allow whatever is going on within me to come to the surface fairly non-defensively, and can also quickly become in tune with the peaceful environment around me. The negative side of this is that I am easily distracted when I try to meditate. Further, there is also a negative effect in the attentional style I use, because after meditation I am highly sensitive. Sometimes after meditation I find myself more easily bothered and annoyed than at other times. Also, an on-rush of inputs often seems quite overwhelming.

In a sense, this is a negative effect occurring from my meditation training. I have had to learn to counter it by a) recognizing my attentional style and situations which make me vulnerable to it, b) building in transition times between formal meditation and external commitments and c) being careful to select appropriate, stimulus-free environments for meditating.

I use the above example as one to illustrate that meditation does condition us in certain ways. There may be unpleasant effects to this conditioning which, if ignored, can be harmful. The case study in Chapter Two gives additional specifies of how to deal with adverse effects in clients.

SUMMARY, CHAPTER ONE

This chapter provides an overview of the structure of the book as embodied in the sentence:

"What effects does the teaching of meditation have on an individual who practices, and why?"

In terms of our microscope analogy, we looked only briefly (and at low power) at effects; somewhat more fully at the issue of what is meditation; and in still greater depth at the individual who might or might not benefit from meditation; the importance of the therapist's orientation; relationship variables; and finally at the issue of practice/adherence. This chapter intended to provide an overview of issues covered in greater detail throughout the rest of the book. In addition to looking at each of these issues separately, as in this chapter, we also need, in subsequent chapters, to look at their interaction with each other. As one way of "grounding" some of the issues discussed in Chapter One, we turn in Chapters Two and Three to two case studies.

Chapter One: Further Reading

ON PARADIGMS

General

Kuhn, T. *The structure of scientific revolutions.* Chic: Univ. of Chic. Pr., 1971.

Tart, C. States of consciousness and state specific sciences. *Science,* 1972, *186,* 1203-10.

Related to Eastern Thought

Walsh, R., Elgin D., Vaughan, F., & Wilber, K. Consciousness disciplines and the behavioral sciences. *American Journal of Psychiatry,* in press.

Wilbur, K. *Spectrum of consciousness.* Wheaton, IL: Theosophical Pub. House, 1977.

ON THE TYPES OF MEDITATION

Books

Carrington, P. *Freedom in meditation.* New York: Doubleday/ Anchor, 1978.

Goleman, D. *Varieties of the meditative experience.* New York: E.P. Dutton, 1977.

Naranjo, C. & Ornstein, R. *On the psychology of meditation.* New York: Viking—Esalen Books, 1971.

Shapiro, D.H. *Precision nirvana.* Englewood Cliffs, NJ: Prentice-Hall, 1978b. (Chapter 1).

Articles

Anand, B., Chinna, E., & Singh, B. Some aspects of electroencephalographic studies in yogis. *Electroencephalography & Neurophysiology,* 1961a, *13,* 452-456. (Reprinted in D.H. Shapiro & R.N. Walsh. *The science of meditation,* [New York: Aldine], 1980).

Brown, D.P. A model of the levels of concentrative meditation, *International Journal of Clinical & Experimental Hypnosis,*

1977, *25*, (4), 236-273. (Reprinted in D.H. Shapiro & R.N. Walsh, [Eds.], *The science of meditation.* [New York: Aldine], 1980).
For components: See Chapter Eight.

ON EFFECTS:

See Chapters Five and Seven.

ON TEACHING:

Orientations:

1. Psychoanalytic
   Shafii, M. Silence in the service of the ego: Psychoanalytic study of meditation. *International Journal of Psychoanalysis,* 1973, *(54),* (4) 431-443.
   Fromm, E. Zen and psychoanalysis, *Psychologia,* 1959, *2,* 79-99.

2. Behavioral Approach
   Woolfolk, R. and Franks, C. Meditation and behavior therapy. In D.H. Shapiro and R.N. Walsh (Eds.) *The science of meditation.* New York, Aldine, 1980, in press.
   Ellis, A. The place of meditation in rational emotive therapy and cognitive behavior therapy. In D.H. Shapiro and R.N. Walsh, *The science of meditation.* New York, Aldine, 1980, in press.

3. Humanistic/Holistic Medicine
   Lesh, T. Zen meditation and the development of empathy in counselors. *Journal of Humanistic Psychology,* 1970, *10,* (1), 39-74.
   Pelletier, K. *Mind as healer, mind as slayer.* New York: Delacourte, 1977.

4. Transpersonal
   Goleman, D. Meditation as metatherapy. *Journal of Transpersonal Psychology,* 1971, *3* (1), 1-25.
   Akishige, Y. The principles of the psychology of Zen in Y. Akishige (Ed.). *The principles of the psychology of Zen.*

Tokyo: Maruzen Co., Ltd., 1977. Reprinted in D.H. Shapiro and R.N. Walsh, *The science of meditation.* New York: Aldine, 1980, in press.

See also Chapters Two and Three for case studies.

On Individuals:

SUBJECT VARIABLES

Smith, J.C. Personality correlates of continuation and outcome in meditation and erect sitting control treatments. *Journal of Consulting & Clinical Psychology,* 1978, *46,* 272-279. (Reprinted in D.H. Shapiro & R.N. Walsh [Eds.] *The science of meditation,* New York: Aldine, 1980).

Beiman, I. et al. Client characteristics and success in Transcendental Meditation. In D.H. Shapiro & R.N. Walsh, (Eds.), *The science of meditation,* New York: Aldine, in press.

ADHERENCE

Glueck, B. & Stroebel, C. Meditation in the treatment of psychiatric illness. *Comprehensive Psychiatry,* 1975, *16,* (4) 303-321. (Reprinted in D.H. Shapiro, & R.N. Walsh, [Eds.], *The science of meditation.* New York: Aldine, 1980.

Marlatt, A. et al. Effects of meditation and relaxation training upon alcohol use in male social drinkers. In D.H. Shapiro & R.N. Walsh (Eds.), *The science of meditation,* New York: Aldine, 1980.

Goldman, B.L., Domitor, P.J., & Murray, E.J. Effects of Zen meditation on anxiety reduction and perceptual functioning. *Journal of Consulting & Clinical Psychology,* 1979, *47,* (3), 551-556.

ON MEDIATING MECHANISMS:

See Chapter Nine.

2

Meditation
and Psychotherapy:
A Case Study—James S.

THE FOLLOWING case studies in Chapters Two and Three exemplify in practical ways how the issues raised in Chapter One can be applied. Both cases are guided by the framework laid out in that chapter and attempt to further help us answer the question, "What effect does the teaching of meditation have on an individual who practices, and why?" The first case study, James S., (Chapter Two) is a clinical case illustrating the use of meditation as a self-regulation strategy; the second case, Deane S. (Chapter Three) illustrates a potential methodology for researching meditation as an altered state of consciousness. Since I am the therapist in the case in this chapter, it is important to include here some remarks on my therapeutic orientation and style. I present my own views within the context of the general issues of "teaching" which need to be addressed in any clinical/therapeutic endeavor. Specifically, these issues, mentioned in Chapter One, include the orientation, beliefs and preconceptions of the teacher and his/her role, the role of the relationship process, and the actual method of teaching.

2.1 *The Orientation of the Therapist*

I REMEMBER being asked my religious orientation in a religious studies class at Stanford. I wrote: a Jewish existentialist with Zen Buddhist inclinations. My clinical orientation is similarly complex. It is behavioral, insofar as that implies belief in the importance of carefully evaluating the efficacy of my clinical work (rather than adherence to a specific body of techniques). It is also behavioral in that it involves an emphasis on action-oriented therapy, a setting of goals with the client, the collection of data, working on change—behavioral or cognitive—i.e. new ways of acting, thinking, feeling about the world and oneself. It is insight oriented insofar as that means that a client's understanding of his/her behavior, thoughts, actions, habit patterns is important, rather than *a priori* assuming historical insight into psychosexual stages is needed. It is relationship oriented—I believe trust, empathy and understanding provide a critical context for therapeutic change. However, I do not believe, in general, that relationship is sufficient, and do not believe it should be the focus of therapy, except as it facilitates changes the client is trying to make outside of the therapeutic context. Finally, it is religious, spiritual, transpersonal, insofar as this means I am committed to my own personal growth and work, believe in working toward developing myself toward the farther reaches of my potential, desire to find a core connection between myself and others, and have experienced feelings of unity and oneness with nature, myself, and others. It does not mean I believe all clients should experience this; that there is only one path to its experience; or that it is an *a priori*, true reality, but rather one which I believe to be true, part of my path of heart: a belief system that, for now, *works* to nourish and sustain me.

Thus my orientation is really a combination of personal, clinical and religious. Interestingly, at the risk of being an overly "general" armchair philosopher, it appears to me that for many, there is a large overlap between the psychological and religious. Scientists and psychotherapists have, for many in our culture, become a type of guru: priests of a technological and secular age.

To label my orientation, we could say I am an applied pragmatic behaviorist who believes in relationship, insight, and spiritual growth, all with appropriate reservations!

Perhaps, true to the behaviorist/existentialist within me, more important than the label, is how I act. So, let us now turn to two different cases, to discuss in more detail the issues raised in the first chapter.

2.2 Therapist's Belief in the Efficacy of the Strategy

I BELIEVE meditation to be a useful self-regulation strategy for certain clients with certain clinical problems. I do not believe meditation to be any more (or less) effective than other self-regulation strategies for a client who wishes some type of stress-management strategy. My decision to use it (rather than other strategies) would depend upon the client's belief system, values and expectations. Further, I do not feel a particular need to call a cognitive focusing strategy "meditation" if a client has a resistance to that term either because of prior religious training, or dislike of its "mystical" association. I am also not convinced, at the level of actual behavior, how different meditation is from other cognitive strategies. As Ted Barber noted, on reading a previous draft of this manuscript (personal communication, January 23, 1979),

> The overlap between self-hypnosis and meditation is tremendous. In fact it seems to me that the variability within self-hypnosis and meditation is almost as large as the variability between these procedures. There seems to me to be so many parallels so that it appears possible to at least conceptualize self-hypnosis as one type of meditation, or vice versa, meditation as one type of self-hypnosis.

It should be noted, however, that for me we are talking here only about meditation as a self-regulation strategy, and its use for clients who wish some form of training for a stress-related problem.

2.3 The Client, and Presenting Problem

JAMES SIDNEY, an Australian male in his mid-thirties, was a short, rather unassuming individual, with a kind and sensitive face. When he introduced himself to me at my private practice office in Portola Valley, California, he shook my hand, but didn't directly make eye contact. Although he had a pronounced accent, his speech was clear and lucid, but his voice was often so soft that I could not hear his words. When we sat down, he said, "I have a problem with insomnia, and wondered if you could teach me meditation." He said he knew of my clinical interest in meditation, and on the recommendation of a mutual colleague on the East coast, presented himself to me to learn an approach to meditation that was not immersed in "cultic" paraphernalia: incense, pictures of gurus, candles, etc.

I told him that yes, I would be glad to teach him meditation and work with him on the issue of insomnia. As one way of doing this, I told him it would be helpful for me to get to know him a bit better—his background—and to learn what he had heard about and expected from meditation.

CLINICAL NOTE

I have three goals in obtaining this information. First, before teaching a technique to a client, it is important to gather information about the client's expectations, hopes, motivation for learning a particular technique. Second, I interact with this information in a way which attempts to build a trusting relationship (cf. Rogers, 1951, 1961; Truax & Carkhuff, 1967) between us. I believe this relationship provides an important context for the teaching of technique and skill training (Shapiro, 1976). Without the trust, the teaching of any technique, whether meditation or a behavioral strategy is more difficult (G. Davison, 1973). Third, I want to obtain some initial background information about the client, as well as a broader profile of what other issues may currently be going on in this client's life that may be relevant to therapy.

OVERVIEW OF THERAPY DURATION

This client was seen for ten months. The first six months we met once a week; the next two months, once every other week, and then I saw him twice at three week intervals. There was a six-month, written follow-up. The sessions were face to face in the office; and involved homework assignments and data collection outside the office.

2.4 Client Expectations

THE CLIENT noted he had heard and read in the newspaper about the scientific experiments showing meditation's effectiveness for stress and felt it would be helpful for him. He said that he was not particularly interested in the "spiritual mumbo-jumbo" that went along with the technique. He noted that although raised a Catholic, he had had no formal religious affiliation for several years. "I consider myself more interested in down-to-earth human concerns than metaphysical issues."

2.5 Client Background

THE CLIENT noted he used to sleep about eight or nine hours a night, but that a couple years ago, for no reason he was aware of, he began to wake up during the night. He began to awaken with increasing frequency per night during the next six months, and finally decided to go into therapy. He noted that he was in therapy for the next six months, and that the therapy focused almost exclusively on trying to understand his dreams. The therapist indicated that the sleep disturbance was only a "symptom." After six months of dream analysis and no improvement, and even some deterioration in sleep, he left therapy. The therapist told him he was not giving the process long enough, and was only leaving now out of fear of confronting the really deep, true material.

Client then began taking valium (5-10 mg. nightly) and had been doing so for the year prior to our first meeting. He came in now because the insomnia problem seemed quite bad, he felt tired and tense at night from fear of going to sleep; and during the day from lack of sleep. He also had read and been told that it was not good for him to continue to use valium every night.

Over the next few therapy sessions, I learned the following information. In addition to the issue of insomnia (Concern #1), he was quite shy and unassertive. He noted that he had almost no contact with either his own or the opposite sex. Further, it was hard for him to be assertive, particularly with his family. He had two brothers, and both parents were living. He felt quite pushed around, "bullied" by the older brother, and ignored and not attended to by the father. The mother was somewhat distant and he had never really felt too close to her. The issue of shyness and assertiveness became Concern #2. The client also noted he was quite self-critical, frequently noting in the session how poorly he did almost everything (Concern #3); felt stress a high proportion of the time during the day (Concern #4), and finally that he was an administrative assistant in business, currently out of work and having difficulty finding a new job, partly because of a poor recommendation from his previous employer (Concern #5).

2.6 Client Motivation

THE CLIENT felt his general weariness and stress from lack of sleep had reached "crisis proportions" and something needed to be done. He noted he was quite willing to learn and practice the technique of meditation.

The client intially appeared highly motivated to me and this was borne out in the course of therapy. Initial concurrent evidence of this motivation and ability to adhere to self-regulation practice was a special diet he was put on by his physician for a phosphorous imbalance. He had to be extremely careful about his eating behavior and monitor closely his intake. He followed this diet meticulously.

During therapy he maintained accurate and complete records of the homework assignments of areas monitored, practiced meditation exactly as instructed, and put a great deal of personal effort and energy into each concern we worked on.

2.7 Baseline Data

BECAUSE OF the behavioral part of my orientation, I felt it important to have the client gather data (i.e. monitor) in diary and/or chart form, on each of the areas of concern: i.e. the frequency, nature, duration of the target behaviors. This baseline data for each of the areas of concern is discussed below.

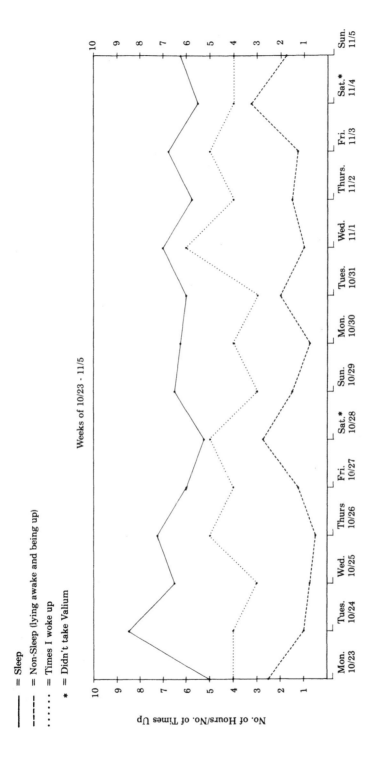

FIGURE 2.1

Sleep: Baseline Data Weeks One and Two

CONCERN NUMBER ONE:
SLEEP BEHAVIOR

As noted, the client stated that he used to sleep seven to eight hours a night, believed he currently was getting only three to four hours of sleep per night, if that; and felt he needed at least six to seven hours. To assess current sleep patterns we monitored length of night, amount of time asleep, number of times awoke, length of time awake, and whether or not he took valium that night.

From a two-week baseline (2.1) we found that this client on an average was sleeping a mean of 5.8 hours, was waking about 4.14 times, and was up 1.53 hours (i.e. twenty-seven minutes per time). The kinds of things that awoke him were: a) anticipation of a noisy neighbor coming in; b) actual noise from a neighbor (e.g., jogging upstairs, loud music); c) a bad dream; d) no actual incident. We also noted that Saturday nights were particularly difficult, partly because of the general noise in his apartment complex. During each week of the two-week baseline, the client took valium on six of seven nights.

CONCERN NUMBER TWO:
COMPANIONSHIP/ASSERTIVENESS SKILLS

The client was asked to monitor the amount of his social interactions not related to job searching. The first week, he noted that his only companionship was a hitchhiker to whom he gave a ride. The next week, it was his brother on the phone, the one he felt nagged him too much—about his health, about not having a job. When asked how he responded, he said he didn't say anything to the brother about the nagging. We discussed the client's fear of being pushed around, being taken advantage of and used both by his family and by potential acquaintances.

The client also noted that he really didn't want to have people back to his apartment because others might think it was sterile and unattractive, "just because it is neat, clean, and totally bare." He said he didn't feel any need to fix it up and artificially put "his stamp on it." He also noted that he seemed to have a response of ignoring (or pretending to ignore) insults or put-downs of other people and then all of a sudden to "snap" (his word) and become aggressive and verbally angry.

CONCERN NUMBER THREE:
POSITIVE AND NEGATIVE SELF-THOUGHTS

The first week of monitoring positive and negative thoughts, the client noted that his thoughts were primarily negative and that every time he had a positive thought (e.g., my piano playing sounds good), he followed it with a negative statement (e.g., who cares?).

CONCERN NUMBER FOUR:
STRESS/RELAXATION EXPERIENCES

A fourth area of monitoring was stress—times when he felt stress (antecedents, behavior consequences). He felt he was always pushing himself—what's going to happen next; how will I cope with tomorrow? Stress for him included physical symptoms of tight jaws, back, and shoulders. Mentally, he would block everyone out and ignore them. Stress frequently occurred for him when he felt there was too much to do with too little time. We also looked at times when he felt relaxed: when he was walking alone, sometimes when reading.

CONCERN NUMBER FIVE: JOB

The final area of monitoring was to look at behaviors he did toward finding a new job and how that process felt to him.

2.8 Interventions

THUS, AFTER the first few weeks, a more complete picture of this person began to emerge, and we began to work together to set goals in each of the areas of concern and develop appropriate intervention strategies to help him meet these goals.

MEDITATION

In structuring a treatment intervention, I try to relate the client's concern to the research literature, to see what interventions have and have not been effective with this type of problem.

To my knowledge there is only one study in the clinical literature on meditation and insomnia. (Concern Number One). Although there are methodological problems with the study (measuring sleep onset and sleep duration) meditation was shown to be as effective as progressive relaxation in treating insomnia, and both were more effective than a non-treatment control (Woolfolk, et al., 1976). Further, as there are problems with drug dependence (Coates & Thoresen; 1978) and as the client requested to learn meditation, it seemed to be the treatment of choice for the sleep problem. Further, it was hoped, with appropriate cueing and practice, that the relaxation aspect of meditation would generalize to other high-stress times in this client's life (Concern Number Four: Stress).

CLINICAL NOTE:
CLIENT BACKGROUND INFORMATION

Before actually teaching meditation, the therapist should have made a careful assessment of the client's feelings, hopes, and expectations. Why did the client come into therapy? What is his/her concern? Is the client willing to take responsibility for that concern? How committed is the client (i.e. how motivated to change)? What is the client's vision of what might (can) happen if he or she does try to change? Does the client fear failure? Why? What are ways the client might sabotage his or her own efforts to change? Does the client fear success? Why? What are the client's reactions to "meditation"? Is there a fear of it, e.g., as mystical? Why? Does the client fear being controlled or losing control? Is there an attraction to meditation? Why? Is the client motivated by the idea of learning to yield and let go of thoughts? A cognitive avoidance? Or a hope for growth? Is the client willing to trust him or herself with an essentially non-analytical technique?

After this assessment, the therapist should determine whether meditation is indicated or contraindicated.

CHARACTERISTICS OF THIS CLIENT
WHICH SUGGEST INDICATION
FOR MEDITATION

First, the client requested meditation. Second, the research literature suggests its effectiveness for insomnia (Woolfolk et al., 1976) and stress management (Shapiro & Giber, 1978). Third, the client's anxiety was primarily cognitive (Schwartz, Davidson & Goleman, 1978). The client was highly motivated and once he made a decision would stick to it and therefore would probably score high in internal locus of control (Beiman et al., in press, 1980); and also fit a personality profile of inward directed, relatively neutral affect (one which correlates with success in meditation; cf. Smith, 1978).

POTENTIAL CONTRAINDICATIONS

The client seemed shy and of low affect. Meditation as a sole strategy might merely reinforce that behavior pattern. Further the client was a "perfectionist" and might apply these same standards to the technique, perhaps being too self-critical.

If an individual has negative association to the term, "meditation," I feel no need to try to convince the client that it is an effective strategy and that they should change their beliefs. Rather, as noted earlier, I would rather change the label—e.g., a relaxation technique, a cognitive (attention) focusing strategy, etc.*

Assuming the client does want to learn meditation, what do I then tell them in terms of outcome results and practice?

CLINICAL NOTE: "DEMAND" CHARACTERISTICS
OUTCOME RESULTS AND PRACTICE

In Chapter Five we discuss in some detail the research literature on meditation's effects. Because I believe it therapeutically beneficial to create positive expectancies, I often find it useful to share in lay terms these results. In this particular case I noted, "I think your choice of meditation for dealing with insomnia and general stress is a good one, for it has in fact been found to be effective for these types of concern."

---

*Earlier, before I would screen clients for their reactions to meditation, I had an interesting experience teaching meditation as part of a relaxation group in a psychiatric ward at the V.A. Hospital. A patient leaped up and ran out of the room shouting, "You're trying to steal my mind with Eastern witchcraft."

However, I also feel it important to state that meditation is not a magical panacea, and that the effects from meditation are a result of practice. I ask if the client is willing to give it a chance to work. "Normally, you should begin to feel a significant reduction in stress and anxiety within four to ten weeks (e.g., Smith, 1975). Are you willing to practice the technique on a regular basis for at least that period of time?" If the answer is yes, I spend some time talking about, planning when, and visualizing where the person might have an opportunity to practice on a daily basis. If the answer is equivocal, I spend some time on this issue, again stressing the importance of practice and talking with the client about how much effort they are willing to expend to deal with their concern. Before teaching a strategy, I do try to get some form of commitment from the client.

RELATIONSHIP ISSUES

By this time there should also be at least the initial development of trust and rapport between the therapist and client. As noted, the therapist should be aware that techniques appear to be more effective if offered within a context of trust and support (Davison, 1973). Because exploring one's self, with any strategy, can be frightening, the therapist's gentleness and encouragement in this process, I believe, are crucial.

SELECTION OF A MEDITATION TECHNIQUE

The research literature on this point is not yet very helpful. For example, we do not yet know whether individuals with certain strong perceptual representational systems (e.g., visual, auditory, tactile, etc.) would be better off with an object of meditation which either is or is not in that same representational system (e.g., should an "auditory" person utilize a mantra or a mandala?). The biofeedback literature indicates that relaxation is facilitated if the feedback is in the non-preferred mode: i.e. biofeedback is more effective for an auditory person receiving visual feedback than for an auditory person receiving auditory feedback (Branstrom, Note 7). However, Davidson and Schwartz (1976) suggest that an object of concentration in the same mode as the problem is preferred. If a person has too many thoughts, they should attend to verbal focus such as mantra, koan, etc. Further, there is some question about whether individuals would be better off learning concentrative versus mindfulness meditation, or both; and if both, in which sequence. The classical literature says first concentration, then mindfulness (e.g., Goleman, 1972). But what about beginning clients? We do not yet have any data which speak to this issue.

INSTRUCTIONS

This client was initially instructed in breath meditation, including counting one through ten, and asked to practice twice a day, twenty minutes each session. Why breath meditation? There is no empirically valid rationale for choosing this particular meditation technique over any other. Personally, it is the one I was taught in the Orient, and clinically, it is the one with which I am most experienced. I hope that further research, as suggested in Chapters Eight, Nine, and Ten of this book, will allow for a less personally biased determination of treatment choice. However, at this point, there seems no clear cut reason not to utilize the meditation technique with which a clinician feels most comfortable.

I generally spend part of two or three sessions instructing the client and having them practice the technique in the office. There are particular signs of "correct" practice I look for, and particular areas of the "teaching" that I believe important to emphasize. These are discussed in detail in Chapter Four where practical instructions for a breath meditation technique are given.

Another question often raised is when in relation to the therapy session should the person meditate? Carrington and Ephron (1975) have described having individuals meditate right before a treatment session so that whatever material may surface would be available for that therapeutic session. I have a meditation room next to my office where individuals can meditate prior to the session, for reasons similar to Carrington and Ephron's, as well as after the session, as a way of attempting to make sure that anything which is dealt with in the therapy session, which may be painful, might just be observed for a certain period of time during the meditation session without undue analysis. Meditation sessions before and after, even though brief, seem to serve also as a helpful transition, both preceding therapy and following therapy before returning to the "real world."

WHY A TAPE, TOO?

In addition to the verbal instructions and practice in the office, I also often give clients a tape to utilize at home. The tape follows the instructions in the office and provides a time frame of twenty minutes. I do this as a way of facilitating practice at home. There are two potential advantages to the tape. 1) The tape repeats the office instructions, and thus provides clients an opportunity to re-check in case they feel they have forgotten or are not practicing correctly. This helps avoid the statement the following week of "I didn't remember exactly how to do it so thought I would wait till our next appointment." 2) The tape is structured with a successive approximation to silence. The first part contains dialogue of instruction followed by a thirty-second silence, then re-instructions to keep focused on breathing, followed by a ninety-second silence; then briefer re-instructions, followed by a ten-minute silence. Many people find this gradual approach to silence more comforting than just abruptly sitting down and counting breaths. Some people, however, find the instructions a disruptive, external intrusion. Therefore, in my instruction to the use of the tape, I note that some people find the tape helpful to facilitate their practice, by keeping them from having to worry about time boundaries, etc. I ask them to try it and if they find it helpful initially, to continue to use it. I note, however, that once they feel comfortable they can practice on their own schedule and time, using the tape only as a checkup when and if they feel it appropriate.

JAMES S's EXPERIENCES DURING MEDITATION

A general description follows of the issues that occurred during the nine months of meditation practice and how they were dealt with.

FIRST MONTH

After the first week of practice, he noted tension in his face that he had not realized was there and also how hard it was for him to be attentive and relaxed. In the morning he felt his heart beat slowly and heavily, but not in the evening—then he got restless. He noted that the tape kept him sitting. This points out one of the potential initial issues in working with a client in meditation: that initially a certain discipline is necessary to give it a try. Generally, he said, by the end of the tape, even though he was not aware of the process by which it happened, he felt more relaxed and refreshed. He noted, "It's easier with the tape than without it." Without it he said he felt too time conscious.

Several times in the first month he noted that he felt "energetic" during meditation—a positive contrast to the lethargy he often felt during the day. The nature of the thoughts that occurred were generally of a "planning ahead" nature, such as people he had talked to or he was planning to talk to. Nice images included flowers, trees, mountains, birds. Sometimes he said he felt sad, lonely and withdrawn.

CLINICAL NOTE

The above comments raise several important issues. First, what should you instruct a client to do with thoughts—either positive ones or aversive ones? I agree with the recommendation of Glueck and Stroebel (1975) that when ideas that seem important to the therapeutic session come up during meditation, the meditator is to treat them like any other thought and return to the meditation focus or "anchor."

In other words, the client is instructed to merely observe the thought, notice any feelings associated with it, watch it and when s/he is ready, to return the focus to the breathing. In the therapy session, we then would spend time discussing issues or insights resulting from meditation. For example, the client's strong awareness of his/her feelings of loneliness became part of the incentive and motivation for him to decide to risk practicing social skills. The positive images gave us helpful information about useful competing responses to the aversive, fearful images in the evening of not being able to fall asleep.

It should be noted that the East says we should let go of thoughts when we meditate. They criticize the Western approach of thinking about thoughts and say that many Westerners believe they are meditating when in fact they are only performing therapy on themselves. My feeling is that a balance is needed. During meditation I believe, as noted, that it is best to let the thoughts go. In meditation as a clinical self-regulation strategy, we can learn to see what issues come into awareness, feel how salient they are (i.e. how attached we are to them); watch them with equanimity and then let them go. However, I believe that after meditation, in therapy, the talking about, discussing, analyzing the issues, antecedents, consequences, etc., is important to facilitate change. The East would say let it all go. The West would say analyze it when it comes up. I think, sequentially, both are possible and useful.

A second important issue is the "anxiety about anxiety" that often can occur when a person initially meditates. They become aware of how tense they are (e.g., face tension for this client); how restless, how inattentive their mind is. Here therapist reassurance that "this is part of the process" is important.

Third, it should be noted that there is a certain discipline needed for the practice of meditation. For this client the tape helped, i.e. kept him sitting, so that by the end he felt more relaxed.

NEXT FOUR MONTHS

These were generally positive sessions for the client in which he experimented with a variety of cognitive strategies—self instructions, imagery, etc. The client noted that the best way for him to let go of thoughts was an image of a window in his mind's eye. He meditated on one side of the window in the room (in his mind); outside the window was a pasture with cows. He opened the window and let the thoughts fly out to pasture to graze with the cows, or let the thoughts "drift away" like kites without a string.

He also said he generally looked forward to the meditation practice, felt it refreshing, that it gave some structure to his days, and to him, a sense of competence. He learned about his thought process, realizing which thoughts he felt were more important (i.e. he was more attached to) because these thoughts had a higher emotional charge and it was harder to let them go.

SIXTH TO NINTH MONTH

At the start of the sixth month of meditation he said he was attaining deeper levels of meditation; that he liked it, in general, and yet he was noticing more thoughts and he felt he was more distracted than when he had initially begun. After six months of meditating, we shifted from counting one through ten to just counting one after each out-breath. He said he did not like this as much as there was too little structure and so we returned to counting one through ten. He noticed, however, that there was still a constant stream of thought and he was becoming angry at himself for this, feeling a failure every time a thought occurred.

We discussed the importance of acceptance. I re-emphasized that "if thoughts come, that's okay, if they do not, that's okay, too." I tried to get the client to view meditation as a process of acceptance of what is and help him become aware how he was bringing "old" behavior patterns to the practice, applying "perfectionist" (goal oriented, accomplishment oriented) standards to meditation. We explained how this could, in fact, just be a way of setting himself up for failure. The image he liked was one which recognized the discipline it takes to practice meditation while trying to stay calm: "A fighter who meditates acceptingly." After two more months, he noted that he was fighting the meditation less and becoming more accepting of where he was with the process. He still noted that at times he felt inundated by his mind, "I can only turn it off . . . so seldom, it feels keyed-up, planning, worrying, finding chores to do." During the positive times he said his hands felt warm and good. They turned into furry, soft, heavy paws.

At this point I suggested he choose his own length of meditation. If he felt distracted and not able to meditate well, not to force it. It was all right to just stop after a few minutes. Again, it was a process of acceptance, not a goal of "reaching the end of the tape." He found this helpful, and sometimes he meditated more, sometimes less, "Not to fight it, to give up if thoughts get away from me."

CLINICAL NOTE:

It is important to note the issue of balance involved here. Initially, as noted earlier, I believe a certain discipline is necessary to give a self-control strategy like meditation a chance. However, we need to be careful that the discipline does not turn into a compulsive rigidity: "I must practice twenty minutes or I'm a failure," etc. The therapist needs to be sensitive to when to encourage the discipline, when to encourage the letting go, of "rigid" standards, i.e. you "should," "it is 'better' if you can practice twenty minutes twice a day." Further, as noted, the therapist can utilize this information to explore with clients their psychological patterns and style as an aid to therapeutic learning.

NON-MEDITATION INTERVENTIONS, BY CONCERN AREAS

Let us now turn to each of the five specific concerns of the client and note how other interventions, in addition to meditation, were utilized to help this client accomplish his goals.

CONCERN NUMBER ONE: INSOMNIA

The client's general insomnia-related goals, on coming into therapy, were to lose his dread of going to sleep at night, increase sleep to at least six to seven hours per night, stop taking valium, and as a by-product, feel more relaxed and rested during the working day.

After the two-week baseline, the client realized he was getting much more sleep that he had thought. This self-observation in and of itself, therefore, became an intervention, and helped the client to feel more confident about his sleep problems. A second intervention was my telling the client, "When you are lying in bed, either initially or after awakening, you should remember that resting quietly is as good as sleeping. So don't worry about being awake. Just let yourself lie there and relax." The client noted that it really helped him to say this statement. (This cognitive restructuring was a strategy taught to me by my father when I was a child!) As the client noted, "I'm not dreading going to sleep as much. It's good to know I'm getting an adequate amount of sleep."

In addition to the regular meditation practice twice a day, the client used the focused breathing and counting as a general relaxation strategy while lying in bed beginning to go to sleep. Besides meditation, the baseline observation and the cognitive restructuring strategy, this client also used humming, listening to an ocean record, and pep-talks (self-instructions) to deal with the anxiety and fear associated with sleep and the racing future-planning thoughts that would keep him tense and lying awake.

Another sleep-related issue the client had which we monitored during the initial few weeks was the amount of valium that he took. The first two weeks he went one night each week without it; the third week, two nights; the fourth week, three nights. The fourth week of three nights without valium was quite difficult for the client and in the following few weeks he resumed taking it every night. However, since the client was sleeping between five and six hours per night and felt comfortable with this, the sleep issue faded into the background and, with only minor spot checking (weeks six through ten, week fourteen), we turned to the other areas of concern (see Figure 2.2).

At week twenty-one, we returned to the sleep issue, particularly in relation to valium consumption. The client was feeling quite confident about his sleep patterns and wanted to work on stopping the valium. We decided to take a "successive approximation approach," beginning by not taking it two nights of the week.

While going off valium he gave himself the following self-instructions, "I am practicing relaxing, meditating, so I'm getting pretty good at this. I am not taking that much valium anyway; don't force it; let it go. If I can't get to sleep right away, it's not a big thing. Practice and be gentle on yourself as you try something new."

Weeks twenty-one through thirty-one involved working on increasing the amount of evenings in which no valium was taken. Figure 2.3 shows that he gradually tapered off valium, until in the last two weeks, he took it only twice.

This felt like a comfortable level to the client—to take it if he needed it, or felt in trouble but to first practice the strategies mentioned above.

Interestingly, the sleep data (Table 2.1, Figure 2.4) revealed that often the client slept as well with or without valium. These data charts helped him realize that in many ways the valium was merely a "psychological" aid, one which in fact did not seem to help him on a regular basis—many nights he would sleep better (i.e. more sleep time, less awakenings, less time up per awakening) without valium than with it. However, we agreed that

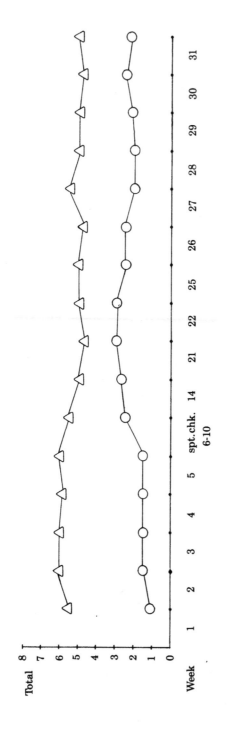

FIGURE 2.2
Weekly Mean of Sleep and Non-Sleep
(Hours)

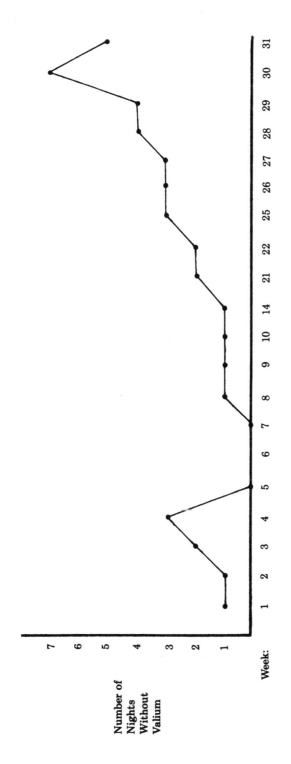

FIGURE 2.3

Nights Per Week Without Valium

TABLE 2.1
Weekly Mean of Sleep, Non-Sleep, (in hours) and Number of times Awoke Total, With Valium, and Without Valium

	WEEK	1	2	3	4	5	6-10	14	21	22	25	26	27	28	29	30	31
Total	Sleep (hours)	5.6	6.0	6.2	5.8	6.3	5.5	5	4.9	5.2	5.3	4.8	5.5	5	5.1	4.9	5.2
	Non-Sleep (hours)	1.5	1.6	1.5	1.7	1.6	2.5	2.9	3.1	3.2	2.3	2.6	2.3	2	2.3	2.5	2.4
	No. Times Awoke	4	4.3	4.9	4	4.7	3.8	4.3	5	5.7	5	4.8	4.7	4.4	3.6	4.3	4
	No. of Nights Mean Based On	7	7	7	7	7	14	7	7	7	7	7	7	7	7	7	7
With Valium	Sleep (hours)	5.6	6.1	6.1	6.2	6.3	5.6	5.2	5.3	5.4	5.4	4.9	5.5	4.8	5.1	—	5.2
	Non-Sleep (hours)	1.3	1.4	1.1	1.1	1.6	2.5	2.9	2.9	2.8	2.4	2.5	2.3	2.1	1.8	—	2.5
	No. Times Awoke	3.8	4.3	4.8	4.5	4.7	3.7	4.5	5	6	5.5	4.8	5	5	4	—	4
	No. of Nights Mean Based On	6	6	5	4	7	11	6	5	5	4	4	4	3	3	0	2
w/o Valium	Sleep (hours)	5.3	5.5	6.4	5.4	—	5.4	4	4	4.6	5.3	4.8	5.5	5.1	5.2	5.0	5.2
	Non-Sleep (hours)	2.8	3.3	2	2.4	—	2.3	3	3.5	3.9	2.2	2.8	2.1	2	2.7	2.5	2.4
	No. Times Awoke	5	4	5	3.3	—	4	3	5	5	4.3	5	4.3	4	3.3	4.3	4
	No. of Nights Mean Based On	1	1	2	3	0	3	1	2	2	3	3	3	4	4	7	5

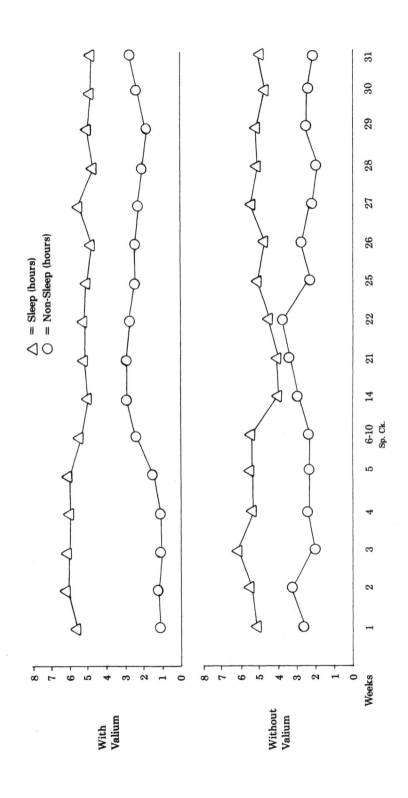

FIGURE 2.4 *Mean Hours of Sleep and Non-Sleep: With and Without Valium*

sometimes, when needed, there was certainly no problem with taking it.

In summary, for this client in the area of concern about sleep, the following observations are in order. The actual amount of sleep per night, on the average, did not change throughout the course of therapy, ranging from a low of $\bar{x} = 4.8$, week twenty-six, to a high of $\bar{x} = 6.28$, week five. If anything, visual inspection of Figure 2.2 suggests that there is a slight, though non-significant downward trend in the data indicating slightly less sleep per week. However, the client reported feeling quite pleased about this area of concern, noting his fear of going to sleep had lessened, his ability to stay relaxed when he woke up during the night improved, and he was able to substantially reduce his valium intake.

CONCERN NUMBER TWO:
ASSERTIVE-COMPANIONSHIP

After several sessions of not dealing directly with this issue because it was too anxiety provoking, we began to talk about companionship and meeting other people. The client got in touch with the "dread" of meeting other people, the fear of being taken advantage of, the fear of getting into hassles with other people, and not wanting to snap, and yet not wanting to be passive either. Yet, he acknowledged that he did have a desire to meet new people. Therefore, we made lists of places where there would be the opportunity of meeting new people. He refused to go to bars, so we came up with the YMCA, a dance-movement class, a singing and music appreciation class. After exploring several options, he did join a music appreciation class. There he noted that he had a "freedom reflex," i.e. if somebody approached him, his "gut response" was to hide, to feel trapped, and to abruptly end the conversation.

Over the course of the music class, he was able to approach and initiate conversation with several people of both sexes. In addition, he was able to stand up in front of the group and sing, a risk-taking behavior he had not believed possible.

Another issue he raised was his feeling that all the people he seemed to meet were merely acquaintances (superficial)—E level on Lazarus' inner circle* (Lazarus, 1971). He also realized how lonely, depressed, and withdrawn he felt and decided it was worth the risk to try to meet other people.

Our goals for companionship were two-fold: 1) to increase the number of people (quantity) from the baseline of zero to three or four, and 2) a later goal was added of increasing the depth of intimate experience (quality) from an E level of self-disclosure to a C or even B level of self-disclosure and closeness.

We made weekly tasks, beginning with inviting one acquaintance to lunch. We made a list of current acquaintances—there were three—and several times in the office we role-played asking each of them out to lunch. After three months he had gone out with each several times and felt comfortable about it. However, he felt the conversations were still too superficial, so we began, at least "loosely," to operationalize what was meant by a "more intimate conversation." We started by discussing how he had heretofore avoided B-level conversations: "I just say nothing about myself; be super-polite and super-cooperative." In order to have a B-level conversation, he and/or his partner would have to share some intimate, less comfortable part of themselves—a vulnerability or fear (or affection).

It should be noted that at the same time I agreed to work cooperatively with this client on the goal of developing "deeper" relationships I also requested that we spend part of our sessions acknowledging the enormous progress that had been made over baseline in even asking people to lunch!

The client felt, by the end of therapy, that he was able to improve the depth of sharing with two of his "acquaintances," and felt a B-level intimacy was occurring with greater frequency in their conversations.

Toward the end of the therapy session he noted that in general he felt more natural being with people, although he still had a gut feeling that he did not contact people very well and they would not really be interested in getting to know him. He admitted that although he could do it, he still did not enjoy taking the initiative and felt it an enormous strain on him. The

---

*Lazarus' inner circle is a concentric circle of A to E on which one can plot the "intimacy" of a conversation. E represents the most superficial conversation, B a self-disclosure of great intimacy, and A an area so sensitive that it is never revealed.

reason he was willing to take the risk is that he balanced strain against the fear and the dislike of the isolation. He also noted that he did feel *more* confident and more able to non-defensively take criticism than before.

Finally, on the issue of assertiveness, he confronted his parents and expressed his feelings of hurt and not feeling cared for; and was able to tell his brother tactfully please not to nag him about his health problems, his job, or lack thereof, and to explore other areas to communicate about. Although he noted relapses, a falling back into "my old docile, trying-to-please self," he generally was able to behave much more assertively, both with his family, and at work, to "not be afraid to say what *I* feel."

CONCERN NUMBER THREE:
POSITIVE AND NEGATIVE SELF-STATEMENTS

This was a theme that ran throughout this client's life. His critical perfectionistic standards got in his way whether trying to learn to meditate, meet new people, or perform a job correctly. Here we worked on increasing positive self-thoughts, in particular, and on "sprucing up" his appearance and environment.

He agreed to "fix up the apartment" for himself—a candle, a couple of green plants, flowers, a Sierra Club calendar. He also decided to take more pride in his appearance: new clothes, getting his hair cut stylishly, grooming himself. He noted, "I am beginning to feel more confident more often although it is so hard for me to justify 'pampering' myself, am I really worth it?" We worked on catching the "critical" self and using these statements as cues for positive ones. We made a list of the positive qualities he had: intelligence, sense of humor, thoughtfulness, musical, with a good sense of rhythm. Homework for a while was at least one positive thought per day more than the number of critical thoughts.

He also realized a need to be gentler on himself—not to be always pushing for meeting new people. Sometimes it was all right to feel comfortable being alone, a self-retreat or a self-nurturance; to walk, to swing, to play the piano, or to read. Or, as we discussed earlier with meditation, not needing to have a *perfect* "empty" mind.

CONCERN NUMBER FOUR:
STRESS/RELAXATION

Because the general strategy of this area has been covered in detail elsewhere (Shapiro, 1978b, 1978c) only a few comments are necessary. First, we worked on generalizing the relaxation from formal meditation to other times throughout the day. We did this by recognizing antecedents to stress, and also by using the behavior of stress as a cue for relaxation (focused breathing, coping self-instructions, and imagery).

CONCERN NUMBER FIVE: JOB

He did get a job in May after eight months of conscientious searching. It included several different simultaneous demands: phoning, typing, filing. His perfectionist side rebelled. We worked on generalizing the "accepting" attitude of meditation, and stress-management strategies of focused breathing, coping self-instructions, etc. At work he found it easier to set limits on what he could accomplish by being more assertive with others and more accepting of his own limits. He found that people did not reject him when he did set the limits.

2.9 Did Meditation and Therapy Work Effectively for this Client?

THE CLIENT noted at the end of therapy that he was smiling more, seeing more colors in the world, holding his head higher, hearing the wind, taking the time to look at things. A six-month *follow-up* revealed that the client still felt good about his sleeping patterns; was using valium only infrequently (once every two or three weeks); continuing to see the friends he had made on a weekly or more frequent basis; practicing meditation at least once, and generally twice a day; and still feeling much less stress throughout the day.

WHY?

He attributed this success both to meditation and to his excitement at working on the companionship area. Yet I could also, with a certain justification, add the issue of dealing assertively with his familial relationship, increased pride in his appearance, finding a job. Meditation did seem a useful and powerful therapeutic tool for this client. However, we must recognize it as one technique among many. On an applied clinical and empirical level, we do not really know too much more than that.

However, some clinical speculations and observations may be worthwhile. These observations are refined and discussed in more detail in Chapter Nine, *Mediating Mechanisms.*

First, let us look at meditation. The client learned the skill of being able to observe thoughts, watch them with relative equanimity and eventually let them go out to pasture. In this way, high affect issues were diffused. This is a mechanism involved in many therapeutic approaches. For example, the task of the therapist, as Freud noted, in his *Studies in Hysteria* (Breuer & Freud, 1893), is to help the patient assume objectivity to his own dilemma, a crystal ball attitude by the patient toward himself. This was done by making the patient into an intellectual collaborator, by showing the patient that he had nothing to fear by revealing the true memories. And Rogers (1957) noted that by fulfilling certain conditions of interpersonal warmth and acceptance, the therapist creates an interpersonal situation in which material may come into the client's awareness and in which "the client can see his own attitutdes, confusions, ambivalences and perceptions accurately expressed by another, but stripped away of their complications of emotion. This allows the client to see himself objectively, to see that these feelings are accepted and are acceptable, and paves the way for acceptance into the self of all these elements. The therapist helps the client to see that the client is a person who is competent to direct himself and who can experience all of himself without guilt" (p. 41). From a behavioral perspective, classical systematic desensitization (Wolpe, 1958) involves having a person observe, in a relaxed way, issues that normally cause distress. This results in extinction of the maladaptive affective charge associated with the fear or phobia.

Similarly, meditation helped give this client a perceptual clarity on events in his life, and with a lessened affect. This may have allowed him to face so many aspects of himself as quickly as he did. As Vahia stated, (Vahia et al., 1973), emphasis on meditation therapy is on detachment (objective assessment) and not a manipulation of environment. This increased equanimity may have helped in the decrease of negative thoughts (Concern Three); the reduction of stress (Concern Four); and the ability to deal more calmly and acceptingly with the number of job-related inputs. This affect-reduction and acceptance might have also been helpful in giving the client the inner strength to be more assertive with others. Further meditation in many ways seemed to help give this client a sense of mastery and control, a sense of increased self-esteem at his success. It also afforded him a "portable" relaxation technique to help him cope with his "generalized anxiety," and a technique which he could use any place at any time (i.e. contingent informal meditation—see Chapter Four).

But I believe meditation was only part of the reason for the therapeutic success. Another part was that the client, feeling more confident, was willing to have his affect *raised* and to take risks. He was willing to be assertive with his family, take the initiative to invite people to lunch or to talk with them. The social-skill and assertive-skill training also seemed a critical element in this case. Further, the baseline data and goal-setting seemed to help with his perfectionist style. It showed him the progress he had made so that he was literally forced to acknowledge improvement, even though his preference would have been to ignore (forget) improvement and only focus on the next mountain. Finally, the client himself was very highly motivated, the therapeutic relationship was an accepting one, and the therapist seemed to be both trusted and respected.

2.10 Summary Clinical Notes

IN THIS CASE there were several areas of concern, individual strands of this person's life. They were not all tackled simultaneously. Sometimes more time in a session would be spent on one issue, sometimes another. However, all of the areas of concern together were important in the fabric of this person's life, and to have had the focus of therapy exclusively on only one would, I feel, have done a therapeutic injustice to this individual.

The following points, illustrated by the case of James S., need to be kept in mind when using meditation as a self-regulation strategy with a client.

The client initially presented a problem area of insomnia and requested meditation; however, meditation was not offered as a technique until the context of his life was better understood and his reasons (expectations) for wanting to learn it were made clear. Clinicians need to gather such contextual information to insure that they understand the full scope of the problem and that there are not reasons why meditation might be contraindicated. Second, meditation was not taught as a unimodal strategy for insomnia, but one technique among many. Third, meditation was taught within a therapeutic context of trust. Fourth, additional techniques, which seemed useful for other areas of this person's life (ranging from assertiveness training to role-playing social skills) were also utilized. I do not believe that meditation alone would have been sufficiently therapeutic for this client. Clinicians need to be careful in matching therapeutic interventions individually and as appropriate to the presenting concerns. Finally, careful evaluation and assessment seem important to determine whether the technique-therapy is having its desired effect. If not, why not? What changes can be made? The above comments are standard operating procedures for all good therapists. If meditation is to be considered as a therapeutic treatment, the same guidelines need to apply.

3

A Content Analysis of the Meditation Experience

~~~ MOST RESEARCH on meditation carried out in Western laboratory and field settings has focused on physiological and overt behavioral changes: meditation as a self-regulation strategy (see Chapter Five). Recently, however, Western investigators have begun to call for a more detailed phenomenology of the meditation experience in order to assess subjective changes during meditation more precisely (Tart, 1975; Shapiro & Giber, 1978; Walsh, 1977): meditation as an altered state of consciousness (see Chapter Seven).

There are three primary reasons for this. First, from a social learning or cognitive psychology standpoint, the role of internal events, thoughts, and images has become an increasingly important area of study (Homme, 1965; Mahoney & Thoresen, 1974; Meichenbaum & Cameron, 1974; Ellis, 1962; Shapiro & Zifferblatt, 1976). Since meditation is a technique purported to bring about strong subjective experiences in practitioners, experiences which involve radically new perceptions of their relationship with themselves, others, and the world around them, it becomes crucial to understand what goes on "internally."

Second, several research studies which have focused primarily on the physiological and overt behavioral changes resulting from meditation have found no differences between meditation and other self-regulation strategies (e.g., Michaels, Huber, and Mc-Cann, 1976; Beiman et al., in press; Marlatt et al., 1980, in press). However, in some cases, although there have been no physiological or overt behavioral differences between meditation and other self-regulation strategies, subjects have reported their experiences of meditation as more profound, deeper, and/or more enjoyable than the comparative control groups (Morse et al., 1977; Cauthen & Prymak, 1977; Travis et al., 1976; Curtis and Wessburg, 1975-6). Thus, even though there may not be overt behavioral and/or physiological differences between meditation and other self-regulation strategies, subjective differences occur, and from a clinical or research standpoint these may be critical.

Third, although there are many different conceptual definitions of meditation, it seems important to attempt to identify what "covert behaviors" actually occur during meditation. In other words, what kinds of thoughts and images does a person have while meditating? what kinds of statements does a person make prior to and after meditating? By investigating these questions, the "internal behaviors" of meditation may be compared with the "covert behaviors" of other cognitive self-regulation strategies to determine where similarities and differences exist.

3.1 Previous Research on the Phenomenology of Meditation

THERE HAVE BEEN several ways that previous researchers have tried to gather information about the phenomenology of meditation. Since these are reviewed in detail in Chapter Seven, we will only mention them briefly here. One way to gather information is by looking at the classical texts, such as the *Abhidhamma* and its summary by Buddhaghosa, the *Visuddhimagga*, (Goleman, 1972, 1977) and the classical root texts of the Mahamudra tradition (Brown, 1977). These texts provide phenomenological reports of the experience of advanced meditators.

A second experimental methodology is to have individuals meditate and then to give them the opportunity to describe their meditation experience. In this approach the meditator and the experimenter/investigator are different individuals. This methodology has been used by several investigators (Van Nuys, 1973; Kubose, 1976). They had individuals push a button during the meditation experience to determine frequency of thought intrusion, and later asked subjects about the nature of their thoughts. Corby et al., (1978) looked at physiological changes and compared those changes with the subjects' accounts of their subjective experiences. Banquet (1973) had subjects push buttons signaling different types of subjective experience and tried to correlate that with EEG data.

Other techniques used to understand phenomenological content include a retrospective content analysis of the meditation experience in terms of thought intrusions (Kanas & Horowitz, 1977); rater coding of the meditation experience (Maupin, 1965; Kornfield, 1979; Lesh, 1970); a factor analysis of self reports about the meditation experience (Osis et al., 1973; Kohr, 1977); and verbal report from the client after meditation focus (Deikman, 1966).

A third approach involves having the subject be both the meditator and the experimenter. This approach, suggested by Tart (1971) involves training individuals in behavioral science skills and then having them be their own subjects in an experiment to look at internal experiences. Tart himself has utilized this approach (Tart, 1971), describing a one year experience with Transcendental Meditation, and Walsh (1977; 1978) has utilized this approach describing a two year meditation experience.

Each of these approaches has advantages and disadvantages. The experience of long-term, proficient meditators described in the classical texts is useful because it provides first-hand accounts of individuals who have had extensive meditation experience. However, one of the potential limitations of this approach is these individuals' lack of behavioral science skills and the resultant inattention to non-specific placebo effects such as expectation effects and demand characteristics.

The second approach—with the experimenter and subjects separate—gives some useful information about subjective experiences, but those experiences are susceptible to certain contaminating variables. First, they are retrospective accounts (except in Banquet, 1973) and thus subject to the vagaries of *post hoc* subject "memory." Second, the subjects' experiences are filtered through hypotheses generated by different individual experimenters who may or may not be sensitive to subtle nuances of meditation experience. Further, as with factor analytic research (Osis et al., 1973; Kohr, 1977), the factors are an artifact of and are limited by the experimenter's initial coding questionnaire.

The third approach, having an individual subject/experimenter, has the advantage of allowing for immediate access of material between subject and experimenter, though presenting a greater potential for problems of experimenter bias (Rosenthal, 1962) and demand characteristics (Orne, 1962). This is the primary reason Tart recommends that the experimenter be someone well trained in the behavioral sciences.

The current study utilizes this third approach. Using the self as subject in an N=1, intensive-design phenomenological methodology, it attempts to refine and extend earlier studies of this nature (Tart, 1971; Walsh, 1977, 1978). The previous studies provided global, retrospective accounts of the meditation experience and its effects. The current study attempts to record thoughts, feelings and images *during* the meditation experience by having the subject report every such intrusion aloud. In this way, precise information can be obtained about the covert behaviors actually occurring moment by moment during the meditation sessions. Second, a coding instrument was developed in order to determine what type of intrusions occurred during these meditation sessions as well as their relative frequency. Third, a comparison was made between length of time of the meditation session in which thoughts, feelings, and images were present; and the length of time for which they were not present.

Although this study was primarily exploratory and heuristic in nature, several hypotheses were formulated.

3.2 Within Session Hypotheses

HYPOTHESIS 1.* Breathing is shallower and quicker (therefore of shorter duration) during a thought period than during a period of non-thought.

Hypothesis 2. Breathing is deeper and longer (fewer breaths of longer duration) at the end of the meditation session than at the beginning.

*These hypotheses are not stated in null terms.

Hypothesis 3. There are fewer thoughts at the end of a session than at the beginning.

Hypothesis 4. There is a higher percentage of negative thoughts (and conversely, a lower percentage of positive and neutral thoughts) at the beginning of a session than at the end; the percentage of negative thoughts decreases and the percentage of positive and/or neutral thoughts increases during the course of a session.

Two types of meditation were practiced: counting one through ten, and counting one. Counting one through ten was practiced for five sessions; then counting one was practiced for five sessions. Because the subject had been meditating for over seven years at the time of the experiment, there were no hypotheses related to practice effect. However, with naive subjects, the following hypotheses would be plausible:

BETWEEN SESSION

Hypothesis a. The fifth session involves fewer and longer breaths, more positive and neutral thoughts, and fewer negative thoughts than the first session.

Hypothesis b. Counting one is more difficult than counting one through ten, and therefore subjects have more distractions and shallower, more frequent breaths in counting one sessions than in counting one through ten sessions.

3.3 Subject and Setting

SUBJECT:

In Chapters One and Two I argue for the importance of gathering intensive historical information about subject's background before meditation, including initial motivation, belief systems, expectations, as well as background during meditation, including length and frequency of meditation, the maintaining of commitment, and adherence and compliance. As a brief model of how to do this, information is included about various aspects of the subject.

BACKGROUND

TYPE AND LENGTH OF MEDITATION:

At the time of the experiment, September, 1977, the subject was a twenty-nine year old psychologist who had begun meditating in 1970. Although the data are not precise, the subject noted that he had been meditating consistently for the seven years prior to the study. The length of meditation varied from a maximum of three hours per day (three half-hour periods in the morning and three half-hour periods in the afternoon) to several minutes (three to five minutes once or twice a day).

The subject varied the type of meditation he engaged in though all were within the Zen framework. Sometimes he counted breaths, one to ten, particularly in the earlier years of his training, and also in later years when he needed the "goal" of reaching ten as a transition from his external commitments into the session. Often he would switch from counting breaths (one through ten) to counting breaths (one, one, one) within the same session. With greater frequency in the middle years, he practiced (and continues to practice) this counting-breaths technique (one, one, one). More recently, the subject also practiced, with greater frequency, a type of meditation in the Soto Zen tradition known as Shikan-taza, or just sitting: choiceless awareness. Here he would not count breaths, but try to sit and be mindful of any event which entered his field of awareness. Generally, his goal during the sessions, regardless of specific technique, was a type of mindfulness. Eyes were open and directed a few feet in front of him (or, in case of a mirror meditation, on his navel in the mirror). When thoughts arose, an attempt was made to note the thought, but not engage in dialogue with it, and return attention back to the breathing or to just sitting. All three of these techniques may be seen as a successive approximation of achieving mindfulness within the meditation session (cf. Shapiro, 1978a).

ADHERENCE AND COMPLIANCE:

Off and on since 1972, the subject had kept records of his formal meditation frequency. These records indicated that he meditated formally approximately seventy-five percent of the days, not meditating formally approximately twenty-five percent of the time. In retrospect the subject noted on days when he did not meditate, it sometimes seemed purely from laziness or an excuse like "I don't have the time," or he felt himself so caught up in the external activities (such as giving talks on meditation!) that he did not take the time to meditate. On the other hand, the subject noted that some of the days on which he did not formally meditate were actually an experiment to see how well he could generalize "mindfulness" to all aspects of the day. On these days he practiced no formal meditation and tested himself by trying to informally meditate and be mindful all day. Thus the subject noted that he probably was practicing some type of formal or informal meditation with about eighty to eighty-five percent compliance.

MOTIVATION AND COMMITMENT:

Here we need to look at two factors: first, the subject's initial belief system about what meditation would or would not give him. In other words, why did he begin meditating? Second, we need to look at commitment, which involves specific expectations and beliefs to maintain the practice on a daily basis: e.g., cognitive statements made prior or subsequent to meditation which influence the continuation of the practice.

INITIAL MOTIVATION:

The experimenter thinks the following material, taken from the subject's journals may be the best way to describe his initial motivation.

> I was quite motivated and ready when I began the practice of meditation. During my junior year in college, a variety of interpersonal and personal "crises" in my life raised for me a series of religious existential questions of meaning and purpose.

> I began to question whether the path I had chosen for myself—a combined law and business career—was one that would give me the most personal meaning and fulfillment. This path heretofore had been what my significant others had wanted for me. But because of my own questioning at that time, I began to reconsider that direction and to read existential writers and religious thinkers such as Camus, Kierkegaard,

Buber, and Dostoevsky. This reading led me to Israel, to a study of the Old and New Testaments, and ultimately to the Orient.

As I conceptualized it to myself, I was on a spiritual search, in Ouspensky's words "in search of the miraculous." I found myself unable to make decisions between graduate school in law or perhaps a career in religious studies until I could first solve some of these larger personal questions for myself. It was no longer sufficient to just pursue advanced degrees for their own sake. I needed the time out in order to reassess. Part of the reassessment had to do with the content of my professional direction and part of it had to do with the process of pursuing that direction. I felt that the upwardly mobile, very competitive, ambitious lifestyle in which I had been brought up, and in which I very much believed, was causing me a great deal of difficulty. I was looking for an alternative to that.

Therefore, for me, the contextual framework within which I turned to the Oriental disciplines, in general, and meditation in particular, was twofold: 1) I was looking for some larger value and philosophical framework which would give me a sense of meaning and purpose in my own life; and 2) I was looking for alternative values to the ones in which I had been raised. I felt that this larger sense of meaning and purpose in my own life was necessary before I could continue with other "societal duties." Therefore I was highly motivated, as I felt in many ways that I was really searching for a foothold into my own life.

COMMITMENT: MAINTENANCE OF THE PRACTICE

Commitment, as noted, refers to what the subject says before he sits down to meditate or when s/he is planning a time to meditate. These are more specific statements that occur on a daily basis about what s/he believes meditation does for him/her. From reviewing the subject's journals, it can be seen that these thoughts were of two types. One type of statement involved a need to get away from the external environment when he was feeling a "sensory overload." These types of thoughts included:

I really need a cooling-out space; I've had too many inputs and need to withdraw; I've lost my perspective and feel confused.

Still other times the subject noted that he meditated because he felt he "should"; he knew it would be "good for him" yet it felt as though it was "just another task" he had to do in a day.

Other statements involved the value which the subject placed on meditation and what it might do for him. These statements included:

> This is my time to let go and accept. This is the time to drop all the ego games and just let myself be; this is a special time for me to allow that yielding, soft, delicate side to be there; this is a time for opening myself up, cleansing myself; this is a time for feeling the harmony with all that is around me and within me; this is a way of practicing the values that I believe in in a pure way.

3.4 Setting:

THIS EXPERIMENT took place during the month of September, 1977 in the subject's home-office, where he had a meditation room. The subject was on vacation during the month of September and was not in Menlo Park the full time. Therefore, the ten days in which meditation sessions were recorded were the ten days that he was actually meditating at the Menlo Park office. The meditation room consisted of a Japanese style (tatami) floor, shoji screens, and green plants. A large floor-to-ceiling mirror covered one wall.

PROCEDURES:

TECHNIQUE

The first five tape-recorded sessions were Zen breath meditation, counting breaths one to ten, and the last five sessions recorded were counting the number one over and over again. Given the method of data gathering described below, Shikan-taza was not done because it would not have been possible to collect comparable information on thought blocks versus non-thought blocks.

METHOD OF DATA GATHERING

Two types of data were gathered in this experiment. One type refered to thought blocks vs. non-thought blocks. The second type involved the coding of the thoughts into different categories.

THOUGHT BLOCK VS. NON-THOUGHT BLOCK

The subject was instructed to count out loud the numbers one through ten or the number one between the end of the inhalation of a breath and before beginning the exhalation of a breath. Subject was asked to state aloud any thoughts, images, verbalizations, feelings, emotions, or sensations that were noticed or discriminated. Thus, as a working definition, a thought block referred to a statement aloud, made about discriminated feelings, images, sensations, or internal verbalizations. If, between any two numbers, there was no aloud verbalization then it was assumed that this was a period of "mindful" blankness or no thought—"Non-Thought Block." If there was verbalization aloud, then that period between numbers was referred to as a "Thought Block." It should be noted that the label "Thought Block" subsumes any aloud verbalization of a noticed intrusion into a blank, or "empty mind," including, but not limited to thoughts, images, sensations, etc. Since we do not really know how long an intrusion takes—the verbalization of the intrusion is different than the experience of the intrusion itself—(hereafter referred to as "thought")—it was decided to make thought blocks an all-or-none proposition. If a "thought" occurred between numbers, the entire time was counted as the thought time whether there were one or more thoughts between the numbers. Thus, there may be an error in that there is an appearance of more thought time than there actually is. In addition, most individuals who have spent time meditating or been involved with some technique which involves a sensitive discrimination of internal cues will recognize that often thoughts or internal sensations seem as though they hover just beneath awareness. If the subject noticed such "activity," he was instructed to state aloud "noticing activity." This was considered a "thought block" even if he could not recognize the actual words or images that were occurring.

CODING OF THOUGHTS

There were many possible ways to approach the developing of a coding instrument. First, past coding instruments were reviewed. Maupin (1965) used a five-point discrimination of subjective experience in hierarchically descending order of depth of experience: concentration, detachment, pleasant body sensations—vivid breathing, relaxation, and dizziness. Kubose (1976) had five different categories: bodily sensations, present situation, past situation, future situation, not involving a time component. Banquet (1973) had individuals push a button depending upon whether they were having body sensation, involuntary movement, visual images, deep meditation, or transcendence. The classical root text of the Mahamudra tradition divides "thoughts" into reasoning, memory, anticipation, and categorizing (Brown, 1977) and the Vipassana tradition of meditation discusses remembering, sensing, worrying, thinking, judging, hearing (Goldstein, 1975).

The current instrument is derived in many ways from a combination of the above instruments. Six different categories were used. Category I refers to general, philosophical thoughts of a non-temporal nature. Category II refers to thoughts related specifically to the meditation task at hand. Category III involves thoughts about the future. Category IV involves temporally current thoughts, and Category V thoughts about the past (memories). Category VI is for miscellaneous, uncodable responses. Each category (one through five) is followed by a + (positive affect), a 0 (neutral affect), or − (negative affect). The categories and some examples are found in Table 3.1.

The actual determination of which category a thought fit into (I-VI) or what affect was associated with it (positive, neutral, negative) was a rating made by the subject. This procedure departs from traditional scientific practice in that external raters were not trained and rater reliability was not obtained prior to the coding. However, a decision was made to depart from traditional practice for two reasons. First, it was felt that the subject would know better than an external rater what his affect was to a given thought. Because of the heuristic nature of this study, the subject's own report, therefore, seemed critical. Second, at the beginning of the experiment, it was realized how important

TABLE 3.1: *Coding Instrument*

I. General/Philosophic
    Example: What is the exact role of responsibility in psycho-
    therapy? 1.1 0 (neutral)

II. Related to the task at hand
    2.1 *Body sensations*
         Example: Sweat on the right side. 2.1 0 (neutral)

    2.2 *Self-Statements*
         Example: feeling myself yield more + (positive state-
         ment); Just relax and let go (self-instruction) 0 (neutral
         affect); Thoughts are running wild; I can't control them
         − (negative affect).

    2.3 *Images*
         Example: external image (seeing windchimes in mind) +

    2.4 *Miscellaneous* insights, ideas, related to task at hand
         Example: You've got to be highly motivated to do
         precise meditation (0).

    2.5 a stopped and looked at time
         a′ would like to look at time
         b writing down ideas

III. Future
    +   +a=ego competitive "thought" e.g., I think that soon I
             will be able to ace out Mr. X in terms of visibility and
             that makes me feel good.

             +b=a nice positive thought, e.g., I like the image I've
             planned for myself.

    0   =neutral, I might want to use Johnston's book in my
             research class next month.

    −   =I'm confused about where I'm heading.

IV. Current Situations, Events
    +   +a=ego/competitive/positive
             +b=nice thought
             c=neutral (non-self related)
    0   =affectless
    −   =competitive feelings, out of control, anger

V. Memories (Past)

VI. Uncodable
    6.1 Can't hear
    6.2 Preverbal — can't code
    6.3 Makes no sense — noncodable

honesty would be in the subject's reporting of his internal experience. It was believed that if the subject felt others were going to listen to the tape, there could easily occur a censoring of information which would, in effect, defeat the purpose of the study. Therefore, the subject rated the thoughts.

3.6 Results

 THOUGHT BLOCKS VERSUS NON-THOUGHT BLOCKS

The data for the ten sessions were grouped according to time spent in thought blocks and time spent in periods of blankness—non-thought blocks. This information is reported in Figure 3.1. The x̄ percent of non-thought time was 73.3% across the ten sessions; and x̄ percent of thought time was 26.7%. Although the mean percent between sessions 1-5 (counting 1-10) involved a slightly higher non-thought time (75.2%,) than sessions 6-10 (counting one) (71.3%), the difference is not significant.

The longest time the subject spent without thoughts was 160.7 seconds, spanning thirteen breaths. The shortest and longest breaths without thoughts were 6.0 seconds and 65.0 seconds.

The longest time spent in continuous thought was 82.5 seconds, consisting of five breaths. The shortest and longest breaths with thought were 6.7 and 62.3 seconds.

HYPOTHESIS ONE

Visual inspection of Figure 3.2 and t-test calculations (Table 3.3) show that the mean length of a breath was significantly longer in a thought segment ($\bar{x}$ = 18.8; S.D. = 7.7) than in a non-thought segment ($\bar{x}$ = 12.7; S.D. = 2.5) for all ten sessions.

This directly refutes hypothesis number one, which posited that breathing would be shallower and of shorter duration during thought periods than in non-thought periods.

Further inspection of Figure 3.2 and Table 3.3 suggests that there was no significant difference between the breath lengths for the five sessions counting one to ten and the five counting just

TABLE 3.2 *Percent of Breath Blocks: Thought and Non-Thought (By Session)*

	1	2	3	4	5	1-5	6	7	8	9	10	6-10	1-10
									Session				
◁ % ▽	28.3	24.2	21.1	18.6	27.9	24.8	32.5	33.6	29.7	19.1	17.6	28.7	26.7
	71.7	75.8	78.9	81.4	72.1	75.2	67.5	66.4	70.3	80.9	82.4	71.3	73.3

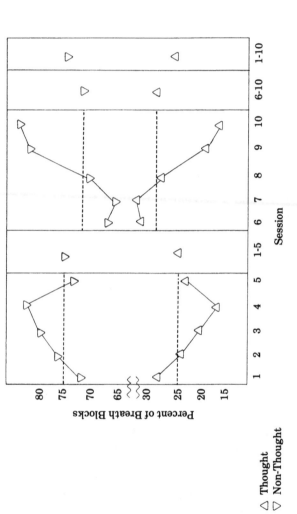

△ Thought
▽ Non-Thought

FIGURE 3.1 *Percent of Breath Blocks: Thought and Non-Thought*

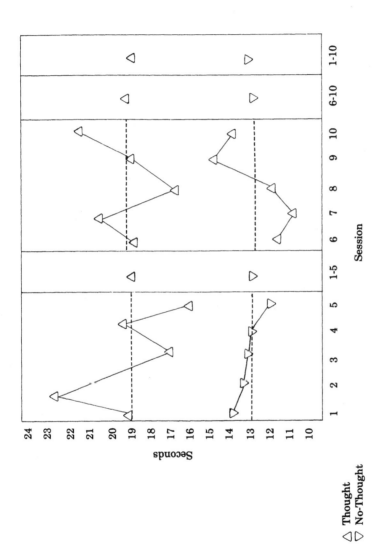

FIGURE 3.2

Mean Time of Breaths in Thought and Non-Thought Blocks/Session

TABLE 3.3

Mean Time of Breaths in Thought and Non-Thought Blocks/Session

		Session												
		1	2	3	4	5	1-5	6	7	8	9	10	6-10	1-10
$\bar{x}$	△	18.7	22.3	16.9	19	15.6	18.5	18.5	20.1	16.7	18.8	20.7	19	18.8
	▽	13.8	13.3	13	12.8	11.7	12.9	11.7	11	12	14.7	13.5	12.6	12.7
s.d.	△	6.5	9.2	10.2	5.3	4.4	7.4	7.2	6.7	7.1	3.5	14.9	7.9	7.7
	▽	2.7	3.1	3	2.1	3	2.9	2.5	1.4	1.8	2.1	2.9	2.1	2.5
τ		5.8	8.4	4.1	5.6	6.4	6.1	8.5	12.5	5.9	1.6	3	6.3	6.2
δ		.01	.01	.01	.01	.01	.01	.01	.01	.01	—	.01	.01	.01

~ — Insignificant

τ —Test for difference between thought and no-thought breath time

δ —Significance level of the above t-test

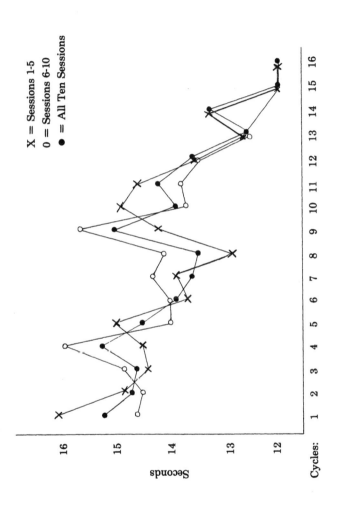

FIGURE 3.3

Mean Time of Breaths, In Seconds:
Comparison of Cycles Within Session

TABLE 3.4

Mean Time of Breaths in Seconds: Comparison of Cycles, within Session

Session

Cycle	1	2	3	4	5	1-5	6	7	8	9	10	6-10	1-10
1	18.7	13.4		18	14.2	16.1	13.2	17.1	13.7	15.9	13.9	14.7	15.3
2	14.6	15.4	12.7		17	14.9	11.2	13.3	13.8	16.9	18	14.6	14.8
3	19.8	14.4	12	12.8	13.3	14.5	16.3	13.8	14.6	16.6	13	14.9	14.7
4	17.7	13.3	13.8	14.2	14.1	14.6	15.9	16.3	18.1	16.4	13.5	16	15.3
5	16.8	13.4	16	15.3	14.1	15.1	12.5	13.5	13.8	14.5	15.7	14.1	14.6
6	14.5	13.7	14.9	12.4	13.7	13.8	14.7	12.8	14.6	13.4	15.2	14.1	14
7	18.5	15.3	14.1	11.1	11	14	13.6	15.6	12.9	15.5		14.4	12.7
8	14.4	14.2	13.1		11.6	13	16.2	10.6	15.7			14.2	13.6
9	16	16.1	13.3		11.6	14.3	18.1	16.2	12.7			15.7	15.1
10	12.6	20.3	15.8		11.4	15	12.4	14.9	14.1			13.8	14
11	14.2	16	16		12.5	14.7	13.7	15.1	12.9			13.9	14.3
12	14.1	15.5	14.5		10.7	13.7	12	15.9	12.8			13.6	13.7
13			15.3		10.1	12.7	11.7	13.9	12.9			12.8	12.8
14			14.4		12.5	13.4							13.4
15					12.2	12.2							12.2
16					12.2	12.2							12.2

one. This was as predicted, given the experience of the subject
(see the preface to hypotheses a and b).

HYPOTHESES TWO AND THREE:
TRENDS IN BREATHS AND
NUMBER OF THOUGHTS

Each meditation session was divided into periods of ten breaths,
and within-session comparisons were made to determine if
meditation became "deeper,"—characterized by fewer breaths of
longer duration (hypothesis two) and fewer thought blocks
(hypothesis three), as a session progressed. Table 3.4 and Figure
3.3 suggest that breathing did not become deeper as a session
progressed. In fact, there is a steady tendency for the mean
length of a breath cycle to drop over cycles for the average of all
sessions. Typically, breathing becomes slightly more shallow as
each session progresses. Therefore, hypothesis number two is rejected. No noticeable differences appear between one through ten
counting in sessions one through five and one, one, one, counting
in sessions six through ten.

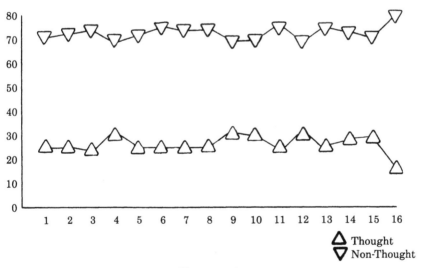

FIGURE 3.4

Percentage of Thought and Non-thought Blocks/Cycle:
Mean Across All Ten Sessions

TABLE 3.5
Thought and Non-Thought Blocks per Cycle

Cycle		1	2	3	4	5	6	7	8	9	10	Frequency Across 1-10	% Across 1-10
1	◁	3	1		3	3	4	3	4	2	1	24	.27
	▷	7	9		6	7	6	7	6	8	9	65	.73
2	◁	4	3	1		7	1	3	3	3	2	21	.25
	▷	6	7	9		3	9	7	7	7	8	63	.75
3	◁	4	1	1	1	4	4	3	3	1	0	22	.22
	▷	6	9	9	9	5	6	7	7	9	10	77	.78
4	◁	4	3	1	3	2	4	5	4	2	2	30	.30
	▷	6	7	9	7	8	6	5	6	8	8	70	.70
5	◁	3	2	2	1	4	3	3	3	2	4	27	.27
	▷	7	8	7	9	6	7	7	7	8	6	72	.73
6	◁	1	3	3	1	2	3	2	4	2	0	21	.23
	▷	9	6	7	9	8	7	8	6	8	1	69	.77
7	◁	1	3	1	2	2	4	2	3	1		19	.22
	▷	9	7	8	8	8	6	8	7	7		68	.78

Session

8	◁▷	2 / 8	2 / 7	1 / 9	4 / 6	3 / 7	2 / 8	4 / 6	18 / 51	.26 / .74
9	◁▷	5 / 5	3 / 7	1 / 9	3 / 7	5 / 5	5 / 5	0 / 10	22 / 48	.31 / .69
10	◁▷	2 / 8	3 / 7	2 / 6	2 / 8	4 / 6	4 / 6	4 / 6	21 / 47	.30 / .70
11	◁▷	2 / 8	2 / 8	2 / 7	2 / 8	4 / 6	4 / 6	2 / 8	18 / 51	.26 / .74
12	◁▷	3 / 7	3 / 8	2 / 8	4 / 6	6 / 4	6 / 4	2 / 8	22 / 49	.31 / .69
13	◁▷			4 / 5	2 / 8	1 / 5	1 / 4	2 / 8	10 / 30	.25 / .75
14	◁▷			1 / 4	3 / 7				4 / 11	.27 / .73
15	◁▷				2 / 5				2 / 5	.29 / .71
16	◁▷				1 / 6				5 / 6	.14 / .86

The maximum number of thought blocks in one complete cycle (i.e. ten breaths) of any given session was six, cycle twelve, session seven; the minimum, zero, session eight, cycle nine. Conversely, the maximum number of non-thought blocks in one complete cycle of one session was ten, session eight, cycle nine; the minimum, four, session seven, cycle twelve. Visual inspection of Figure 3.4 shows that there is no discernable trend in the percentage of thought versus non-thought blocks over cycles. Therefore, hypothesis three is rejected.

TYPES OF THOUGHT — GENERAL INFORMATION

An effort was then made to determine more precise information about the nature of the thoughts. Thoughts were coded for all ten sessions, as per the temporal coding categories and were given an affective rating of positive (+), neutral (0), or negative (−). Across all ten sessions there was a total of two hundred and eighty-six thoughts. Visual inspection of Figure 3.5 and Table 3.6 and 3.7 shows that across all ten sessions, the S's attention was most occupied with neutral thoughts (N = 159.5* thoughts, 56%), second with negative thoughts (N = 61.5 thoughts $\bar{x}$ = 22%), and least with positive thoughts (N = 45.5 thoughts, $\bar{x}$ = 16%).

As can be seen from Table 3.7, most of the subject's thoughts were either focused on the task at hand (Category II, 117 thoughts = 41%) or current situations or events (Category IV, 82.5 thoughts = 29%). There were more future thoughts (Category III, 47.5 thoughts = 16%) than general, philosophical (Category I, 17 thoughts = 6%) or past (Category V, 3 thoughts = 1%).

Among categories, the highest frequency of positive thoughts occurred in Category II, task at hand, and the highest frequency of negative thoughts occurred in Category IV, current events.

In Category II where a more precise coding of thoughts was made, (see Table 3.8) the largest amount of thoughts was in

---

*The .5 (½ thought) results from the coding system. If two different thoughts (e.g., a positive and a negative one) came up within the same "thought block," each thought was coded in the appropriate category as ½ thought.

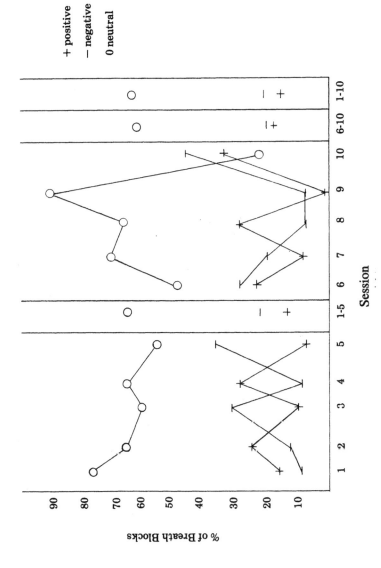

FIGURE 3.5

Percent of Breath Blocks/Session of Positive, Negative, and Neutral Thoughts

TABLE 3.6 *Percent of Breath Blocks/Session of Positive, Negative, and Neutral Thoughts*

	1	2	3	4	5	1-5	6	7	8	9	10	6-10	1-10 %	No. for Sessions 1-10
+	14.7	24	9.6	27	6	14	22.6	9.3	26.3	0	33.3	18.3	16	45.5
−	9	12	30.7	9	36.6	22	28.6	19.8	7.9	7.7	44.4	19.7	21	59
0	76.4	63.8	59.6	63.6	57.3	64.2	48.8	71	65.8	92.3	22.2	62.1	63	159.5

Session

TABLE 3.7 *Number of Thoughts (and Percentage) Across Ten Sessions, Per Coding Category*

	No. Thoughts	Percentage	Positive		Neutral		Negative	
			Number	Percent	Number	Percent	Number	Percent
Category I (General, Philosophical)	17	6%	3	1%	13	5%	1	<1%
Category II (Task at Hand)	117	41%	27.5	10%	81	28%	8.5	3%
Category III (Future)	47.5	16%	5	2%	30	11%	12	4%
Category IV (Current)	82.5	29%	9	3%	35.5	12%	38	13%
Category V (Past)	3	1%	1	<1%			2	1%
Category VI (Uncodable)	17	7%						
Total Number	286	100%	45.5	~16%	159.5	56%	61.5	~22%

Category 2.4, miscellaneous thoughts: (55.5 thoughts = 47%), all generally analytical and related to the task at hand. (For instance: "Does this type of talking magnify the thought and actually cause it—verbalizing what may otherwise disappear?" "The last thought could be called a persona-type thought," etc.) The majority of these were neutral (82%). The "looking-at time," or "writing-down-notes" instrusions (Category 2.5) occured sixteen times (1.6 times per session); all were neutral.

The remaining instrusions (45) were a combination of body sensations, images and self-statements. Of these, self-statements (Category 2.2) were the most frequent, 25 thoughts = 21%, followed by kinesthetic (body sensations) (Category 2.1) 11 = 9%, and images (Category 2.3) 9 = 8%. Of these three categories, the highest percentage of positive instrusions occured with images (66%) and self-statements (58%). Examples of the former include both internal and external visual images (windchimes, green plants, wind swaying the trees, myself peacefully meditating in my mind's eye); examples of the latter include, "feeling peaceful and relaxed, getting deeper, nice calm breath, more centered." Positive body sensations were sexual, erotic feelings. Examples of neutral intrusions for body, self-statements, and images respectively were: "right side sweaty" (2.1 0); "remain centered" (2.2 0); and "focusing on my nose" (2.3 0).

Negative examples for the three include: "strong pain in my feet" (2.1 −); "amazed at my inability to stop thinking" (2.2 −); "imagining someone watching me meditate, makes me feel self-conscious" (2.3 −).

HYPOTHESIS FOUR:
AFFECTIVE TRENDS WITHIN SESSION

To support hypothesis four, each session was again divided into "cycles" of ten breaths to determine whether the percentage of negative thoughts decreased and the percentage of positive and neutral thoughts increased from the beginning to the end of the meditation session. Although hypothesis three—fewer thoughts at end of a session than at the beginning—was rejected, it would still be possible for the affective nature of these thoughts to change, to become less negative, and more positive and/or neutral.

TABLE 3.8

More detailed breakdown of Category II:
"Thoughts Related to Task at Hand"

	No. Thoughts	Percentage	Positive		Neutral		Negative	
			Number	%	Number	%	Number	%
Body Sensations (2.1)	11	9%	2	18%	8.5	77%	5	4+%
Self-Statements (2.2)	25	21%	14.5	58%	9.5	38%	1	4%
Images (2.3)	9	8%	6	66%	1	11%	2	22%
Miscellaneous (2.4)	55.5	47%	5	9%	45.5	82%	5	9%
Time looking and Idea writing (2.5)	16	14%	0		16.2	100%	0	

TABLE 3.9 *Percent of Positive, Negative, and Neutral Thoughts in Each Cycle*

Affect	1	2	3	4	5	6	7	8	9	10	11	12	13	14	15	16
+	21	20	14	16	17	14	24	13	18	25	6	23	23	0	0	0
−	52	65	76	60	67	59	56	38	61	35	76	63	64	100	33	0
0	26	15	10	24	17	27	21	50	21	40	19	15	14	0	66	0

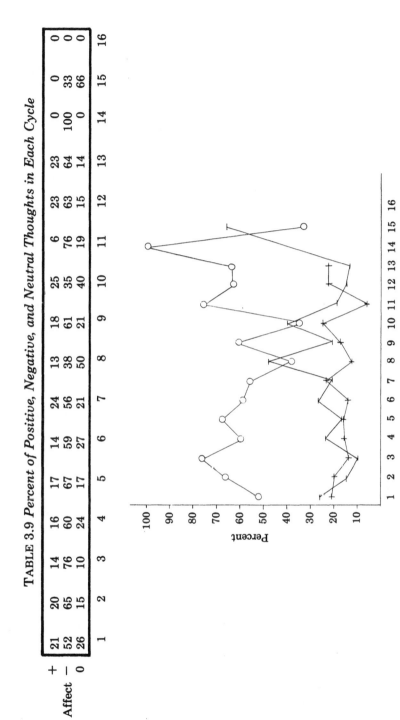

FIGURE 3.6 *Percent of Positive, Negative, and Neutral Thoughts in Each Cycle*

A summation of thoughts for all ten sessions, by cycles, was calculated and divided into positive, neutral and negative thoughts. Visual inspection of Table 3.9 and Figure 3.6 show that no significant trends appear, and therefore hypothesis four is rejected.

3.7 Discussion

INTERESTINGLY this study led to the complete rejection of all four hypotheses. My years of meditation practice, familiarity with the traditions, and training in "scientific observation," made me expect my hypotheses to be right on target. It was a humbling experience to miss in every case. Let me offer one example of the learning that occurred from this.

For example, hypothesis one predicted that breath-time during thought-time would be shallower and shorter than during non-thought time. The data showed a totally different picture. Neither the experimenter nor the subject really believed this. However, the next time the subject meditated after reviewing the data, he noticed that when he was thinking during meditation, he braced slightly and held his breath. This would account for the longer time interval during "thought-times." In non-thought times he reported his breathing as smoother and more regular. The subject also noticed that when he could keep his breathing regular during a thought, it substantially lessened the "affective" charge of the thought. In this case, the data were like a feedback machine, showing the subject an error in his practice of which he was not aware. This particular finding, as did the others, surprised me, and stressed the importance of "data" as a check on our belief systems and our behavior. The subject *knew intellectually* he should keep breathing slowly and easily during intrusions, and was not even aware of bracing.

As noted in Table 3.7, when a thought occurred about the meditation task (Category II), there was the highest probability, relative to any other category, that the thought would be positive. When a thought about the subject's current life situation occurred, (Category III) there was the highest probability, relative to any other category, that the thought would be negative. Extrapolating from this, meditation seemed to serve as a decompression chamber for this subject. His thoughts from current-life situations, which were generally of negative affect, "spilled" into the meditation session. Some of these were "diffused" during the course of the session. Although not statistically illustrated by the quantifiable data (hypothesis four), the subject noted that often there was a change in the valence of a given thought within a meditation session. For example, in one session he noted he was struggling with an issue. Initially, each time it came up, he had a negative charge. However, by the end of the session, he said he could view the issue with equanimity—it had become "neutral." Another example he noted was:

> An image occurred this session which helped me to dissolve (counter-condition) a problem I was having with one of the students where I work. I had an image of that person coming at me with a huge, bloated, angry, attacking face, arms flailing and fists clenched. I became, in the scene, an atom, and that person just passed right through me—between my electrons and my nucleus. I felt the issue took on a perspective—and that rather than rising to confront the attack, or backing away from it, I could just be there, calm and centered—without having to respond angrily or with annoyance, or without having to feel put down or unjustifiably slandered. I felt calm, delicately embracing and caring. The attack no longer threatened me.

Thus, meditation seemed to help the subject diffuse negative affect "spilling" into the session from current events. The task of meditation itself, when reflected upon, provided an opportunity for competence, harmony, relaxation; and thoughts associated with the task were generally positive. From informal "conversations" with the subject, this experimenter would suggest that this may be one of the primary reasons why the subject often felt slightly "out of balance" if he went too many days without meditating.

Regarding the coding instrument, "positive self-statements" were divided into two types, reflecting an experimenter bias that needs to be made explicit. While meditating, all positive thoughts were, in fact, perceived by the subject as positive and later coded as such, 2.2+. However, given the value system of the experimenter, these thoughts were divided into competitive, ego-oriented, positive thoughts (e.g., Dr. X used to ignore me and now I am getting more famous) coded as 2.2+a; and other non-competitive positive ego thoughts (e.g., I like the gentleness I am sensing more and more in myself) as 2.2+b. Theoretically, given the values and demand characteristics of the meditation tradition, ego-oriented self-aggrandizing thoughts eventually decrease. However, for this subject, at that time, these thoughts still occurred and still gave him a positive and powerful feeling.

In a different vein, the subject, upon reviewing the data, noted the difference between the "quantifiable" data and his subjective experiences. For example, during the ten sessions, he reported having many experiences in which he reported "contacting my center." During these experiences "I felt a harmony with myself, 'pure,' in touch with my place in the world." On the data sheet, these came out as positive self-statements (2.2+), e.g., "I am my house"; "feeling the windchimes"; or a positive image (2.3+): e.g., "light filtering through trees"; "shadows and visions of my body at peace."

The subject also noted that meditation seemed to make things more "true" for him. As he recounts,

> "When I am talking to someone, I'll say, 'Well, this came up for me more while I was meditating,' " implying that that must be *really, really* real. Or before I begin to meditate, I am implicitly saying, "Let's see what's really going on with me." Now, this may be true. Meditation may in fact be allowing the most salient thoughts to occur. However, I am also aware of this as a strategy, implicitly saying to the other person: "How can you argue with my meditation experience — it would be like blasphemy!"

The subject also expressed interest at the specific breakdown of the thoughts in Category Two (Table 3.8). He reported that these data provided a confirmation of his own observations, that his primary representational system was verbal/cognitive; followed by kinesthetic and then visual. Of the forty-five thoughts in these three categories (2.1, 2.2, and 2.3), 25 intrusions were cognitive self-statements (55%); 11 intrusions were kinesthetic (24%), and nine were images (20%).

This subject, in retrospect, seemed to be an excellent candidate for meditation. He was a highly motivated individual who wanted to channel his energy, which had heretofore been directed toward competitive, upwardly mobile tasks, into his own growth and quest for personal meaning. This subject also had high control needs, and yet had to face that, in reality, there are a great many situations and events one cannot control. Meditation provided him with a vehicle by which he could learn to accept what he could not control. It fit into his world view, therefore, in that through cognitive restructuring, he could feel that he was in fact controlling reality at least in terms of his ability to react acceptingly.

Some comments need to be addressed to the role of the teacher (or lack thereof) for this subject. This subject did not have the qualities of a very good long-term pupil.

By his own admission, he is in many ways a loner by temperament and an independent person without too much respect for formal rules and regulations. As he noted, "I found the Zen monastery in Japan, with its rules and procedures and bowing, too rigid for me. On the one hand, I've had to learn over the last ten years a willingness to surrender and bow to 'oneness.' On the other hand, although I am often attracted to individuals as models of how I would like to live, I haven't ever found one whom I feel has arrived sufficiently to totally instruct me. So, I am skeptical of living teachers. I use the image of idealized teachers—Gandhi, Hesse's Siddhartha; I ask advice from, confide in, share with people I admire; that feedback is critical to me. But having a long-term teacher has not yet worked for me. It may be adolescent rebellion or fear of surrender. Both, I'm sure, are partly true. But, (of course!) I also feel it is a healthy skepticism for me. Ultimately, as Buddha said, it is our own task to find the path."

There are some methodological and interpretive problems which need to be mentioned. First, there may be problems with the reactive effect of the observation. Initially, the subject noted that having to state a thought aloud was a hindrance and caused a greater dwelling upon thoughts per se, as well as thoughts such as, "I wonder how intrusive this has been," or "What a pain this is to have to say this aloud." Also there were thoughts about who was going to transcribe this, should he be totally honest, etc. Second, the meditation literature suggests that there is a slowing of thoughts during the later phases of meditation (e.g., Brown, 1977). If that is so, are periods of "blankness" merely an absence of accurate discrimination of thoughts and a result of lowered awareness? Further, the objective of mindfulness meditation is to be "choicelessly aware," so fewer intrusions do not necessarily mean a more "effective" meditation. In addition, there is an assumption that when an intrusion occurred, he was mindful of it. The subject believed he was generally "mindful." The only concurrent evidence comes from the taped record of the counting 1...2...up to 10. I reviewed the tape to determine how many times the subject skipped a number, e.g., (1...2...4) or repeated (1...2...2) a number without being aware of it. Of 594 numbers counted in sessions one through five, there were thirteen times he either skipped or repeated a number. Therefore, 97.9% of the time the subject counted accurately without losing track or being distracted.

In terms of the process of meditation, the subject noted that "I initially take in my surroundings in a broad sweeping awareness. Soon, I reach a homeostasis with the environment, and remain relatively quiet and empty-minded until a new thought arises." The specific interpretation of the blankness must, of course, take into account the subject's experience of it, level of practice and attentional focusing skills. The subject also noted:

> My body feels like a tight looseness: tight in that my mind and parts of my body posture are in a good way firm and rooted. Looseness in that my stomach and breathing feel spontaneous and nice. I am aware that I need quiet space. I enjoy the visual feedback of myself in a mirror, that I am together in one piece. I enjoy best meditating at sunrise or sunset, feeling a natural movement of the earth.

> Sometimes I noticed that I had high affect over trivia. It was as if there was a "pool" of high affect in me, and it was looking for something to attach itself to, to rationalize itself. If there was an important issue then the high affect made it a *very* important issue. If it was an unimportant issue the high affect *made* it an important issue.

"I also noticed that in the last five meditation sessions in which I counted one, one, one, that it felt like there were more thoughts, yet also I had more positive feelings of deep relaxation and peace. As usual, counting one, staying more in the moment, was both more difficult for me, but, when it worked, more enjoyable."

There are several different areas future research could profitably pursue. First, it would be important to determine whether the types of thoughts that occur during a meditation or quiet period of time are different than the thoughts that occur during a random section of the day. Second, it would be useful to refine the role of counting a "number": does it become a cue to remember; to be mindful; a thought in itself; a cue to center; a distraction; a labeling of breathing? Does breathing out and stating a number become a discriminative cue for noticing whether intrusions have occurred, are occurring? A signal for stopping that talk? A signal for returning to the task at hand?

An additional consideration concerns the multi-step process involved in reacting to intrusions. For example, the subject noted that many times there were "rumblings" which were not always conceptualizable. "This research task made me bring these thoughts into awareness, recognize them, label them, discriminate them. If I had just been meditating, I may have let these go as unsalient." Thus, the first step was recognizing and verbalizing the intrusion. The next step, via the coding instrument, was to determine whether the intrusion was of a positive, negative, or neutral affect. A third step would be to determine whether the subject was able to discriminate positive, negative, neutral and *still* maintain equanimity. In other words, how did the subject respond to intrusions.

Regarding additional research, to reduce the intrusiveness of "outloud talk," future studies might have the individual cite specific words (rather than sentences, as in the present study; cf. the Vipassana tradition). Further, it would be interesting to compare the cognitive experiences of beginning and very advanced meditators in the dimensions of this study. Finally, the experience of individuals practicing different self-regulation therapies, as well as different spiritual practices, should be compared for the nature, type and frequency of the "internal behaviors."

4

Practical Instructions

〰️ IF THE THERAPIST, after taking into consideration his/ her own therapeutic orientation and belief system, the client's value system, the presenting concern and the relevant empirical literature, decides that meditation would be a useful therapeutic strategy to teach the client, what alternatives are available?

For those therapists who do not want personally to teach their clients a meditation technique, there are two alternatives: tapes or a specific teaching organization. I often recommend individuals to organizations such as the Transcendental Meditation group. This has the advantage of group support, instructors who can check to ensure that meditation is going properly, frees up more time in therapy sessions, and is therefore useful for beginning instruction. However, a caution must be added — any organization has a tendency toward evangelism and promoting a particular type of meditation as the *one* right path. In a sense, we need to separate the Madison Avenue sales pitch from the essence of the technique being used.

As far as taped instructions are concerned, a number are available and several are listed at the end of this chapter. Some therapists may wish personally to teach the client meditation and then use the tape to facilitate the practice as described in Chapter Two. For the therapist who wishes to learn meditation, there are

similar options: taped or written instructions or a specific program/
workshop from a "meditation" teacher or organization.

Below is a specific instruction in the practice of Zen Breath
Meditation, the technique used in the case studies in Chapters
Two and Three. In addition, instruction in a meditation technique for more advanced practitioners is offered (as used in
Chapter Three), as well as a way in which formal meditation may
be practically combined with behavioral self-management skills
(as used in Chapter Two).

The instructions are in three parts: 1) the introduction of the
technique to the client; 2) the actual training in and practice of
the technique; and 3) generalization of the new response. This
model is similar in conceptualization to the one presented by
Meichenbaum (1976) on cognitive factors in biofeedback therapy.

4.1 Introductory Talk to Client

PURPOSE: The purpose of this *introductory* talk is to
give clients a clear, simple overview of what meditation
is, and what are some of the results they might expect. No
specific journal articles are cited, and the *introductory* talk is *not*
delivered in the structured form *presented here,* although most of
the points discussed below are covered in some manner.

Content: In the past fifteen years, a new conception of the individual has begun to emerge within the Western scientific community. This conception has involved a new view of the nervous
system, and a new view of the individual's potential for self-
regulation. Because of reports from India and the Orient detailing extraordinary feats of bodily control and altered states of
consciousness by Zen and Yoga masters, Western science has
begun to explore Eastern religions to determine whether some of
their techniques, such as meditation and yoga, might have
medical and therapeutic value in a Western setting.

Zazen (Zen Meditation) The word Za means "sitting" and the
word Zen comes from the sanskrit word dhyāna meaning meditation. This "sitting meditation" is not a passive technique, but
rather an active exercise which requires hard work. Its goal is
not a contemplative life withdrawn from the cares of the world,
but a state of mind which can give renewed strength and
calmness to deal with daily events. For example, the samurai

warriors of Japan meditated to gain strength for battle. The Japanese martial arts of fencing, jujitsu, and aikido require the centeredness which meditation can give.

Studies have shown that Zen monks during meditation are significantly more sensitive than ordinary subjects to sounds around them. At the same time, the monks are able to produce both alpha and theta waves (measured by EEG). These waves are thought to be indicative of states of calmness and restfulness. Thus, the monks have attained simultaneously a state of intense awareness of their environment and of deep rest and quiet.

It seems important at this point to clarify some possible misconceptions about meditation. The effects of meditation have been compared to the effects of psychedelic drugs. It is true that often people have images, thoughts, and sometimes even hallucinations while meditating. These images, however, are not the goal of meditation. Second, meditation is nothing magical. It takes patience and practice. You have to work at it; and, all life's problems will not be solved just by meditating.

On the other hand, meditation is potentially a very powerful tool, and it is equally important to suggest what you might expect from meditation if you practice it. Studies have shown that Zen meditation can have an effect within the first two to four weeks and generally does have an effect within four to ten weeks. Some of these effects can be measured physiologically—e.g., slower brain waves, slower breathing, slower heart rate. These all contribute to a state of relaxation and inner calm. Meditation may help you become more aware, both of what is going on outside you and what is happening within you—your thoughts, feelings, hopes and fears. Thus, although meditation will not solve all your problems, it can give you the calmness, awareness, and self-control to actively work on solving those problems.

CLINICAL NOTE:
CULTIC VERSUS NON-CULTIC MEDITATION

It should be clear that these instructions are meant for beginning meditators. A question which is often asked is, "Is meditation a religion? Is the technique you are going to teach me a type of prayer?" This is an interesting question. Legal opinions (e.g., Malnak vs. Yogi, New Jersey, 1977), states that Transcendental Meditation is based on religious doctrine and as such cannot be taught in schools.

For an individual who is interested only in the clinical self-regulation aspect of meditation (Chapter Two) or who has some concern that meditation may interfere with his or her religious beliefs, I emphasize the non-cultic aspect of meditation. I discuss the scientific literature, the actual behaviors involved (e.g., attentional focusing, calm breathing) and point out that we can utilize the technique separate from its cultural context.

For an individual who is interested in the religious or spiritual aspect of the technique (e.g., Chapter Three) this issue ·becomes less important and may even be an enhancement.

4.2 Formal Zen Meditation Instructions:*

1. CHOOSING A SETTING: It is best to pick a quiet room, where there will be few distractions. Let the other members of your household know that you would like a few moments to yourself, and ask them to please pick up the phone for you. You may also want to meditate outside, in a place in nature which is special to you. The natural setting can provide a way to remove you from the distractions of daily routine.

2. *Choosing a Position:* Find a comfortable position—probably in a chair, or on a pillow on the floor. Loosen your clothing. Unbuckle your belt if you'd like, take your shoes off, and let yourself relax. It is best not to lie down because in meditation you do not want to go to sleep; you want to be relaxed but alert. Settle in for a second. Let go. Feel the floor or the chair holding you up. Put your legs in a comfortable position. If you are sitting on a chair, let them dangle uncrossed over the sides of the chair. If you are sitting on the floor, you may want to sit cross-legged. Put your hands in your lap so they too feel comfortable. Your back should be straight, but not tightly erect. The important thing is to find a posture that is comfortable for you. Although the research suggests that the full or half-lotus

*Adapted from Maupin, 1965; Weinpahl, 1964; Lesh, 1970; and Kapleau, 1967.

position* is the posture with the least muscle tension for experienced Zen masters, it is usually not the most comfortable for those in the West who are beginning to practice meditation.

Further, the studies of Akishige and his colleagues have suggested that the attitude of the meditator is more important than the actual physical posture or the environment. Alpha brain waves occurred in subjects who had the "right" attitude, even if they were not in the lotus position. Conversely, those who were in the lotus position, but without the right attitude, did not evidence alpha brain waves.

3. *The Process of Meditation: Attaining the Right Attitude.* Take a deep breath. Feel yourself controlling your breathing. In meditation, *you do not want to control your breathing;* you want to let it go—very naturally, just as you have been breathing all day. The only difference between the way you have always breathed and the way you are breathing now is that now you are focusing on your breathing. Yet, at the same time, you continue to breathe naturally. Breathe through your nose, letting the air come in by extending your diaphragm. Do not draw it in, do not try to control it, rather allow it to come to you—slowly—letting your diaphragm expand naturally, letting the breath in as much as you need. Then, allow the breath to go out slowly, letting all the air out of your lungs. As you exhale slowly, count one. Now inhale again, just letting the air come to you. Then exhale and count two. Continue focusing on your breathing, letting the air come in, letting the air go out. Take a few minutes to focus on the breathing, letting the air come naturally, exhaling, and as you exhale, count from one to ten. Do this up to ten, and then begin at one again. Do not pay attention to anything but your breathing. If your attention begins to wander, or thoughts arise, just watch the thoughts, let go of them, and return to observing your breathing. If you get lost and lose count of breaths, just

---

*Two successive approximations to the full lotus position are the half and the quarter lotus. In the half lotus, the left foot is placed over the right thigh and the right foot is placed under the left thigh, with both knees still touching the mat. In the quarter lotus, the left foot rests of the calf of the right leg, and again both knees are supposed to rest on the mat (After Kapleau, 1967).

return to your breathing and the count of one again.* If you begin to feel anxious, watch this anxiousness. If you feel pleasant, watch this feeling also, while continuing to focus on your breathing. Eventually you will be able to be quiet in both mind and body. There is no goal in meditation, there is nothing you have to do except be in the moment, and let yourself relax.

4. *The End of Meditation Sessions:* As you feel comfortable doing so, gradually begin to open your eyes. Do not rush to do anything, just sit quietly for a bit and notice what you are feeling.

You may want to stop and practice a brief ten or fifteen minute meditation before reading any further. Following is a checklist that may be helpful.

CHECKLIST FOR MEDITATION

1. Find a quiet setting with few distractions.

2. Sit comfortably, with your back erect, but not taut, hands in your lap, legs in a comfortable position and with your eyes closed.

3. Breathe through your nose, letting the air come to you; do not draw it in; exhale slowly and completely, and as you exhale, count one; inhale; exhale slowly to the count of two—up to ten, then start at one again.

4. Keep your mind on the breath and numbers, and do not count absentmindedly or mechanically.

5. If your mind wanders, let thoughts rise and vanish. Do not become involved with them; merely watch them. Relax, let go, and continue to focus on your breathing.

6. At the end, gradually and gently open your eyes, and sit quietly for a few moments.

After you have practiced a brief meditation, notice what

---

*A device borrowed from behavioral self-observation strategies, helpful in focusing the individual's attention on the task of breathing, is the wrist counter. The individual is told to hold the wrist counter in his palm and is instructed as follows, "Every time you find yourself caught up in some thought or other, punch the wrist counter. Then, continue to relax, let go, and focus on your breathing." In this way the wrist counter becomes a cue for returning to the task of breathing (cf. Van Nuys, 1971). The wrist counter may also help facilitate generalization in learning from formal to informal meditation.

you are feeling. Notice what you thought about, the images you had. There is a space below in which you may want to record your feelings and thoughts. Just quickly jot down a few words or phrases to describe your reactions to your first meditation experience.

_____

_____

_____

_____

At first it may be best to practice meditation for not more than forty minutes a day. Twenty minutes in the morning and twenty minutes in the evening is usually suggested. If you are interested in practicing meditation, it might be worthwhile to take a minute or two to write down where (i.e. home, office, specific site in nature, etc.) and when would be a good place and time to do so.

First Meditation

Where_____ When: from _____ to _____

Second Meditation

Where_____ When: from _____ to _____

It may seem somewhat arbitrary and formal to put down precise times and places to practice obtaining a state of awareness that is not time-oriented. However, my personal experiences, as well as those of clients and students to whom I have taught meditation, suggest that this is important for two reasons. First, it helps us arrange our schedule, thereby preparing us ahead of time for the practice. Second, we often place doing something nice for ourselves, such as meditation, low on our priority list. Therefore, if we are not careful, it may become the first thing to be omitted in our busy schedules. Usually schedules that are filled with pressing external demands do not provide the time or the reinforcement for our internal demands. This planning of time for ourselves suggests the interrelationship between the two modes of awareness: precise chronological time is used to structure experiences that can help us attain a non-time-oriented altered state.

CLINICAL NOTE

Generally, when teaching this strategy, I emphasize and practice two instructions in detail in the office: 1) abdominal (diaphragmatic) breathing; 2) just letting air come in (rather than forcing it in). Research does suggest that abdominal (as opposed to chest or thoraxic) breathing is most highly correlated with a relaxed state (Timmons, et al., 1972), and yet is often difficult for beginning meditators, as is the concept and practice of both being aware of breathing and "letting air flow in."

4.3 Generalization

OVER THE YEARS I have found it helpful to provide a gradual transition from the formal meditation practice back into "daily" life. An effective strategy for this is to have the client engage in a few moments of walking meditation. In a Zen monastery, this involves rising after meditation, and walking in a slow, methodical manner around the sand garden. I instruct clients, after they have formally meditated, to rise, and, keeping the "centeredness" of the meditation practice, to walk slowly around the room. Reports of clients and my own personal experience suggest this is a helpful strategy. It provides a way to generalize the quietness of formal meditation into movement and activity. In the words of the *Bhagavad Gita*, it is to see action in inaction (formal meditation) and inaction in action (walking meditation). Another strategy for enhancing generalizability, "contingent informal meditation," is described later in this chapter.

4.4 *Adherence*

〰️ I REEMPHASIZE often to the clients that the effects of meditation depend on practice. If the clients seem to be having difficulty continuing the practice of meditation, I generally would want to recheck the following:

1) Have I worked with them in the office to plan when and visualize where they are going to practice.

2) Do they understand the technique.

3) If 1 & 2 have been accomplished, I review with them their (our) reasons for learning the technique. Are they still motivated? I stay with this issue until the client says s/he is willing to recommit to the practice. If not, I explore in the therapeutic context the possible resistance to change and/or to the technique itself. As noted in Chapter Two, if clients are not willing to learn the technique, I do not feel any need to "thrust" it upon them.

4) If the clients are willing to learn and practice the technique, I have them monitor what they say to themselves when they do not practice. This provides us with a list of "excuses" which can then become part of our therapy process. We can either therapeutically work through the excuses and facilitate continued adherence; or, as may happen, the client may decide that the effort required to change is more difficult than learning to accept the clinical concern they are having.

4.5 *More Advanced Formal Meditation Techniques*

〰️ I GENERALLY BEGIN by having clients focus on breathing and counting breaths, as described, one to ten. When appropriate, and "appropriate" at this point in our knowledge is a function of client interest, and therapist intuition, I instruct the client to just count one. This is usually a more difficult technique for individuals educated in the West because the goal of "reaching ten" is removed. However, it can be more effective in helping an individual center more in the "here and now." Eventually, if the client is quite committed, I teach the Soto Zen's technique of Shikan-taza, or "just sitting," a mindfulness technique where neither breaths nor counting are focused upon.

Each of these techniques represents a successive approximation to a non-goal-oriented living in the moment.

INFORMAL MEDITATION PLUS
BEHAVIOR SELF-CONTROL STRATEGIES:
"CONTINGENT" INFORMAL MEDITATION*

Introduction to Clients: We have been talking about formal Zen meditation, which may be practiced twice a day at specific times. Meditation can also be useful at other times during the day, especially at times of stress. We will work now on ways of understanding what events make us tense during the day, and then on ways to relax once we become aware that we are anxious.

Awareness: List below current problems, difficulties, or concerns which you are having or have had that cause you to become tense and anxious:

(a)_____

---

*Contingent informal meditation involves training in behavioral self-observation and functional analysis (cf. Kazdin, 1974) which provides as an initial part of the procedure. Then the procedure combines behavioral self-control strategies such as relaxation (Jacobson, 1929), thought stopping (Wolpe, 1969), covert self-modeling (Cautela, 1971), and covert self-instruction (Meichenbaum & Cameron, 1974) with the practice of informal meditation (Weinpahl, 1964; Rahula, 1959). This procedure has been called "contingent informal meditation" because its performance is made contingent upon certain antecedent cues like tension, anger or stress. This process of anxiety management has been conceptualized within a social learning framework as follows (Shapiro, 1978; modified from Homme, 1965, Mahoney, 1971):

1. Target behavior (TB) stimulus occurs which causes tension, such as an argument or an inability to control the external environment. Cues are either external and/or internal.

2. Awareness: Discrimination plus labeling of target behavior as antecedent to maladaptive behavior chain. Accurate functional analysis of environment facilitated by formal meditation.

3. Kwat! aversive imagery, verbal statement or physical action to interrupt maladaptive response, for example, covert self-statement "No! Stop!"; physical action, such as clenching jaws and fist.

4. Contingent informal breath meditation which functions as a competing response incompatible with tension.

(b)_____

(c)_____

Focus on situation (a) now, and see if you can make it as specific
as possible. Who is present; where are you; what kinds of things
are you doing, saying, and thinking? Now close your eyes and
imagine yourself in that situation, and allow yourself to experience the tension that you normally feel. Observe your tension. It
is all right to let yourself feel anxious. You are in a safe place
here, and the tense scene is not actually happening. Continue to
observe your tension, noting where in your body you feel tense:
is your heart beating faster; is your breathing more rapid; how
does your stomach feel? What kinds of images do you have in
your head? What sort of things are you saying to yourself? Are
you saying things such as: "I am helpless; I am not competent
to handle this situation?" Let yourself go and just experience all
that is happening to you.

Interruption of Sequence and Competing Response: Once you
have observed these thoughts and actions, say to yourself
"Stop!" and clench your fist and your jaw.* Then relax your
fingers and your jaw and imagine yourself beginning informal
breath meditation: you are closing your eyes and beginning to
focus on your breathing. Now, actually take two deep breaths
through your nose, and as you exhale let your "center" sink into
your stomach.

Say to yourself: 1) Your name: "I am _____ ."

    2) "I am breath," (and take another deep
breath).

    3) "I am calm and relaxed and am in
control," (and take two more deep breaths,
letting your "center" sink to your
stomach as you exhale).

*In effect, this "Stop!" is an attempt to interrupt the maladaptive
behavioral sequence long enough to begin the competing response of informal
meditation. In behavioral terms this "Stop!" is referred to as the technique of
thought stopping (Wolpe, 1969). In Zen, it can be conceptualized in terms of a
symbolic kwat! applied by the individual to him/herself (Shapiro, 1978b).

Now imagine yourself becoming more and more relaxed. Image yourself meditating, feeling calm, and in control. At the count of ten you may open your eyes, and you will feel calm, relaxed, and wide awake.

A final note: Breathing is the most simple and basic action we do. If we did not breathe, we would not be alive. If we were not breathing, we would not be able to get angry or tense or upset. When you get anxious, remember that you are "just breath" and return to that simple behavior.

IN VIVO: AWARENESS PLUS PRACTICE:

In vivo awareness: Before actually teaching the skills of formal and contingent informal meditation, normally one or two weeks are spent in self-observation training. Clients are given a wrist counter (or a similar type of counting device) and asked to monitor the frequency of anxious feelings. They are also given a self-observation form, varying from an unstructured journal to a more structured data collection sheet. They are asked to note on this form the following: a) antecedents to tension: what was happening right before; who was present; where were you? b) behavior of tension: where did you feel tense; what did you say to yourself during the time you were tense; do you get tense in the same way in every situation? and c) consequences of tension: what did you do to relieve the tension; how did you act differently as a result of the anxious feelings? This self-observation usually provides helpful information in making up the list of anxiety-related situations during the awareness component of contingent informal meditation training.

In vivo practice. Clients are normally instructed to practice formal meditation for fifteen to twenty minutes, two times a day. They are instructed to practice contingent informal meditation skills throughout the day whenever they become aware that they are feeling tense, anxious, or stressed.

CLINICAL NOTE: ON EVALUATION

As discussed in Chapters One and Two, therapists should closely monitor the client's practice, including frequency, length, and nature of experience. If the client experiences troublesome feelings during meditation, these should be discussed in the therapy sessions. If the client has trouble meditating, this can be discussed in terms of the issues mentioned under adherence. Similarly, if in the therapist's opinion the client seems to be meditating too much, this too should be discussed in the therapeutic context. Further, as with any clinical intervention, close evaluation of treatment outcome effects should be evaluated in order to determine whether the technique is beneficial to the client.

FOR MEDITATION INSTRUCTIONS:

Books:
Benson, H. *The relaxation response.* New York: William Morrow, 1975. A useful, secular technique for those interested in meditation as a self-regulation strategy.
LeShan, L. *How to meditate.* New York: Bantam Books, 1975.
Shapiro, D.H. *Precision nirvana.* Englewood Cliffs, NJ: Prentice-Hall, 1978b. Also includes instructions for meditation.

Tapes:
Goleman, D. *Meditation instructions.* New York: *Psychology Today, Consumer Service Division,* 1976. Provides a useful set of instructions.
Shapiro, D.H. *Instructions for meditation and behavioral self-management strategies.* In C. Franks (ed.) *Behavior therapy tape series,* New York: BMA, 1977. Provides instructions in meditation and behavioral self-management strategies.

5

Meditation as a Self-Regulation Strategy: The Empirical Literature

5.1 Self-Control and Self-Regulation Strategy: Toward a Working Definition

IN A PREVIOUS WORK, I defined self-control as "the ability to decide what one wants to do, and the skills to follow through with that decision" (Shapiro, 1978b, p. 246). In order to decide what one wants to do, one must first learn to become aware of when one is acting by habit and reflex (i.e. nonconscious decisions). Second, one must have the skills to perceive increased alternatives, new ways of perceiving and acting in the world. Third, one needs the skills to carry the decision through.

A self-control or self-regulation technique, therefore, is a cognitive or behavioral activity generated by an organism and maintained over time in order to facilitate the attainment of certain goals that the organism defined as desirable.*

---

*The process by which this definition was arrived at and comparison with other definitions of self-control is not included here as it is outside the primary scope of this book. It is discussed in detail, however, in my forthcoming book, *The Psychology of Self-Control.*

"ROUND-ONE STUDIES"

Almost without exception the studies viewing meditation as self-regulation strategy have focused on its relaxation (stress reduction) component. This is true in the stress studies, therapy studies, the majority of the addiction studies, and the hypertension research.

The "first-round" of studies viewing meditation as a self-regulation strategy helped establish interest in the field. These early studies suggested that meditation may be quite promising for a variety of clinical problems.

Generally these "first-round" studies consisted of anecdotal case reports, intensive design studies containing "non-specific variables," and/or combining techniques for treatment and/or comparing meditation to control groups, but not to other, similar techniques. Because this "first-round" literature has been reviewed at length elsewhere (including both clinical/therapeutic effects [Smith, 1975; Shapiro & Giber, 1978] and physiological effects [Woolfolk, 1975; Davidson, 1976]), only a brief summary is provided here. As this first-round literature is generally quite flawed methodologically, I have confined myself to general comments on methodological issues. Specific criticisms of individual studies may be found in the tables accompanying the discussion. The clinical tables (5.1-5.3), based on Shapiro and Giber (1978), have been updated by David Giber; the physiological tables (5.4-5.6), based on Woolfolk (1975), have been updated by Roger Walsh. Tables 5.1-5.3 are particularly addressed to descriptions of independent variables such as therapist contact, length of training, description of techniques; method of subject selection; descriptions of dependent variables for clinical problems; methods of data collection, the nature of data collected, be it physiological, behavioral, subjective, overt-concurrent; types of follow-up; and the quality of control procedures. Tables 5.4-5.6 give a systematic basis for 1) comparing physiological changes such as oxygen consumption, skin response, blood pressure, heart rate, EEG resulting from different independent variables like yoga, Zen, transcendental meditation (TM); and 2) looking at methodological issues within each study: experience of meditators, type of design, and quality of control procedure.

5.2 Stress and Stress Disorders: Round-One Fears, Phobias, Stress and Tension Management

THERE HAVE BEEN twenty round-one studies concerned with the reduction of fears and phobias and stress and tension management.* These studies suggest that meditation may be a promising clinical intervention technique for several stress-related dependent variables. All studies reported successful outcomes on dependent variables ranging from fear of enclosed places, examinations, elevators, being alone (Boudreau, 1972) to "generalized anxiety" (Shapiro, 1976), anxiety neurosis (Girodo, 1974), pain due to bullet wounds, back pain (French & Tupin, 1974) and fear of heart attack (French & Tupin, 1974), rehabilitation after myocardial infarct (Tulpule, 1971), and bronchial asthma (Honsberger, 1973). Many of these studies involved within-subject design (Boudreau, 1972; Shapiro, 1976; Girodo, 1974; French & Tupin, 1974) and a combination of meditation and other techniques, with meditation sometimes first (Girodo, 1974), sometimes second (Boudreau, 1972), sometimes concurrent (Daniels, 1975; Shapiro, 1976) with other modes; the data were gathered by subjective measures (patient verbal self-report). Girodo (1974) also used an anxiety symptom questionnaire and Shapiro (1976) had the patient monitor daily feelings of anxiety using a wrist counter.

The study by Vahia et al., (1972), the first to use control groups, reported a consistent and greater reduction in anxiety for the treatment group. The control group consisted of a "pseudo-yogic treatment" with only superficial use of postures and breathing exercises. Data were gathered from patient notebooks, from Taylor's Manifest Anxiety Scale, and from relatives, friends, and colleagues. Its conclusions will be discussed in greater detail in the following section: Meditation and Psychotherapy.

---

*Lazar et al., 1977; Berwick & Oziel, 1973; Otis, 1974; Boudreau, 1972; Shapiro, 1976; Girodo, 1974; Vahia, Doongaji, & Jeste, 1972; Vahia, Doongaji, & Jeste, 1973; Smith, 1976; Goleman & Schwartz, 1976; Hjelle, 1974; Linden, 1973; Woolfolk, Carr-Kaffashan, McNulty, 1976; Tulpule, 1971; French & Tupin, 1974; Dillbeck, 1977; Daniels, 1975; Berwick & Oziel, 1973; Honsberger, 1973.

TABLE 5.1 Studies on Fears and Phobias, Stress and Tension Management

Investigator(s)	Clinical Problem	S's (N; age; sex, prior experience)	INDEPENDENT VARIABLE — Type and Length of Treatment/Training	Frequency of Therapist (T) Contact	DEPENDENT VARIABLE — Subjective Effects	Behavioral	Physiological	Overt, Concurrent (e.g. medical)	Follow-up	Type of Design, Quality of Control, Methodological Problems
Boudreau 1972	Case One: fear of enclosed places; examinations; elevators; being alone. Duration of problem: 5 years.	N=1, 18 yrs, male, not stated specifically "adept at TM"	Systematic desensitization and massed desens. first (3 days x 3 hrs.), then since no improvement Transcendental Mediation (one month). TM practiced both non-contingently and contingent upon imagining phobic scenes.	Sys dens. and massed desens. done with tape recorder	Self-reported tension decrease	Avoidance behaviour had disappeared.	None	None	None	N=1 case report; an in-vivo assessment pre and post of fears would have been useful.
	Case Two: excessive perspiration. Duration of problem: 35 years.	N=1, 40 yrs, female, took summer course in Yoga	Intervention #1: Relaxation practice w/paired anxiety-arousing imagery (6 months) provided partial symptom alleviation. Intervention #2: Yoga practice (3 mos. x ½ hr. daily) plus additional practice during tense moments.	Not stated	Not reported	None	None	Daily Perspiration: mild/excessive. Intervention #1: mild perspiration decreased from 12 hrs. to 5 hrs. on average; excessive from 3 to 1 hr. Intervention #2: excessive disappeared; mild is below 1 hr. per day.	6 months: perspiration maintained at below 1 hr. daily	N=1 case report; relative effects of relaxation and Yoga not clear. Operationalizing of mild and excessive perspiration good and follow-up admirable.
French and Tupin 1974	Case One esophagitis. Duration of problem: 20 years.	N=1, 65 yrs, male, not stated	3 phases: (1) slowed breathing and (2) muscle relaxation followed by (3) focusing on pleasant images. (In this case for 10-15 min.)	Not stated	Self-reported decrease in pain and relief of sleep disturbance	None	None	None	Patient reported successful use of method for 6 months	N=1, within subj.; case report, pre and post ratings of pain severity and sleep disturbance would have been useful.
	Case Two: severe pain due to bullet wounds; anxiety and depression during 3 mos. hospitalization; poor eating; weight loss.	N=1, 22 yrs, male, not stated	Same method as above (in this case, used for 30 min. according to patient self report)	Not stated	Self-report of improved ability to manage pain and sleep; also improvement in general mood and eating.	None	None	None	None	Same as above
	Case Three: widely disseminated oatcell carcinoma of the lung; sleep disturbance; pain; relief through narcotic use.	N=1, 53 yrs, male, not stated	Same method as above	Not stated	Found focusing technique "frightening and distressing"; used daily muscle relaxation. If pain controlled by relaxation, patient could sleep without use of hypnotic.	None	None	None	None	Same as above
	Case Four: referred for psychiatric succs; panic, neurotic fear of heart attack, used 120 mg. diazepam per day; severe sleep disturbance.	N=1, 50 yrs, male, not stated	Same method as above	Not stated	Used method to monitor heart beat and control fear of heart attack. However, fear resumed when after patient's death of myocardial infarction, patient returned to use of technique 10 min./daily for "relaxing"; no soporific effect.	None	None	None	None	Pre and post ratings of fear would have been useful.
	Case Five: hospitalized for chronic back pain.	N=1, 45 yrs, male, failed at hypnotic induction.	Same method as above	Not stated	Method unsuccessful in inducing relaxation, subsequent surgery revealed herniated disc at L4-5.	None	None	None	None	Case report.
Vahia, et al 1972;1973	Psychoneurosis and psychosomatic disorders that failed to respond to conventional treatment.	Stage One: N=165 Stage Two: N=37 Stage Three: treatment N=21; controls N=18; age range for all S's 15-50 yrs. experience not stated	Nine year study Stage One: psychophysiologic therapy based on concepts of Patanjali (yoga): (1) postures; (2) breathing exercises; (3) withdrawal from senses; (4) concentration on object; (5) identification with object) practiced one hr. 6 days/week for 6 weeks Stage Two: treatment compared with controls who receives similar pseudotreatment with "superficial" postures, breathing exercises, and no interpretation or insight to help steps 3-5 practiced one hr. each weekday for 4-6 weeks.	Not stated	Stage One: biased clinical assessment at 3 and 6 weeks; for target symptom (inkal) 70% of patients rated relieved from neurosis, hysteria and bronchial asthma showed improvement. Stage Two: patients self-reported intrusive thoughts during treatment; and at 3 and 6 weeks showed greater and consistent anxiety reduction for treatment group; MMPI and	Self-reported increase in work efficiency on the job and objective global improvement reported by patient's as friends, spouse, other relations, and colleagues.	None	Bronchial asthma assessed	None	Double blind used; stage two groups matched for age, sex, diagnosis and duration of illness. Same therapist used for total treatment and pseudotreatment introducing possible experimenter effect (Smith, 1975).

TABLE 5.1 Studies on Fears and Phobias, Stress and Tension Management (cont'd.)

Investigator(s)	Clinical Problem	S's (N: age, sex, prior experience)	INDEPENDENT VARIABLE — Type and Length of Treatment/Training	Frequency of Therapist (E) Contact	DEPENDENT VARIABLE — Subjective Effects	Behavioral	Physiological	Overt, Concurrent (e.g. medical)	Follow-up	Type of Design, Quality of Control, Methodological Problems
(Vahia et al. 1972-1973 continued)			both groups given placebo tablets, support and reassurance. Stage Three: treatment compared with controls using anxiolytic and antidepressant drugs (e.g. Amitriptyline and chlordiazepoxide).			Rorschach tests given pre and post-treatment. 73% of S's in total therapy showed improvement of at least 50% on basis of clinical assessment, while 42% of S's on "pseudo-treatment" showed significant improvement. MMPI showed greater overall improvement for total therapy group. Those who showed greater ability to meditate to total therapy group displayed more clinical improvement than those who did not. Stage Three: pre-treatment, 3 and 6 week assessment with Taylor's Anxiety Rating Scale, Hamilton's Depression Rating Scale, and Bell's Social Adjustment Scale. treatments equally effective on depression rating; psycho-physiologic therapy showed greater reduction than drug therapy on anxiety scale, and psychophysiologic therapy patients showed reduction on social adjustment scale.			
Girodo 1974	Patients diagnosed as "anxious," "neurotic," length of illness: 5-71 months.	N=9, 7 male, 2 female, ages 18-42 years, not stated	"TM like" meditation on mantric sound used 20 min., twice per day used for all patients. Combined with imaginal flooding procedure for 4 patients who failed to show anxiety decrement after 8 sessions with meditation alone (total length of treatment: 6-8 months)	Patients seen every 7-14 days	Anxiety symptom questionnaire (administered every 2 weeks) showed reduction in anxiety symptomatology by 8th session of meditation. 4 patients found meditation unbeneficial, but experienced relief of symptoms with flooding. Note: late analysis showed difference in group successful with meditation treatment (mean group duration of symptoms—14.2 months and mean "cognitive" symptom severity of 9.5) and group successful with flooding (mean group duration of symptoms—44.2 months and mean "cognitive" symptom severity of 16.4)		Degrees of somatic symptoms reported in questionnaire	None	6 month mailed follow-up questionnaire	Patients as own controls, patients told to expect "calm relaxation", etc. from technique introducing expectation effect, no control group.
Shapiro 1976	Complaining of "free-floating anxiety."	N=1, female college student, no prior experience	(1) 2 weeks: monitoring of anxiety with counter. (2) weekend Zen workshop teaching anxiety contingent Zen breath meditation plus covert self modeling (3) 3 weeks with instructions to meditate 10 min. 2x per day, to continue anxiety monitoring and practice informal breath meditation when anxious	Therapist (E) did not contact patient during 3 week meditation period.	Significant decrease in feelings of anxiety during intervention phase (3 weeks) and positive self perception change on semantic differential	Wrist counter used as anxiety monitor	None	None	None	N=1 design, relative effect of formal vs. informal meditation on relief of anxiety not clear; also possible reactive effect from initial self monitoring.
Smith 1976	Anxiety (isolating effect of TM from expectation of relief and daily sitting.)	Exp. 1: N=139, college students, mean age 22 yrs. 70 male, 69 female, no prior meditation experience Exp. 2: N=54, college students, mean age 21.5 yrs. 27 male, 27 female.	Exp. 1: 1) Pretreatment: Elaborate placebo procedure with control treatment. Rationale given. Assessment included SIAI A-Trait Inventory, Epstein-Fenz Manifest Anxiety Scale, and other supplementary measures including test of skin conductance reactivity. 2) Random assignment of S's to: 1) Standard' TM training (N=49) 2) Control treatment called (PSI) "Periodic Somatic Inactivity" (sitting, eyes closed) (N=51) 3) No treatment - (waiting list) (N=39) Exp. 2: 1) No treatment controls, Exp. 1 (N=24) and others (N=30) given similar pretreatment assessment (cf. Exp. 1) (placebo procedure 2) Random assignmt. of S's to: 1) TM-like meditation called "Cortically Mediated Stabilization" 2) "Anti-meditation" exercise involving sitting with eyes closed, actively generating pos. thoughts	Exp. 1: Placebo treatment matched with that procedure for similar amount of therapist contact and treatment credibility. Exp. 2: Both treatments taught in similar fashion by experimentor with elaborate treatment rationales given.	Subjective Exp. 1: TM and PSI groups did not differ significantly on post-test SIAI-A Trait Scale (trait anxiety) scores; symptoms of striated muscle tension and autonomic arousal (Epstein-Fenz Manifest anxiety scale). Both TM and PSI post-test means significantly lower than No treatment on all dep. var. Exp. 2: Groups did not differ significantly on dep. var. measures. T-test of within group differences reveal significant impact on SIAI-A Trait and symptoms of autonomic arousal for both groups.	None	None	None	Exp. 1: No treatment S's post-tested at 3.5 mos., TM and PSI S's post-tested at 6 mos., including assessment on drug use and subjective responses to treatment. Exp. 2: Same post-tests (Exp. 1) given at 11 weeks.	Useful study is beginning to isolate aspects of treatment variance.

TABLE 5.1 Studies on Fears and Phobias, Stress and Tension Management (cont'd.)

Investigator(s)	Clinical Problem	S's (N: age, sex, prior experience)	Type and Length of Treatment/Training	Frequency of Therapist (t) Contact	Subjective Effects	Behavioral	Physiological	Overt, Concurrent (e.g. medical)	Follow-up	Type of Design, Quality of Control, Methodological Problems
						INDEPENDENT VARIABLE				
Goleman and Schwartz 1976	Ability to reduce stress in lab situation in response to stressful film.	Group One N=30, avg. age approx. 25 yrs. more than 2 years TM experience. Group Two N=30, avg age approx. 23 yrs. non-meditators interested in TM or Yoga. Note: Difference in "life-style" found: meditators reported reduced usage of licit and illicit drugs, coffee, and dietary changes (e.g. less meat and candy).	Experimental Procedure - Note: S's assigned serially to 1 of 3 experimental conditions 1) 4 min. baseline 2) 20 min. treatment - 3 conditions a) Meditation: eyes closed (not using mantra) b) Relaxation: eyes open c) Relaxation: eyes closed 3) 5 min. rest 4) 12 min. exposure to stressful film		Pre and post treatment testing on State-Trait Anxiety Inventory A State Form (Spielberger, 1970) showed meditators reported less state and trait anxiety before and after treatment. Affective Adjective Checklist (Zuckerman 1960) showed meditators reported feeling more positive upon entering lab and throughout treatment. Activity Preference questionnaire (Lykken & Katzenmeyer 1960) administered post treatment found S's in meditation condition were less anxiety prone after leaving lab though no between group differences. Post treatment testing on Eysenck Personality Inventory showed meditators significantly less neurotic and more stable than non-meditators.	None	Physiological: Meditators heart rate less than controls during treatment, increase heart rate more than controls to anticipation of stress or impact, then recover more quickly post impact. On phasic skin conductance—all groups decrease equally in response frequency during treatment; meditators increase more in anticipatory minute prior to stressor impact and decrease more during post impact minute. Meditators compared to controls had higher skin conductance response freq, peaks and lower troughs.	None	None	Treatment conditions randomized and controlled, eyes open/closed factor. "Life-style" differences between groups suggest importance of other factors besides meditation in stress response.
Linden 1973	Test anxiety, field independence, and reading ability.	N=15 male and 15 female randomly assigned to each treatment condition. S's drawn from upper half (in reading ability) of third grade classes of school in disadvantaged urban areas.	Group One: Taught Zen breath meditation (Maupin, 1965) and visual fixation task (Deikman, 1963), practiced 2x per week x 13 weeks for 20-25 min. Group Two: Given guidance counseling focusing on improving study skills, met 45 min. per week for 18 weeks in 3 groups of 10 S's. Controls: Controlled for by guidance condition		Pre and Post treatment test Results: Meditating group showed gain in field independence (Children's Embedded Figures Test) and decrease in test anxiety (Test Anxiety Scale for Children over controls). There was no effect on reading achievement	None	None	None	Follow-up to be reported.	Well designed study, between groups design.
Lazar, Farrow and Farrow 1977	Anxiety	Group A: N=12, 7 male, 5 female, mean age 23.66 yrs. 4 weeks meditation experience. Group B N=11, 5 male 6 female, mean age 24.10, prospective meditators.	Same as above		IPAT anxiety scale questionnaire administered pre and post-(after 2 weeks) meditation instruction found mean group average reduction from 80th to 66th pop. percentile (Group B). Mean posttest score of Group A (50th percentile) was significantly lower than pretest score of Group B and nonsignificantly different from posttest score	None	None	None	None reported	Employed recurrent institutional Design (Campbell & Stanley, 1963).
Woolfolk et al. 1976	Chronic insomnia	N=24, mean age approx. 44.3 yrs. 6 male, 18 female. Avg duration of trouble with insomnia — 14.1 yrs.	All S's suspended sleep medication. Group One: N=8. Taught meditation technique involving immobility, closed eyes and a passive focus on breathing. Breathing: focus shifted (session 2) to mantra and then to focus on a specific image (session 3). Group Two: N=8. Taught in 4 weekly 1 hr. sessions in groups S's instructed to practice 30 min./2x daily at home. Group Three: Waiting list controls, asked to keep records of sleep patterns with promise of treatment at end of experiment	4 wks. x 1 hr. treatment	S's retrospective rating initial belief in potential effectiveness of treatments revealed no significant differences in treatment groups. College students asked to rate credibility of treatment procedures and rationale on same scale showed no significant differences between treatments.	Behavioral Treatments reported on— (1) Latency of Sleep Onset Means (in minutes) Pretest / Post-test / Follow-up Meditation 74.08 / 34.19 / 24.51 Progressive Relaxation 65.01 / 29.20 / 26.73 Control 67.21 / 66.61 / — Treatments equally effective. Both meditation and Progressive Relaxation groups showed significant improvement over pretreatment, while pretreatment and follow-up means for control group did not differ. (2) Rated Difficulty of Falling Asleep (10 — extremely difficult) Pretest / Post-test / Follow-up Meditation 5.92 / 2.91 / 2.94 Progressive Relaxation 6.35 / 3.48 / 3.28 Control 5.38 / 5.79 / —	None	None	6 month follow-up in form of 1 week of daily sleep records.	Techniques called "self-control" skills protecting against meditation placebo effect. Excellent study.
Tupule et al. 1971	Ischaemic Heart disease patients with history of myocardial infarct. Period from infarction to time of study ranged from 1 to 10 yrs. Group One: all but 2 patients with history of relief from antianginal drugs. Group Two recent myocardial infarct	Group One N=23, avg age= 48.5 yrs. male, all of high economic class with sedentary habits except 1 farmer. Group Two N=21, avg. age=32.4 yrs. 19 male, 2 female. all except 1 belonged to a sedentary occupation	11 Hatha Yogic positions (asana) practiced until patient was symptom free (e.g. stable heart rate and blood pressure, and absence of complications of E.C.G.). Positions practiced daily	Not stated specifically	Group One Patients who performed exercises regularly expressed "feeling of physical well-being" and ability to work without fatigue. Group Two: Similar subjective feelings reported. Ambulation achieved during 2nd week in 10 cases and 3rd week in 10 cases. Rehabilitation achieved during 5th week in 8 cases and before 9th week in others	None	Physiological: Group Two: 150 observations made before & after exercise on heart rate, B.P. & respiration Behavioral: Group One: Report states: "Patients unable to return to their full occupation, even after a year from infarct, could be rehabilitated after about a month of starting these exercises."	None	One month to 7 years	Patients in group one had been treated by one of experimenters in past. "general" measure of "well-being" not reported. no controls. no statistical data reported.
Honsberger and Wilson 1973	Bronchial asthma	N=22, no prior experience with TM	Treatment Group (N=11). Practiced Transcendental Meditation for 3 months Control Group (N=11) read related material daily x 3 months	Not reported	74% of patients reported TM has benefited their asthma. 69% thought it had helped their general health. 63% reported TM assisted their emotional life. None reported worsening on these parameters.	None Reported	Pulmonary function data obtained at baseline, 3 & 6 months. GSR showed 79% of patients effectively meditated. 94% of patients had improved airway resistance after TM in comparison to control values.	None	At 6 months 80% of patients, still meditating only 60% thought it was helping their asthma.	Parameters of "general health" and emotional assistance from TM vague.

Other studies, using control-group designs, have also reported a consistent reduction in anxiety for the meditating treatment group. The data have been gathered primarily by pre-test and post-test questionnaires, including Speigelberger's State-Trait Anxiety Inventory (Smith, 1976; Goleman & Schwartz, 1976; Davidson, Goleman & Schwartz, 1976; Ferguson & Gowan, 1976; Dillbeck, 1977), the IPAT anxiety questionnaire (Lazar et al., 1977; Ferguson & Gowan, 1976) the Bendig anxiety scale (Hjelle, 1974), and the Test Anxiety Scale for Children (Linden, 1973). Other data measuring anxiety-related behaviors include heart rate and phasic skin conductance (meditators recovered more quickly after viewing a stressful film [Goleman & Schwartz, 1976]) and insomnia (meditators showed substantial improvement on variables of sleep onset and rated difficulty of falling asleep [Woolfolk, Carr-Kaffashan & McNulty, 1976]).

5.2A *Meditation and Psychotherapy*

THIS MATERIAL FOLLOWS the section on stress because the two "control group" studies researching meditation and psychotherapy have focused on the stress-reduction aspect of meditation. Further, it should be noted that most of the studies detailing meditation's potential psychotherapeutic stress-reduction effects have been done with normal subjects. Although the results are provocative, generalization to clinical populations must proceed cautiously. In addition to the anecdotal case reports (e.g., Kondo, 1958; Boudreau, 1972; Girodo, 1974; Deathridge, 1975), there have been two "control" group designs to assess meditation's effectiveness as psychotherapy (Vahia et al., 1973) and as an aid to psychotherapy (Glueck & Stroebel, 1975). As noted above, the theoretical rationale for the use of meditation in both of these studies involves the role of stress as a mediating variable. Vahia et al. (1973) noted that the exercises of Patañjali teach one to develop internal standards and to rely less on the views and standards of others. He noted that as long as the individual is vulnerable to external standards or internalized "conscience" standards, he will be vulnerable to stress. Therefore, stress is seen as the mediating variable which these exercises correct. Similarly, Glueck and Stroebel (1975) suggested that many psychiatric patients activate the emergency response system, (Cannon's [1932] fight or flight; Selye, [1956]), at inappropriate times and with inappropriate or misperceived stimuli. They suggest that training in self-regulation techniques like meditation may help in dealing with those problems.

The Vahia study (1973) was done with patients diagnosed with psychoneuroses or psychosomatic disorders. The treatment was based on the concepts of Patañjali. The techniques were a graduated series of five Yoga meditation exercises beginning with attempts to gain voluntary control over the musculature (asana exercises—selected postures for relaxation); followed by attempts to gain voluntary control over the autonomic nervous system (prānāyāma—breathing exercises); to restrain the senses by voluntary withdrawal from the external environment (pratyahara); and still later a gaining of control over thought processes themselves (e.g., four, dhāranā—selection of an object for concentration). Finally, development of total concentration on the selected object and eventually union—dhyana—was sought. There was significant improvement on psychological tests, such as MMPI, Taylor's Manifest Anxiety Scale, and Rorschach, for individuals who practiced the complete series of meditation exercises, compared to a control group, matched for age, sex, and diagnosis, who practiced only the first three exercises.

A second study, more elaborate in scope, was done by Glueck and Stroebel (1975). Initially, they had three groups of psychiatric in-patients: an autogenic training group, a biofeedback group, and a TM group. The initial two control groups dropped out of the study, so a comparison group matched for age, sex, and level and kind of psychopathology, as measured by the MMPI at the time of admission, was used. Diagnoses included schizophrenia, neurosis, personality disorder, alcoholism, drug dependence, adjustment reaction. Patients practicing TM showed a statistically significant greater degree of improvement upon discharge (based on the report of the treating psychiatrist) than that of the hospital's other patients and also a significantly better level of improvement than their comparison twins.

5.3 Addiction and Drug Use

 THERE HAVE BEEN eight first-round studies evaluating meditation's effectiveness in treating various types of addictions and drug use.* The research design of these studies falls into two categories: retrospective polling and longitudinal design. Seven of these studies indicate that meditation may be a promising preventive and/or rehabilitative strategy in decreasing the use of addictive substances. In the one study showing negative results (Anderson, 1977), it was noted, that motivation and adherence to treatment seem to be an important variable in determining the success of treatment. It is hard to make more definite claims for meditation's effectiveness at this point because of a number of methodological problems. For example, the retrospective questionnaires in the first group of studies (Benson, 1969; Benson & Wallace, 1972b; Shafii, Lavely, & Jaffe, 1975) are subject to several criticisms. Subjects were asked to recall daily drug use patterns as far back as two years. There are three possible problems with this type of questionnaire: 1) A subject's report on a paper and pencil questionnaire may be inadvertently inaccurate; we may not be aware of how we in fact act, 2) A subject's memory of two years ago may be faulty (Benson & Wallace, 1972b), and 3) Subjects may try to deceive the experimenters to gain experimenter approval—i.e. demand characteristics.

With regard to demand characteristics, the most experienced meditators noted that they had "strong positive feelings about the experience of meditation" (Shafii, Lavely, & Jaffe, 1974). This positive feeling about meditation, coupled with the instructions in the TM initiation that drug use adversely affects TM performance, may have contributed to an exaggeration on the retrospective questionnaire about the decrease in drug use and the magnitude of prior drug-use patterns. As Shafii, Lavely, and Jaffe (1974) noted, meditators retrospectively reported using twice as much marijuana prior to their TM initiation as nonmeditators.

A second problem with the retrospective questionnaires is one of sample bias (Marcus, 1975). In the above studies, the questionnaire was only given to long-term meditators. The TM initiates who stopped meditating (thirty percent of the original sample) were not considered (Shafii, Lavely, & Jaffe, 1974). Therefore, there may have been a subject selection bias in that the surveyed

*Benson, 1969; Benson & Wallace, 1972b; Shafii, Lavely, & Jaffe, 1974, 1975; Shapiro & Zifferblatt, 1976; Lazar, Farwell & Farrow, 1977; Brautigam, 1971; Anderson, 1977.

group had a commitment to meditation.

Finally, the earliest two studies (Benson, 1969; Benson & Wallace, 1972b) had no control group. Shafii, Lavely and Jaffe's (1974; 1975) studies on marijuana and alcohol abuse added a control group; TM meditators provided their own matched control. However, the control group does not effectively control for possible variance of treatment due to subject's motivation and/or expectations.

Because of the methodological problems inherent in retrospective sampling, the more recent drug studies have employed prospective longitudinal designs (Shapiro & Zifferblatt, 1976; Lazar, Farwell & Farrow, 1977; Brautigam, 1971). In these studies, self-report of drug use was obtained on a daily, ongoing basis. Although there is still the possibility of deception in two of the studies (Lazar, Farwell & Farrow, 1977; Brautigam, 1971), the possibilities of inadvertent inaccurate reporting and of memory lapses are minimized. The most effective means of data gathering thus far have combined drug-use information from self-report with the concurrent validity of random urinalysis checks (Shapiro & Zifferblatt, 1976a). Thus, these longitudinal within-subject (Shapiro & Zifferblatt, 1976a) and group designs (Lazar, Farwell & Farrow, 1977; Brautigam, 1971) improve on previous studies, though not definitive because of their own methodological problems including self-report without concurrent validity (Lazar, Farwell & Farrow, 1977; Brautigam, 1971); combination treatments (Shapiro & Zifferblatt, 1976); and lack of control for demand, expectation effects, and subject motivation (Shapiro & Zifferblatt, 1976; Lazar, Farwell & Farrow, 1977; Brautigam, 1971).

Further, all seven studies suffer from the lack of a clear theoretical rationale linking their independent and dependent variables. For example, Brautigam (1971) divided the dependent variable into two groupings: light drugs (hashish) and heavy drugs (LSD, amphetamines, opiates), though lumping LSD, amphetamines, and opiates together clouds several issues. First, amphetamines and LSD do not produce physical addiction, whereas opiates do. Second, possible reasons for using LSD and amphetamines—e.g., self-knowledge, creativeness, spiritual enlightenment and expansion of consciousness (Cohen, 1969)— could be quite different from the reasons for opiate use such as

TABLE 5.2 Studies on Addictions: Drugs/Cigarettes/Alcohol

Investigator(s)	Clinical Problem	INDEPENDENT VARIABLE Ss (N: age, sex, prior experience)	Type and Length of treatment/training	Frequency of Therapist (T) Contact	DEPENDENT VARIABLE Subjective Effects (unless otherwise noted)	Follow-up	Type of Design, Quality of Controls, Methodological Problems
Benson, 1969	Drug abuse	N=20, male, age 21-38	Standard TM training	None: study done by retrospective survey	19 claimed to have stopped drug abuse ranging from marijuana to LSD, heroin, amphetamines, and barbiturates. Ss reported drug induced feelings became "extremely distasteful" compared with those during TM.	None reported	No control group; subject self selection bias; subject were only those who had continued to meditate more than 3 months; and were motivated to attend a one-month training session; no concurrent validity; retrospective questionnaire.
Benson and Wallace, 1972b	Drug abuse, alcohol and cigarette consumption.	N=1950 (original sample) f=1862 (final no. of respondents). 50% between 19-23 yrs. 1080 men, 781 women. Avg. experience: 20 months. Minimum: 3 months	Standard TM training. Ss were attending one month TM teacher training course	Same as above	With three mos. TM, Ss reported marked decrease in abuse of all categories of drugs (marijuana, LSD, narcotics, amphetamines, tobacco and liquor). With continued TM, Ss report progressive decrease of drug use. After 21 mos. most Ss completely stopped using drugs. In 6-mo. period pre-TM 80% of Ss reported marijuana use, 28% heavy use (once a day or more). After 6 mos. TM, 37% reported marijuana use, 6.8% heavy use. Marked decreases in LSD and narcotic abuse. Also Ss reported stopping former drug-selling and discouraging others from drug use. After TM. Most Ss felt TM important in curbing their drug abuse.	None reported	Same as above
Brautigam 1971	Drug abuse, pathological behavior and anxiety	N=20, 6 light drug users (e.g., hashish) and 4 heavy drug users (e.g., amphetamines, LSD, opiates) in each group; no prior actual experience.	Group One: N=14. TM instruction 2 hrs. per day x 4 days. Checking one a week for first month. Group Two N=18: controls group counseling 4 hrs. per week	Not stated specifically	Hashish use dropped from approx. 20x/mo to 3x/mo. among experimental group and 18.2x/mo. among controls. After 3 mos. hard drug usage decreased among meditators, increased with controls. Reduction in pathological behaviors and anxiety self-reported by meditators. Behavioral Data Tension-restlessness; flaccidity; psychomotor retardation reported improved by outside observers. Ratings and Ss self-estimate.	None reported	Possible expectation effect; Ss informed of probable subjective benefits; effect of motivation. In experimental group, only 6 Ss meditated regularly. Dependent variables lumped together: hashish, LSD, and opiates. These should be treated as separate. Other effects— e.g. "meeting a new group of non-drug using peers"— may be part of treatment variance.
Shafii, Lavely and Jaffe 1974	Marijuana use	Ss provided their own matched control N=60. Ss placed in 5 groups according to length of TM practice (range from 1-39 mos.). N=125 (original sample) N=115 (final no. respondents)	Standard TM training	None: study done by retrospective survey	1) 92% of meditators (2 yrs. or more exp.) reported significant decreased marijuana use, 77% reported stopping of usage. 2) In above group, 69% reported stopping marijuana use during first 3 mos. post TM in contrast to 15% stoppage among controls. 3) In Group I (0-3 mos. TM) a 46% decrease and a 23% stoppage reported in marijuana use during first 3 mos. post TM instruction. Controls reported 15% stoppage. 4) In Groups II (4-6 mos. TM), III (7-12 mos. TM) and IV (13-24 mos. TM) reported significant decrease and stoppage marijuana use during first 3 mos. post TM instruction. 5) The longer group practiced meditation, the more they reported a decrease or discontinuation of marijuana use. 6) Mean frequency marijuana use per month for meditators pre TM was 7.3. The control group's mean was 3.6. Following TM, mean of the meditators dropped to 2.8 whereas the control group's mean stayed the same.	None reported	Control group does and control for possible variance of treatment due to Ss motivation. Margin same.
Shafii, Lavely and Jaffe 1975	Alcohol abuse	Same as above	Standard TM training	Same as above	No control Ss reported discontinuation of beer and wine use. 40% of Ss meditating for more than 2 yrs. reported discontinuation of wine and beer use within first 6 mos. After 25-34 mos. of meditation, 60% reported discontinuation, with 54% discontinuing hard liquor use. 6-20% of Ss reported discontinuation of beer and wine in first 3 mos. 11-40% of Ss reported discontinuation of beer and wine in second 3 mos.	None reported	Control group picked by the meditators. This control group, however, does not control for possible variance of treatment due to Ss's motivation. Also, dependent variables gathered by retrospective questionnaire.
Lazar, Farrell and Farrow 1975	Anxiety, drug abuse, cigarette smoking, and alcohol consumption	Study Two: Group 1: N=24, 8 male, 16 female. mean age 25.29 yrs., (S.D. 7.37) Controls Meditators Group 3: N=13, 9 male, 4 female. mean age 20.85 yrs. (S.D. 4.41) Study Two: Group 3: N=9, 2 male, 7 female. mean age 29.11 yrs., (S.D. 0.75) Group 4: N=14, 6 male, 8 female. mean age 23.5 yrs. (S.D. 7.88)		Not stated specifically	Study Two: IPAT anxiety scale and questionnaire concerning drug abuse, cigarette and alcohol consumption. Group one controls administered a few days prior to TM instruction. Group one controls administered a few days prior to TM instruction and 4 weeks (group 2), eight weeks (group 3), or twelve weeks (group 4) after instruction. Showed progressive decreases in anxiety among meditators and use of drugs, cigarettes and alcohol. drug use showed initial rapid decrement then continuing gradual decline.	None reported	
Shapiro and Zifferblatt 1976	Methadone addiction	N=2 Case One: 25 yrs. male no prior experience Case Two: 29 yrs. male no prior experience	Clients taught behavioral functional analysis to monitor drug abuse; covert behavioral rehearsal and formal Zen breath meditation. Practiced one month	Overt. Concurrent	Case One: Drop in dosage from 30 milligrams methadone to complete detoxification. Case Two: Drop in dosage from 40 milligrams methadone to complete detoxification. Concurrent validity random urinalysis to monitor possible drug use.	Case One: 2 yrs. Ss self-report free of all opioid use. Case Two: 6 mos. + 2 yrs. Ss self-report: free of all opioid use.	Within subject design relative effects of varying treatments unclear.

social pressure, rebellion against authority, primary reinforcement, escape from social and emotional problems, and relief of
withdrawal symptoms (Shapiro & Zifferblatt, 1976). As
Brautigam's (1971) report now stands, it is impossible to tell who
stopped taking which "heavy drugs" for what reasons.

5.4 Hypertension

SEVEN FIRST-ROUND studies have involved the use of
meditation in reducing blood pressure (Benson &
Wallace, 1972a; Benson et al., 1974a; 1974b; Patel, 1973; Patel,
1975a; 1975b; Stone & DeLeo, 1976; Datey, et al., 1969). Certainly, from a research standpoint, blood pressure is one of the
"cleanest" dependent variables to measure. These studies consistently indicate a reduction in blood pressure in the treatment
group (Benson & Wallace, 1972a; Benson et al., 1974a, 1974b;
Patel, 1973; Patel, 1975a, 1975b; Stone & DeLeo, 1976; Datey et
al., 1969), in the use of hypertensive medication (Patel, 1973;
Datey et al., 1969), and in reports of somatic symptoms (Datey
et al., 1969). Follow-up data have shown that treatment gains
were maintained during a twelve-month period (Patel, 1975b).

Although the treatment effect seems relatively clear, there are
still several unanswered questions as to what is causing that
effect. The treatment interventions have ranged from a combination of Yoga breathing, concentration, and muscle relaxation
(Datey et al., 1969), the "Relaxation Response" technique (Benson & Wallace, 1972a; Benson et al., 1974a; 1974b), a combination
of Yoga, breath meditation, muscle relaxation, concentration, and
biofeedback (Patel, 1973), to a Buddhist meditation procedure
(Stone & DeLeo, 1976). Future research should attempt to isolate
the variance of treatment success due to different aspects of the
intervention. Further research should also determine whether the
results are maintained. For example, Pollack et al. (1977) found
that changes in blood pressure had disappeared after six months.
For a more detailed discussion of possible variables influencing
treatment outcome, readers are referred to an excellent review of
the literature by Jacob, Kraemer and Agras (1977).

TABLE 5.3 Studies on Hypertension

Investigator(s)	Clinical Problem	Ss (N, age, sex, prior experience)	INDEPENDENT VARIABLE: Type and Length of Treatment/Training	Frequency of Therapist (E) Contact	Subjective Effects	DEPENDENT VARIABLE: Physiological (Note: BP measures given systolic/diastolic, unless otherwise noted)	Follow-up	Type of Design, Quality of Controls, Methodological Problems
Benson and Wallace, 1972a	Hypertension	N=22, no prior experience	Standard TM training by Student's International Society—8½ hrs. Ss instructed to practice technique 2x20 min daily	Not stated	None reported	Found decreased resting systemic arterial blood pressure levels. Mean BP levels prior to meditation—150±17/94±9mmHg. Mean BP levels post meditation—141±11/87±2mmHg (mean ± one S.D.)	4.63 weeks	N=1, Ss as own control pre, during, and post meditation
Benson et al., 1974a	Borderline hypertension with Ss not using anti-hypertensive drugs	N=22, avg. age approx. 43.1 ± 12.3 yr. (mean ± one S.D.) 10 male, 12 female, volunteers from introductory TM lecture group	Same as above	Not stated	None reported	Found decreased resting blood pressure levels. Mean BP levels prior to meditation—146.5±13.7/61±6.9&mmHg. Mean BP levels post meditation—139.5±12.6/90.7±8.8mmHg	Post meditation instruction measurement every 2-3 weeks x 25 weeks	N=1, Ss as own control 6 weeks prior to meditation instruction measurement
Benson et al., 1974b	Hypertension with Ss using anti-hypertensive drugs	N=14, avg. age approx. 53.3 yrs. (S.D.) 8/9, 6 males, 8 females, no prior experience, volunteers from introductory TM lecture.	Same as above	Not stated	None reported	Found decreased resting blood pressure levels. Mean BP levels prior to meditation—145.6±7.38/91.9±1.34mmHg. Mean BP levels post meditation—135.0±8.32/87.0±1.34mmHg Ss's diet and antihypertensive drug use (mean ± one S.D.) monitored by questionnaire	Post instruction measurement 10 days x 20 weeks	1 x 6 weeks prior to meditation instruction measurements taken, study unbiased in regard to alterations in antihypertensive agents or significantly altered diet
Patel 1973, 1975c follow-up	Hypertension with Ss using anti-hypertensive drugs (one or more), Duration of hypertension from 1-20 years (avg. 8 years) Symptomatology ± tiredness (14 patients), headache (13), dyspnoea on exertion (11), dizziness (a), irritability (9), chest pain (6), angina (7), palpitation (6), and nervousness (5).	Group One (N=20, avg. age 57.35 yrs. 9 males, 11 females) Group Two (N=20, controls matched for age and sex)	Patients instructed to practice Yoga, breath meditation, muscle relaxation, and concentration exercises in an order relayed from back of GSR through audio signal of "relaxometer" given continuously. Patients also told pre and post session BP levels.	3x per week x 3 months for ½ hr. relaxation training	Report stated "patients responded favourably" criteria of subjective effects not stated.	1) Alteration in BP over 3 months of Relaxation training "Pre-trial" BP Treatment Group 159.1±15.9/100.1±17.8 Control Group 169.2±20.9/99.9±12.8 "End of trial" BP Treatment Group 138.7±16.0/85.9±8.7 Control Group 162.6±29.4/97.0±12.0 2) End of trial arrival BP End of trial arrival BP Treatment Group 144.6±11.0/86.0±5.74 Control Group 167.7±9.73/97.1±6.54 Final arrival BP Treatment Group 144.4±9.83/86.7±6.33 Control Group 163.6±9.47/98.1±7.83 (12 month)/(9 month)	3, 6, 9 and 12 months (12 month)/(9 month)	Variance of treatment effect attributable to Yoga, biofeedback and role of therapist not clear. with 42% drop in total drug requirement among patients. 5 patients ended use of drugs of four patients who did not control BP then achieved control of migraine and stopped antidepressant drug therapy. BP requirition rates recorded and given to patient pre and post session: also biofeedback of GSR given continuously during treatment.
Patel 1975b	Hypertension with Ss using anti-hypertensive drugs	Phase One (N=34) Group One (treatment) N=17, mean age 55.5 yrs. 6 male, 11 female Group Two (control) N=17, mean age 58.6 yrs. 7 male, 10 female Phase Two control group (2) given treatment	Treatment procedure (2 sessions per week x 6 weeks) 1) Educational discussion about hypertension, physiology of relaxation, etc. and patients 2) Instruction in methodical (yogic) relaxation and slowed breathing 3) After mastery of step 2: Transcendental meditation-like technique taught 4) Biofeedback (e.g. audio signal of GSR level) given continuously by "relaxometer" during steps 2 and 3 5) Ss urged to practice informal relaxation and meditation outside of treatment when tense. (e.g. each patient had a red disc on his watch as a reminder to relax when he looked at the time.	Extensive doctor-patient interaction between doctor and patients	None reported	1) BP before trial Treatment Group 167.5±23.6/99.6±9.3mmHg Control Group 168.3±20.0/100.6±11.4mmHg 2) Mean Final BP Phase 1 Treatment Group 141.4/84.4mmHg Control Group 160.0/96.4mmHg 3) Mean BP Phase 2 Mean initial BP treatment (formerly control) 176.6/104.3 Control (formerly treatment) 148.8/-/87.8 Mean final BP treatment (formerly control) 148.5/89.3 Control (formerly treatment) 146.7/86.2	2 wks. x 3 months after phase one: then 2 month interval prior to phase two, Phase two: single used follow-up examination	Same criterion as above
Datey et al., 1969	Hypertension with chronic hypertensive (essential—32 patients, renal—12, atherosclerotic—3) Symptomatology. Giddiness (30 patients), headache (28), chest pain in 12 (angina 7), palpitation in 12, breathlessness on exertion in 10, exhaustion in 10, insomnia in 8, irritability and nervousness in 8.	N=47, avg. age 46 yrs., 37 male, 10 female Group One N=10, not using antihypertensive drugs. Group Two N=22, BP well controlled with antihypertensive drugs. Group Three N=15, BP inadequately controlled with antihypertensive drugs.	"Shavasana" Yogic breathing concentration and muscle relaxation done 30 min. daily for approx. 30 weeks. EMG feedback of frontalis muscle tension used as check of muscle relaxation.	Not stated specifically	Report states "patients experienced a sense of well-being after exercise. Improvement reported among almost all patients in somatic symptoms (e.g. headaches, giddiness, nervousness, irritability, and insomnia)	Decreases in avg. mean blood pressure. Group One 134mmHg to 107mmHg (reduction 27mmHg) Group Two 102-100mmHg unchanged (since patient's BP well controlled by drugs, therapy aimed at reducing drug dosages. In 13 Ss (59%), req. drug requirement was reduced to 32% of original dosage. For 9 patients dosage could not be reduced, however, 6 of these Ss performed Yogic exercise inadequately. Group Three 120mmHg to 110mmHg, drug requirement reduced to 29% of original in 6 patients (40%), dosage unchanged in 7 patients (of these, 2 were irregular and 2 could not perform exercise correctly), dose had to be increased in 2 patients (regular with exercise). Essential (62.5%), Renal (47%), not statistically significant, atherosclerotic (not favorable response)	to 40 weeks	Placebo tablets given Ss not using antihypertensive drugs and match prior to treatment, data substantiating report of improvement in somatic symptoms needed. also follow-up needed.
Stone and DeLeo 1976	Mild or moderate hypertension (defined as mean arterial BP greater than 105mmHg during at least 50% of 14 pretreatment examination with Ss who had never received antihypertensive therapy	N=19 Group One (controls) N=5, avg. age 28, all male Group Two (treatment) N=14, avg. age 28, (±1 yr.) (mean ± s.e.m.) Baseline BP for both groups similar	"Buddhist" meditation taught (e.g. counting breathing) for 20 min. training sessions 2x for half hour period. Ss told to repeat technique 2x daily for 10-15 min.	Not stated specifically	None reported	Effect of Physiology: Relaxation on Arterial-Blood Pressure (mean ± Standard error mean systolic/diastolic BP in mmHg) Group One (controls) Baseline—Supine 144±6/90±2 Upright 147±7/93±2 6 mo.—Supine 145±7/92±3 Upright 145±3/95±2 Group Two (treatment) Baseline—Supine 141±9/93±3 Upright 132±3/82±2 6 mos.—Supine 146±/95±3 Upright 131±4/85±2 Found lowered mean (by 12mmHg) BP for treatment group over controls. Changes in dopamine beta-hydroxylase (a blood enzyme) showed decrease among treatment group which correlated with BP reduction. Also reduction in fenestedin-stimulated renin activity (PRA) uncorrelated with BP changes. No significant changes in blood volume	6 months	Effect of possible dietary salt reduction, assessed by measuring urinary sodium excretion, but not substantiating with small N, reduction in adrenergic activity (DPH) may be statistically significant but not a physiologically important alteration.

5.5 Physiological Changes

THE STUDIES discussed in 5.1-5.3 suggest that meditation may be a promising therapeutic intervention strategy for several different clinical areas. One hypothesis that attempts to explain meditation's effectiveness in these clinical areas is that meditation helps relax an individual. There seems general agreement that meditation does, in fact, produce a state of relaxation (Smith, 1975; Benson, Beary, & Carol, 1974), variously described as an activity (effortless breathing, [Shapiro & Zifferblatt, 1976b]); a "state" (the hypometabolic state, [Wallace, Benson, & Wilson, 1971]); and a response (the relaxation response, [Benson, Beary, & Carol, 1974]). This relaxation, as a mediating mechanism, is discussed in Chapter Nine.

I would like here to briefly review the round-one physiological changes evidenced during the act of meditation itself: *reduced heart rate*, decreased oxygen consumption**, decreased blood pressure†, increased skin resistance‡, and increased percent time, regularity and amplitude of alpha activity§*. These results, summarized by type of meditation technique, are presented in tables 5.4-5.6.

*Wallace, 1970; Wenger & Bagchi, 1961; Goyeche, Chihara, & Shimizu, 1972; Karambelkar, Vinekar, & Bhole, 1968; Anand, Chinna, & Singh, 1961a; Das & Gastaut, 1955; Bagchi & Wenger, 1957.

**Wallace, Benson, & Wilson, 1971; Wallace, 1970; Wenger & Bagchi, 1961; Goyeche, Chihara, & Shimizu, 1972; Karambelkar, Vinekar & Bhole, 1968; Sugi & Akutsu, 1968; Watanabe, Shapiro & Schwartz, 1972; Allison, 1970; Treichel, Clinch & Cran, 1973; Hirai, 1974.

†Wallace, Benson & Wilson, 1971; Wenger & Bagchi, 1961; Karmabelkar, Vinekar & Bhole, 1968; Bagchi & Wenger, 1957.

‡Wallace, Benson & Wilson, 1971; Wallace, 1970; Wenger & Bagchi, 1961; Karambelkar, Vinekar & Bhole, 1968; Bagchi & Wenger, 1957; Akishige, 1970; Orme-Johnson, 1973.

§Wallace, Benson & Wilson, 1971; Wallace, 1970; Anand, China & Singh, 1961a; Das & Gastaut, 1955; Bagchi & Wenger, 1957; Watanabe, Shapiro & Schwartz, 1972; Hirai, 1974; Akishige, 1970; Kasamatsu & Hirai, 1966; Banquet, 1972; Banquet, 1973; Williams & West, 1975.

TABLE 5.4 Summary of Indian Yogic Meditation Based Partially on Woolfolk (1975)

References	Experience of Meditators	Changes During Meditation	Type of Design	Quality of Control Procedures
Das & Gastaut, 1955	Highly experienced	Faster EEG, increase in HR	Within-subject	Poor, measurements taken in field under highly variable conditions
Anand, Chinna & Singh, 1961a	Highly experienced	Faster EEG, decrease in O₂ consumption, decrease in HR	Within-subject	Excellent, laboratory study
Bagchi & Wenger, 1957	Highly experienced	No change in EEG, increased in SR level, no change in HR, no change in BP	Within-subject	Poor, measurements taken in field under highly variable conditions
Kasamatsu et al., 1957	Highly experienced	Slower EEG	Within-subject	Adequate, laboratory study, meditation period too short
Anand, Chinna & Singh, 1961a	Highly experienced	Slower EEG	Within-subject	Excellent laboratory conditions
Wenger & Bagchi, 1961	Moderately experienced	Decrease in SR level, decrease in respiration rate, increase in HR, increase in BP	Within-subject	Poor, initial readings not comparable before meditation and relaxation periods
Karambelkar, Vinekar & Bhole, 1968	Moderately experienced	No change in SR level, increase in O₂ consumption, no change in HR, no change in BP	Between-subjects	Poor, no control over duration of meditation, sketchy reporting
Corby et al., 1978	—Novice —Intermediate 2.1 years for 3 hours per day —Expert, 4.4 years for 3.4 hours per day	Novices showed autonomic relaxation while meditators showed activation. Meditators showed ↑ alpha and theta power and minimal evidence of EEG defined sleep. One meditator showed sudden EEG activation concurrent with the experience of approaching the Yogic ecstatic state of intense concentration.	Within & between subjects	Good
Elson, Hauri & Cunis, 1977	9-54 months	↑ basal skin resistance ↓ respiratory rate ↓ EEG evidence of sleep ↑ alpha and theta EEG activity	Between-subjects	Adequate

TABLE 5.5 Summary of Studies of Transcendental Meditation Based Partially on Woolfolk (1975)

References	Experience of Meditators	Changes During Meditation	Type of Design	Quality of Control Procedures
Jevning, et al., 1977	4 months & 3-5 years	↓ serum cortisol in long term meditators probably consistent with complete suppression of cortisol secretion during meditation. No change in serum testosterone. Equivalent amounts of stage 1 sleep between groups. No correlation with cortisol secretion.	Within & between subjects	Good use of same subjects before and after learning TM plus a long term practice group.
Jevning, Wilson & Smith, 1977	4 months & 3-5 years	Serum phenylalanine changes in long term meditators. No change in 12 other amino acids.	Within & between subjects	Good use of same subjects before and after learning TM plus a long term practice group.
Jevning, Wilson & Vanderlaan, 1978	4 months & 3-5 years	Plasma prolactin rose in the post meditation period. No effect on growth hormone.	Within & between subjects	Good use of same subjects before and after learning TM plus a long term practice group.
Jevning, Wilson, Smith & Morton, 1976	Average of 1 year	Slight ↑ in cardiac output and blood flow during meditation. Sharp ↓ in renal blood flow in both controls and meditators. Slight ↓ in arterial lactate in meditators.	Within & between subjects	Good use of same subjects before and after learning TM plus a long term practice group.
Younger, Adrianne & Berger, 1975	Average of 3 years	EEG records were rated as showing % time during meditation as: alert −12.7%, predominant alpha −45.9%, asleep −41.4%.	Within-subject	Adequate. Randomized blind scoring.
Pagano, Rose, Stivers & Warrenburg, 1976	Average of 2.5 years	EEG records were rated as showing % time during meditation: wakefulness −39%, state 1 sleep 19%, state 2 sleep −23%, stages 3 or 4, 17%.	Within-subject	Unclear whether EEG records were scored blind.
Bennett & Trinder, 1977	Intermediate	Evidence of shift in hemispheric laterility to the right.	Within-subject	Adequate
Wallace, 1970	Moderately experienced	Slower EEG, increase in SR level, decrease in O₂ consumption, decrease in HR	Within-subject	Excellent, laboratory study, statistical comparisons made.
Wallace, Benson & Wilson, 1971	Moderately experienced	Slower EEG, increase in SR level, decrease in O₂ consumption, decrease in BP	Within-subject	Excellent, laboratory study, statistical comparisons made.

TABLE 5.5 Summary of Studies of Transcendental Meditation Based Partially on Woolfolk (1975) (cont'd.)

References	Experience of Meditators	Changes During Meditation	Type of Design	Quality of Control Procedures
Schwartz, 1973	Moderately experienced	Slower EEG, increase in SR level (these changes not significantly different from those found in controls)	Between-subjects	Excellent, laboratory study, statistical comparisons made appropriate control group.
Banquet, 1973	Moderately experienced	Slower EEG (stages I & II), in some individuals, faster EEG observed during third stage.	Within-subject	Excellent, laboratory study, statistical comparisons made.
Orme-Johnson, 1973	Moderately experienced	Galvanic skin response more stable	Between-subjects	Excellent, laboratory study, statistical comparisons made appropriate control group.
Allison, 1970	Not reported	Decrease in rate of respiration	Within-subject	Adequate, laboratory study, sketchy reporting.
Williams & West, 1975	Average — 31 months	Earlier and more frequent alpha induction. EEG response to intermittant photic stimulation shows alpha blocking.	Between-subjects	Adequate
Fenwick, et al., 1977	Novice	EEG evidence of maintenance of stage "onset" sleep. 10_2 consumption & CO_2 production which were accountable for in terms of traditional physiological mechanisms without resorting to hypotheses of a special hypometabolic state.	Between-subjects	Good design. Excellent use of multivariate statistical analysis.
Pagano & Frumkin, 1977	Novice & experienced (1.4-3 years)	Seashore Tonal Memory Test of right hemisphere function showed improved performance in experienced but not novice meditators both before and after a meditation session. There were no differences between before and after sessions.	Between-subjects	Adequate

TABLE 5.6 Summary of Studies of Zen Meditation Based Partially on Woolfolk (1975)

Reference	Experience of Meditators	Changes During Meditation	Type of Design	Quality of Control Procedure
Kasamatsu et al., 1957	Highly experienced	Slower EEG	Within-subject	Adequate, laboratory study, meditation period too short
Kasamatsu & Hirai, 1969	Moderately experienced & highly recommended	Slower EEG	Within-subject	Excellent, laboratory conditions
Akishige, 1968	Highly experienced	Slower EEG, galvanic skin response more stable, decrease in O_2 consumption, decrease in respiration rate	Within-subject	Excellent, laboratory conditions
Hirai, 1960	Highly experienced	Slower EEG, decrease in respiration rate	Within-subject	Adequate, laboratory conditions
Sugi & Akutsu, 1968	Highly experienced	Decrease in O_2 consumption	Within-subject	Excellent, laboratory conditions
Goyeche, Chihara & Shimizu, 1972	Minimally experienced	Decrease in respiration rate, decrease in HR	Within-subject	Excellent, laboratory conditions, order of meditation and control periods randomized
Malec & Sipprelle, 1977	Novices 1 trial only	↓ Respiration, EMG and transient heart rate; no effect of expectation	Between-subjects	Good control for expectation

5.6 Comparisons with Other Self-Regulation Strategies: Physiological, Metabolic, EEG Patterns

THERE WAS INITIAL enthusiasm that meditation might be a unique strategy (Muchlman, 1977), different from all other self-regulation strategies. It was suggested, on the basis of certain first-round studies that this uniqueness could be measured by the physiological parameters noted in section 5.5. However, Benson (1975, 1977) suggested that this physiological response pattern is not particularly unique to meditation *per se* but is common to any passive relaxation procedure. This view has been supported and replicated by a number of studies which suggest no physiological difference between meditation and other self-regulation strategies, and often no differences between meditation and a "just sit" control group. For example, earlier studies suggested that skin resistance significantly increased within subjects (Wallace et al., 1971; Wallace, 1970) and in a TM group versus a control group (Orme-Johnson, 1973). Recent studies, however,* show no significant difference on galvanic skin response (GSR) between meditation and other self-regulation strategies, including self-hypnosis, Progressive Relaxation, and other instructional "relaxation" control groups. Further, the above studies also show no difference between meditation and other self-regulation strategies on heart rate or respiration decrease.

Curtis and Wessberg (1976) tested differences between a meditation group, a deep muscle relaxation group, and non-experienced individuals and found no difference either between groups or between trials on GSR, heart rate, or respiration. They noted that there was high subject variability, with some subjects "actually increasing their rate of functioning," and that the few measurements approaching statistical significance were in the control group and not in the meditators or relaxers.

In their short report, Cauthen and Prymak (1977) tested five different groups (N=7): experienced meditators (subjects

*Morse et al., 1977; Walrath & Hamilton, 1975; Cauthen & Prymak, 1977; Curtis & Wessberg, 1976; Boswell & Murray, 1979.

averaging five years experience), moderately experienced meditators (fourteen months), novice meditators (seven days), a relaxation group (five days), and a pseudo-TM group that thought about a word. These groups were compared on measures of respiration, GSR, temperature, and heart rate. The authors note that there was no significant difference for any group before, after, or during the experimental period for GSR or respiration, a finding which, as noted, goes counter to previous studies. The Cauthen and Prymak study (1977) does not seem to tease out any particularly unique physiological changes as a result of meditation, even when long-term meditators are tested.

In a related study, Travis et al. (1976) compared subjects who had meditated an average of five to thirty months with a control group which simply relaxed. After a two-minute base line, experimental subjects meditated for twenty minutes and then had a ten-minute post-meditation follow-up. There was no significant change in the meditating group in heart-rate decrease, electromyogram (EMG) decrease, or increase in occipital alpha. The only significant changes were in the control group on decrease in occipital alpha, decrease in heart rate, and decrease in frontal EMG. The authors note that most striking was the lack of changes in alpha and EMG occurring during Transcendental Meditation, compared with those previously reported (Wallace, 1970; Wallace et al., 1971). The changes in the control subjects, the authors note, seem most likely to be the result of sleep or sleep onset that occurred in thirteen of the sixteen control subjects.

In an interesting and complex study, Morse et al., (1977) looked at four experimental groups (trained in TM but not hypnosis, trained in auto-hypnosis but not TM, trained in both, trained in neither). Each of these four groups were monitored under six conditions: alert state, relaxation, heterohypnosis relaxation, heterohypnosis task, autohypnosis relaxation, and meditation. During the meditation session, those who had not practiced TM were given one of the following words: one, om, flower, garden, river, sail. There were four different orders in which the four groups underwent the six conditions. There was significant condition effect between the alert state and the experimental condition, but not among the experimental conditions, according to GSR. There was interhemispheric EEG synchronicity in all experimental conditions: That is, when synchronization of slow alpha occurred, it was not unique to TM but found in all the relaxation conditions. Neither respiration rate, pulse rate, nor systolic and diastolic blood pressure differentiated experimental conditions. The authors noted that the physiological responses of TM and simple word meditation were similar, and concluded that, "It appears that relaxation, meditation, and relaxation hypnosis yield similar physiological responses suggestive of deep relaxation."

The Morse study (1977), in addition to supporting the literature suggesting a lack of uniqueness of meditation on measures of GSR and heart rate, also calls into question its uniqueness in terms of EEG pattern—the synchronization of slow alpha (cf. Glueck & Stroebel, 1975). Further, the above studies suggest that there is not a unique respiratory effect as a result of meditation. This lack of unique respiratory effect has also been replicated by Pagano (Note 14), who found no difference between meditation and a Progressive Relaxation group, and Fenwick et al. (1977), who found no difference between meditation and listening to music. Fenwick et al. (1977) noted that subjects who were tense to begin with showed a greater relaxation effect than subjects who were not, and suggested that the findings of Wallace et al. (1971) may have been due to high initial levels of metabolism and tension. Regarding metabolic change, Fenwick et al. (1977) noted that subjects in the fasting meditation group, a control group used to reduce the level of tension and metabolism to the lowest possible level, "showed that under these circumstances meditation failed to produce any significant change in the metabolic rate."

A similar lack of metabolic uniqueness has also been found by other investigators. Michaels, Huber and McCann (1976) attempted to differentiate meditators from resting controls biochemically. Since stress increases blood catacholamines, the experimenters looked at plasma epinephrine and norepinephrine as well as lactate. Twelve experienced meditators (more than twelve months experience) were compared with controls matched for sex and age who rested instead of meditating. There were no significant fluctuations of plasma epinephrine during meditation. Neither were significant differences observed between controls and meditators. The same held true for plasma lactic acid concentration, thus failing to replicate the earlier findings on TM (Wallace, 1970).

More recent studies further call into question the uniqueness of meditation's effects. In an earlier study, Goleman and Schwartz (1976) showed increased responsiveness of meditators to an upcoming stressful event on a film and their quicker recovery time as compared to a relaxing control group. However, from a cognitive standpoint, in terms of number of post-stress intrusive thoughts, significant differences between meditators and controls have not been detected (Kanas & Horowitz, 1977). Further, earlier theories which suggested that TM was unrelated to sleep have recently been called into question by Pagano et al. (1976) and Young and Berger (1975) who note that at least beginning meditators may spend an appreciable part of their time in sleep stages two, three, and four.

Thus it appears that the original belief that meditation would be able to be discriminated as a unique physiological state has not been confirmed—either on an autonomic or metabolic level, or in terms of EEG pattern. Although it does seem clear that meditation can bring about a generalized reduction in multiple physiological systems, thereby creating a state of relaxation in the individual (Davidson, 1976; Shapiro & Giber, 1978), it is not yet clear from the available data that this state is differentiated from relaxation effects of other techniques, whether they be hypnosis (Walrath & Hamilton, 1977) or deep muscle relaxation (Curtis & Wessberg, 1976; Cauthen & Prymak, 1977; Travis, Kondo & Knott, 1975; Morse et al., 1977, etc.). The constellation of changes is, in most studies, significantly different between meditation and placebo control groups, but not between self-regulation treatment groups.

In conclusion, it should be noted that not everyone would agree with the above interpretation of the findings (e.g., Jevning & O'Halloran, 1980 in press); the results are not unequivocal. For example, Elson, Hauri and Cunis (1977) compared meditation with a "wakefully relaxed" group and a group of ĀnandaMārga meditators. They noted that "meditation was characterized by a marked increase in basal skin resistance and by a decrease in respiratory rate, changes which were not observed in the controls. Further, six of the eleven controls fell asleep, while none of the meditators fell asleep—rather meditators remained in a relatively stable state at alpha and theta EEG activity." Also, Jevning and O'Halloran (in press, 1980) suggest blood flow as a metabolic measure unique to meditation. They believe that

TABLE 5.7 Summary of Studies Comparing Meditation with Other Self-Regulation Strategies: Physiological Measures

Roger N. Walsh

Reference	Type of Meditation	Amount of Meditation	Changes During Meditation	Type of Design	Quality of Control Procedures
Walrath & Hamilton, 1975	TM	> 6 months practice	Meditators, autohypnotizers and controls all showed decreases in heart and respiration rates and GSR activity but did not differ between groups.	Between-subjects	Adequate except for equal amounts of practice for meditators and hypnosis subjects.
Curtis & Wessburg, 1975/76	TM	~ 2 years practice	No effects across trials or between meditation, progressive relaxation and controls, in GSR, heart or respiration rate.	Between-subjects	Adequate.
Cauthen & Prymak, 1977	TM	7 days, 14 months, or 5 years	2 more experienced groups of meditators showed ↓ heart rate during meditation. Relaxers and least experienced meditators showed ↑ skin temperature.	Between-subjects	Adequate. Controls focused on a word.
Travis, Kondo, & Knott, 1977	TM	5-30 months	No differences between meditators and relaxation controls on EEG, alpha, heart rate and frontal EMG. Both groups showed ↓ alpha activity. Meditators showed less EEG sleep patterns than relaxation controls.	Between-subjects	Adequate.
Morse et al., 1977	TM	2 months - 8 years	Measures of pulse rate, respiratory rate, blood pressure, GSR, EEG and muscle activity all suggested significantly greater relaxation in experimental subjects trained in TM, self-hypnosis or both, than in controls. However experimental groups did not differ between themselves except for lower muscle activity in TM.	Between-subjects	Good design and statistical analysis.
Pagano et al., (Note 14)	TM	Experienced average = 3.4 years	Both TM and progressive muscle relaxation subjects showed similar small (2-5%) decrements in O_2 consumption from a resting baseline, which did not differ from eyes closed controls.	Between-subjects	Adequate. Good statistical analysis.

TABLE 5.7 Summary of Studies Comparing Meditation with Other Self-Regulation Strategies: Physiological Measures (cont'd.)

Roger N. Walsh

Reference	Type of Meditation	Amount of Meditation	Changes During Meditation	Type of Design	Quality of Control Procedures
Glueck & Stroebel, 1977	TM	Intermediate	Showed heart and respiration rates ↑ GSR, ↑ EEG alpha. Intrahemispheric alpha and theta synchrony even in inexperienced meditators. Greater intrahemispheric synchrony in thermal and EMG biofeedback subjects than in TM or relaxation response subjects. Evidence of interhemispheric synchrony in TM and relaxation response subjects but not in biofeedback subjects.	Between and within subjects	Adequate.
Boswell & Murray, 1979	Zen	2 weeks	No significant differences between groups in Spiegelberger Trait-State Anxiety inventory, GSR, skin conductance, and heart rate.	Between-subjects	Good. Three control groups: Relaxation, placebo, and no treatment.
Beiman et al., 1980	TM	Seven 1½ hour sessions	No significant differences in effectiveness of TM, behavior therapy, or self relaxation, were detected for self report measures (locus of control, regression sensitization, autonomic perception, trait anxiety, or fear survey schedule), or physiological measures (skin resistance, skin response, pulse rate, EMG). Locus of control accounted for a major proportion of variance in the response to TM.	Between-subjects	Adequate. Good use of multivariate analyses, especially multiple regression to determine amounts of variance accounted for by subject variables.

additional unique physiological response patterns will be found, and that current findings do not reflect this simply because we do not yet have sensitive enough physiological measures to ferret out the unique aspects of meditation patterns as compared to other self-regulation strategies.

5.7 Comparison with Other Self-Regulation Strategies: Clinical

SIMILAR FINDINGS are also now being reported on a clinical level. Meditation appears to be equally but no more effective than other self-regulation strategies for dependent variables ranging from anxiety (Beiman et al., in press 1980; Goldman, Domitor & Murray, 1979; Kirsch & Henry, 1979; Boswell & Murray, 1979; Zuroff & Schwartz, 1978; Smith, 1976; Thomas & Abbas, 1978), anxiety in alcoholics (Parker et al., 1978), to alcohol consumption (Marlatt et al., in press, 1980), insomnia (Woolfolk et al., 1976) and borderline hypertension (Surwit, Shapiro, Good, 1978). Self-regulation strategies compared include Progressive Relaxation (Woolfolk et al., 1976; Marlatt et al., 1979; Beiman et al., 1979; Boswell & Murray, 1979; Thomas & Abbas, 1978), Benson's Relaxation Response (Marlatt et al., in press, 1980; Beiman et al., in press, 1980), a pseudo-meditation treatment (Smith, 1976), anti-meditation treatments (Goldman et al., 1979; Boswell & Murray, 1979; Smith, 1976), self-administered systematic desensitization (Kirsch & Henry, 1979) and cardiovascular and neuromuscular biofeedback (Surwit, Shapiro & Good, 1978; Hager & Surwit, 1978).

As examples of these types of studies involving clinical comparison of self-regulation techniques, let me describe two that seem representative: One on alcohol consumption (Marlatt et al., in press, 1980) and one on anxiety (Kirsch & Henry, 1979).

Marlatt et al. describe a nicely designed study which took heavy social drinkers through a two week pretreatment baseline phase, a six week treatment phase, and seven week follow-up. There were four groups, a meditation group (Benson's method), a Progressive Relaxation group, an attention placebo group practicing bibliotherapy, and a no-treatment control group that was monitored and took all the tests. This study is one of the first in

TABLE 5.8 Summary of Studies Comparing Meditation with Other Self-Regulation Strategies: Clinical Measures

Roger N. Walsh

Reference	Type of Meditation	Amount of Meditation	Changes During Meditation	Type of Design	Quality of Control Procedures
Zuroff & Schwartz, 1978	TM	9 weeks	Only significant difference between TM and relaxation was greater RM reduction in trait anxiety measured by the S-R Inventory of Anxiousness. Another self report measure, the Adjective Check List, and a behavioral anxiety measure did not differentiate between meditators, relaxers or no treatment controls. Similarly there were no treatment effects for psychological maladjustment measured by Rotter's Incomplete Sentence Test, locus of control, or reported alcohol or marijuana use. In subjective reports of benefits in life areas, meditators reported improved academic performance.	Between-subjects	Good—random assignment of subjects. Attempts to equalize expectancies for TM and relaxation.
Goldman, Domitor, & Murray, 1978	Zen	5 days	Meditators reported more altered states of consciousness and relaxation. No significant differences on measures of anxiety (Spielberger's State-Trait Anxiety Inventory, or the Epstein-Fenz Anxiety Scale) or of perception (Holtzman Inkblot and the Embedded Figures Tests). Locus of control did not interact with treatment but volunteer versus course requirement status did, with volunteers reporting greater Zen induced altered states and increasing proficiency across days.	Between-subjects	Very short training period but otherwise good. Employed two control groups, no treatment and placebo. Also controlled and tested for locus of control and volunteers versus subjects fulfilling course requirements.
Kirsh & Henry, 1979	TM like	Unclear	The three experimental treatments (systematic desensitization with meditation replacing progressive relaxation, and meditation only) all effected significant reductions in public speaking anxiety on self report and behavioral measures. Significant reductions in anticipatory pulse rate occurred only in the desensitization relaxation groups. Subjects who perceived treatments as highly credible showed greater improvement on both subjective anxiety and pulse rate than did subjects who perceived treatments as less credible.	Between-subjects	Good. Four groups matched according to level of performance.
Marlatt et al., 1980	Benson	6 weeks	As opposed to the no treatment control group, meditation, progressive relaxation, and the bibliotherapy attention control groups all showed significant reductions in alcohol consumption and increases in internal locus of control. However these three groups did not differ significantly. All three treatment groups reported significant increases in ratings of daily relaxation, with the greatest effect in meditators. At seven week follow-up alcohol consumption in the three treatment groups remained less than pretreatment levels but not significantly so. Most subjects ceased practicing their treatment during the seven week follow up. No significant effect of expectations was found on treatment outcome.	Between-subjects	Good. Subjects matched for baseline alcohol consumption. Attempted control of expectation.

which there was a specific, clearly spelled out theoretical rationale between the independent variables (relaxation procedures) and the dependent variable (decrease in alcohol consumption). Results suggested that the relaxation training, whether it be meditation, Progressive Relaxation or attention placebo had a significant effect on the consumption of ethanol compared to the no-treatment group. However, there were no significant differences between the three different relaxation training procedures.

Kirsch and Henry (1979) assigned thirty-eight "highly motivated" and highly speech-anxious subjects to four groups: 1) a desensitization relaxation group (including Progressive Relaxation, hierarchy construction, imagery relaxation pairing instructions on how to generalize relaxation and coping skill instructions) 2) a desensitization meditation group (identical to group one except meditation instructions similar to Benson's replaced Progressive Relaxation; 3) meditation only, which included meditation plus the coping-skill instruction, but without instructions for hierarchy construction and imagery relaxation pairing; and 4) a no-treatment group. It appears that the treatment phase (conditions one through three) lasted three weeks. Pre- and post-treatment assessment of pulse rate and performance anxiety were taken. Results showed that improvement occurred in all three treatment conditions on self-report and behavioral measures, and that this improvement was significantly greater than the no-treatment control group. However, there were no significant differences in improvement between the three treatment conditions (see Table 5.8).

5.8 Summary and Future Directions

WHAT ARE THE implications of these studies? First, the data from these studies indicate that meditation does not appear to be any more effective than other self-regulation strategies on a wide variety of clinically relevant dependent variables. It should be noted, however, that my interpretation of the data is not without its critics. The critics point to studies of Vahia et al. (1972; 1973) and Glueck and Stroebel (1975) in which meditation was more effective than a pseudo-yoga group (Vahia et al., 1972; 1973) and than a biofeedback group (Glueck & Stroebel, 1975). However, I believe it could be argued that therapists' belief in treatment of credibility may have been a critical confounding factor in Vahia's studies (cf. Smith, 1975). Further the fact that Glueck and Stroebel's study was conducted at the Institute for Living, where a great deal of TM research was being conducted, could have caused strong confounding demand characteristics, possibly accounting for subjects' continuing to adhere to the TM program, while dropping out of the biofeedback treatment group.

What future directions might clinically oriented research profitably pursue? Let me suggest four different approaches, each of which is covered in more detail in subsequent sections of the book. The first involves a *refinement of the independent variable.* What are the active components of meditation (Chapter Eight)? Might these components be profitably combined with other self-regulation strategies (Chapter Six, also Woolfolk, 1979, Kirsch & Henry, 1979; Shapiro & Zifferblatt, 1976a; 1976b; Shapiro, 1978b)?

The second involves a refinement of the dependent variable. For example, Davidson and Schwartz (1976) have suggested that anxiety actually has both a cognitive and somatic component, and meditation may be more effective for reducing cognitive anxiety while doing relatively little for somatic anxiety.

A third approach (Chapter One), involves examining subject variables (Smith, 1978; Beiman et al., 1980, in press). This approach attempts, based on certain pre-test indicators, to develop a subject profile of those for whom meditation is likely to provide a successful clinical intervention.

The above three refinements would enable us to become more precise in choosing the correct clinical intervention (or combination of interventions) for a specific individual with a specific clinical problem.

A fourth suggested approach, not necessarily negating the others, involves looking at the phenomenology of meditation. This approach, valued by the Eastern tradition for centuries, is just beginning to gain favor within psychology. Despite certain problems, researchers are beginning to note its importance. For example, Morse et al. (1977) notes that physiological responses failed to show significant differences between the three relaxation states, but subject evaluation *did* show significance (cf. also Gilbert & Parker, 1975). Therefore, they cite and agree with Tart's remark that "In subject's own estimate of his behavior, an internal state is a rich and promising source of data which some experimenters tend to ignore in their passionate search for objectivity." (Tart, cited in Morse et al., 1977). Similarly, Curtis and Wessberg (1976) noted that there were more positive subjective changes in the meditation group than in the control "relaxation group" even though there was no difference on physiological measures. They noted that if meditation has a unique effect, it seems one which is different from a visceral or neuromuscular effect.

If meditation is a unique technique, its uniqueness may not be as a self-regulation strategy and therefore it will not be seen as different from other self-regulation strategies on either a clinical or physiological basis, but may be seen to be unique in the way the individual experiences it. The literature on phenomenological or subjective experiences during meditation—meditation as altered state of consciousness will be discussed in Chapter Seven.

Chapter Five: Further Readings

REVIEWS OF THE LITERATURE

Clinical

Smith, J. Meditation as psychotherapy: A review of the literature. *Psychological Bulletin,* 1975, *82,* (4,) 553-564. (Reprinted in D.H. Shapiro & R.N. Walsh. [Eds.], *The science of meditation.* New York: Aldine, 1980).

Shapiro, D.H. & Giber, D. Meditation and psychotherapeutic effects. *Archives of General Psychiatry,* 1978, *35,* 294-302. (Reprinted in D.H. Shapiro & R.N. Walsh [Eds.], *The science of meditation,* New York: Aldine, 1980).

Physiological

Woolfolk, R. Physiological correlates of meditation. *Archives of General Psychiatry,* 1975, *32,* 1323-1326. (Reprinted in D.H. Shapiro & R.N. Walsh [Eds.], *The science of meditation.* New York: Aldine, 1980).

Davidson, J. Physiology of meditation and mystical states of consciousness, *Perspectives in Biology and Medicine,* 1976, *19,*

345-380. (Reprinted in D.H. Shapiro & R.N. Walsh [Eds.], *The science of meditation.* New York: Aldine, 1980).

Comparison with Other Self-Regulation Strategies

RESEARCH

Physiological

Walrath, L. & Hamilton, D.W. Autonomic correlates of meditation and hypnosis, *American Journal of Clinical Hypnosis,* 1975, *17,* (3), 190-197. (Reprinted in D.H. Shapiro & R.N. Walsh [Eds.], *The science of meditation.* New York: Aldine, 1980).
Morse, D.R. et al., A physiological and subjective evaluation of meditation, hypnosis and relaxation. *Psychosomatic Medicine,* 1977, *39,* (5), 304-324. (Reprinted in D.H. Shapiro & R.N. Walsh [Eds.], *The science of meditation.* New York: Aldine, 1980).

Clinical

Marlatt, G.A. et al., Effect of meditation and relaxation training upon alcohol use in male social drinkers. In D.H. Shapiro & R.N. Walsh, [Eds.], *The science of meditation.* New York: Aldine, 1980.
Kirsch, I. & Henry, I. Self-desensitization and meditation in the reduction of public speaking anxiety. *Journal of Consulting and Clinical Psychology,* 1979, *47,* (3), 536-541.

Adverse Effects

Otis, L. Adverse effects of transcendental meditation. In D.H. Shapiro and R.N. Walsh [Eds.], *The science of meditation.* New York: Aldine, 1980, in press.
Lazarus, A.A. Psychiatric problems precipitated by transcendental meditation. *Psychological Reports,* 1976, *10,* 601-602.

Refining the Dependent Variable

Schwartz, G., Davidson, R., Goleman, D. Patterning of cognitive and somatic processes in the self-regulation of anxiety: Effects of meditation versus exercise. *Psychosomatic Medicine,* 1978, *40,* 321-8. (Reprinted in D.H. Shapiro & R.N. Walsh [Eds.], *The science of meditation.* New York: Aldine, 1980, in press).

6

A Model for Comparing Self-Regulation Strategies:
Zen Meditation and Behavioral Self-Management, A case in point.

AT THE END of Chapter Five, I noted that one of the promising clinical directions for meditation involved a refinement of the strategy into its "active" components. In this way, we could strip the aura of mystery and mysticism* from those aspects of meditation responsible for successful treatment. Further, we noted, as in the case of Woolfolk (1980, in press), we could, where appropriate, combine meditation with other self-regulation strategies. For example, a combination of two self-regulation strategies—e.g., biofeedback and autogenic training, has become common practice. However, in order to combine meditation with another technique in a sophisticated rather than a haphazard way, we need to develop expertise about what meditation is (see components, Chapter Eight), as well as how it compares with other self-regulation strategies.

Meditation has been compared on a descriptive level with several different self-regulation strategies—hypnosis (Davidson &

---

*Except, of course, for those to whom this is a component responsible for its success!

Goleman, 1977); biofeedback (Glueck & Stroebel, 1975); behavioral self-control (Shapiro & Zifferblatt, 1976b; Shapiro, 1978b); autogenic training (Onda, 1965)—as well as generally with other self-regulation strategies (Davidson & Schwartz, 1976). Hirai, Ikeda, and Watanabe (1977) tried to determine whether previous meditation experience enhanced biofeedback training; and Solomon and Bumpus (1978) have investigated combining meditation with running.

A comparison of the eight most commonly used self-regulation strategies with meditation and with each other, the subject of a forthcoming book (Shapiro, Note 5), would deflect us from the major thrust of this book. Therefore in this chapter, as an example of a methodology for comparing meditation with other self-regulation strategies, it is compared with behavioral self-management; then possible ways and rationales for combining the techniques are discussed.

6.1 Introduction and Background

BASED ON CURRENT biofeedback, meditation, and self-control research, a new paradigm of the individual is emerging within the scientific community, conceptualizing the healthy person as an individual who can pilot personal existential fate in the here-and-now, with far greater bodily self-regulation than heretofore imagined. Concomitant with this new paradigm is an attempt to develop and improve techniques by which people can self-observe their behavior, change it (if desired), and then continually modify and monitor it according to their needs.

This chapter compares self-control techniques developed within the Eastern religion of Zen Buddhism and the Western psychological framework of social learning theory. Because of seemingly different epistemological and cultural frameworks, it might at first appear an impossible task to bridge this gap between an Eastern religious technique, such as Zen meditation, and Western therapeutic strategies, such as self-management skills. There is certainly no doubt that differences both in origin and goals exist.

For example, formal Zen breath meditation (*zazen*) is a technique developed over one thousand years ago as a method of attaining religious insight (Kapleau, 1967; Maupin, 1968; Weinpahl, 1964). Behavioral self-control techniques, on the other hand, involve a constellation of strategies tailored to specific problem areas, and are the product of recent empirical investigations derived from experimental research in Western laboratories and field settings (cf. Goldfried & Merbaum, 1973; Mahoney & Thoresen, 1974). In addition, Zen meditation is a technique within a religious/philosophical framework that has a view of man different from the philosophical view of man on which social learning theory rests (cf. Bandura, 1974; 1977b; Hirai, 1974; Suzuki, 1956). Finally, based on current split-brain research (Galin, 1974), it may be argued that Zen meditation may primarily involve the right side of the brain (i.e. nonrational, nonanalytic, simultaneous integration of material), while behavioral self-control strategies may primarily involve the left side of the brain (i.e. analytical, rational, sequential processing of information).

Despite the fact that the techniques were developed in different eras, for different philosophical purposes, and with different assumptions about the nature of humankind, systematic investigation of the two techniques is fruitful for several reasons. By looking closely at the *behaviors* involved in both techniques, it might be possible to determine when behavioral differences in fact exist between the two, and when the supposed differences are merely semantic distinctions. Where behavioral differences do exist, further research might then document whether unique aspects of one could become profitable additions to the other. Social learning theory employs a naturalistic observation technology to identify and measure behaviors and events (cf. Zifferblatt & Hendricks, 1974). By using these tools of experimental analysis (naturalistic observation), it is possible to gain an understanding of meditation as a series of behavioral events under explicit contingency arrangements. In this way meditation is removed from the realm of mystical practice accessible only to the select few, and is redefined as a technique that, if useful, could be practiced and understood by many people.

6.2 Behavioral Self-Observation

THE CONCEPT OF awareness, so predominant in the literature on meditation, is also critical to behavioral self-change strategies. In the behavioral literature the means of attaining this awareness is called "self-observation." Self-observation is the initial step of a self-change strategy, and involves teaching a person how to monitor his or her own behavior (Kanfer & Phillips, 1966). Other behavior therapists (e.g., Ferster, 1972; Goldiamond, 1965; Thoresen & Mahoney, 1974) also stress the importance of a self-directed functional analysis of the environment as a prerequisite to behavior change. Ferster (1972) has referred to his functional analysis as "outsight therapy," noting that probably the most significant and difficult event to learn to observe is the functional relationship between one's own behavior and the elements of the environment that are controlling it. By recognizing this, an individual takes the necessary first step toward manipulating, rather than being manipulated by the environment (Bandura, 1974b).

Self-observation strategies are not limited to the individual's interaction with the external environment, and may include monitoring covert thoughts and feelings, such as physiological reactions, somatic complaints, and covert images (Cautela, 1967, 1971; Homme & Tosti, 1971; Jacobson, 1971; Kazdin, 1974; Thoresen & Mahoney, 1974; Meichenbaum, note 10). After discriminating and labeling certain specified behaviors in the internal and/or external environment, the individual then examines the antecedents and consequences of the behaviors. In this way the individual learns to recognize antecedent or initiating stimuli; to recognize consequences maintaining the behavior; and to recognize the behavior itself: frequency, latency, duration, and intensity.

Zen meditation also focuses attention both on inner experiences (Maupin, 1965) and on the external environment (Kasamatsu & Hirai, 1966). In Zen, however, the goal is to remain aware of the "ongoing present" without dwelling on it. Therefore, in Zen meditation, unlike behavioral self-observation strategies, no attempt is made to plot data charts, use counting devices, or employ systematic and written evaluation of data gathered from the ongoing present. The contrast might be one of a relaxed awareness, a receptive "letting go" compared to an active focusing and dwelling on data (cf. Deikman, 1971). Furthermore, in Eastern self-observation strategies (cf. Rahula, 1959; Spiegelberg, 1962), the important factor is not what is observed—all behaviors experienced by the individual—but how it is observed, in a non-evaluative way, without comment. In Western self-observation strategies, the important factor is the specific problem area observed, the behavior to be changed or altered.

One of the consequences of behavioral self-observation is that the procedure serves both as a method of gathering data and also as a possible self-change technique. As Kanfer and Karoly (1972) point out, self-observation appears to be intimately linked with self-evaluation and self-reinforcement. And Homme and Tosti (1971) suggest that the "act of plotting on a graph serves as a positive consequence for self-management, and once conditioned, the operation of a wrist counter appears to act as a reinforcer in its own right."

Several recent studies have attempted to verify this reactive effect. Most indicate that self-observation of a behavior does influence the occurrence of that behavior, depending on such factors as the valence of the behavior, the timing of the self-observation, the nature of the response monitored, and the frequency of the observations.*

It was noted earlier how a similar reactive effect takes place during the first step of Zen meditation in which self-observation of the behavior of breathing influences its occurrence (see Chapter One, Figure 1.2). However, the reactive effect in Zen seems to serve no therapeutic value, but rather causes a difficulty in breathing. Because the behavior of breathing is presumably nonvalenced, further research needs to clarify the exact nature and differences between the reactive effects that occur in behavioral self-observation and meditation.

Thus, in summary, although both behavioral self-control and meditation strategies involve the concept of awareness, there are differences in terms of the nature of what is observed, the method by which it is observed, and the types of reactive effects that occur as a result of observation.

6.3 Self-Evaluation and Goal Setting

IN A BEHAVIORAL self-control strategy, after discriminating, labeling, recording, and charting the data, the individual evaluates the data and often sets a personal goal (e.g., Kanfer & Karoly, 1972; Kolb & Boyatzis, 1970).

---

*Cf. Broden, Hall, & Mitts, 1971; Johnson & White, 1971; Kazdin, 1974; McFall, 1970; McFall & Hammen, 1971; Mahoney & Thoresen, 1974).

The goal in Zen, on the other hand, is not to evaluate the effects of self-observation but rather to just self-observe. As Alan Watts (1972) put it: "Zen meditation is a trickily simple affair, for it consists only in watching everything that is happening, including your own thoughts and your breathing without comment" (p. 220). Further, Zen also stresses the importance of living in the present without setting goals. For example, Suzuki, (1956, 1960) discusses the dilemma of modern Western man, who is so busy striving after future accomplishments that he is unable to appreciate the day-to-day beauty right beside him.

However, there is a contradiction in the Zen explanation of nonevaluative self-observation. In fact, two goals are posited: One is the goal of living-in-the-moment without self-evaluation, and the other is the goal of not having any goals. From a behavioral standpoint, a series of techniques are involved that represent a successive approximation toward the "goal of non-goals." For example, beginning meditators are taught, as noted earlier, to count from one to ten. More advanced meditators, however, are taught to just count one over and over again. This represents an attempt to focus the individual meditator more in the present, without striving after the goal of reaching ten. Finally, there is a technique in the Soto Zen sect for the most advanced meditators called Shikan-taza, which means just sitting and involves neither focusing on counting nor breathing. Thus, rather than no goals in Zen, there are a series of sub-goals designed to help the person reach the goal of being goal free and fully in the present.

A similar analysis could be made of the goal of no self-evaluation. In order for an individual to be able to observe himself without comment and without evaluation, he has to be able to discriminate, label, and evaluate those times when he in fact evaluates. For example: "I'm no longer focusing on breathing; I'm being too self-critical, I should stop being so critical and return to just observing myself." Thus, a behavioral analysis, although not denying that Zen in fact has a goal of nonevaluation, raises the question of whether that goal can be reached and maintained without the initial aid of evaluating the effects of one's progress. Seemingly, one must first learn how to evaluate before one can experience nonevaluation.

6.4 Environmental Planning:

ONCE THE INDIVIDUAL has become aware of the target behavior, several self-management strategies are available for him or her to use. The first of these strategies is environmental planning, which occurs prior to the execution of the target behavior. Examples of environmental planning include arranging antecedent or initiating stimuli (stimulus control), pre-programming certain punishments or reinforcements for specified actions (self-contract), self-regulated stimulus exposure (self-administered desensitization), and covert self-verbalizations and imagery (self-instructions).*

STIMULUS CONTROL

The development of stimulus control may be a prerequisite step in successfully implementing a behavioral self-management strategy. The individual must identify and plan changes in relevant situations: ones that will "cue" or set the occasion for self-change responses to occur. Stimulus control strategies may involve the association of desired responses with stimuli likely to evoke them. Examples of successfully implemented stimulus control procedures have been reported in the areas of weight control (Ferster, Nurnberger, & Levitt, 1972), obesity (Stuart, 1967, Stunkard, 1972), study skills (Beneke & Harris, 1972), and smoking (Bernard & Efran, 1972; Shapiro, Tursky, Schwartz, & Shnidman, 1971).

The uncluttered location of the meditation setting may be seen as a type of stimulus control in that the individual pre-arranges the physical environment to reduce unwanted distractions and thereby to help him or her focus attention on breathing. Similarly, the physical posture may be seen as a way of reducing unwanted proprioceptive feedback. Incense may be used as a means to block out other smells or as a discriminative cue for relaxation. The dimness of the lighting may be a method of reducing unwanted visual distractions. All of the above are examples of stimulus control, in that the individual is trying to

---

*Cf. Mahoney & Thoresen, 1974; Thoresen & Mahoney, 1974.

prearrange the physical environment to set the occasion for the proper occurrence of meditation behavior.

Other examples of environmental planning include meditating with a group of people in order to ensure daily practice, a using of social reinforcement to encourage the performance of certain actions. Similarly, in formal Zen meditation, the use of the *kwat*, a slap by the master of a "non-concentrating" student represents a preprogramming of punishment to reduce "nonalert" behavior. These are examples of environmental planning because they occur prior to the execution of the target behavior of meditation, with the individual prearranging relevant environmental cues and social consequences to influence the occurrence of the behavior.

It is important to note, however, that although the meditator prearranges environmental cues, and may use social reinforcement and consequences to influence the occurrence and proper execution of meditation behavior, the long-term goal of meditation is eventually to eliminate the need for social consequences, environmental cues, or even covert self-reinforcement. In the beginning, however, the need for these cues and consequences is both recognized and used.

SYSTEMATIC DESENSITIZATION:

Wolpe (1958, 1969) borrowed from Jacobson's (1929, 1971) relaxation techniques and used them as the first step in his three-step process of systematic desensitization. Wolpe hypothesized on the basis of reciprocal inhibition that the negative affect of a phobic or stressful event would be reduced and eventually eliminated (extinguished) if it could symbolically occur in the presence of an incompatible response such as relaxation. He had the patient construct elaborate hierarchies, labeling the items on the hierarchy in ascending order of subjective units of disturbance. He would then relax the subject using Jacobson's method, and once the subject was relaxed, have him or her visualize the item having the lowest subjective rating of disturbance on the hierarchy. If the subject began to feel tense, Wolpe would instruct him/her to dismiss the image and continue to relax. If the subject felt no tension, the therapist would have him/her imagine the next highest tension-producing item.

Step four of formal meditation (Chapter One, Figure 1.2) has several similarities to the Wolpe paradigm. First, step four of formal meditation may be conceptualized as a type of counter-conditioning (cf. Bandura, 1969; Davison, 1968b) in which responses incompatible with maladaptive behavior are practiced; that is, step three, relaxation or effortless breathing, precedes the feared image, step four. However step four of meditation is different from Wolpe's paradigm in that there is no structured hierarchy of anxiety-producing events, but rather a "global desensitization hierarchy" (Goleman, 1971).

There is still considerable debate, in the literature as to what exactly accounts for the success of systematic desensitization. Wolpe and others have argued on the basis of reciprocal inhibition: an incompatible response causes a counterconditioning to occur (Bandura, 1969; Davison, 1968b). Others have argued in favor of a cognitive refocusing model, suggesting that it is primarily the attention shifts that cause the effectiveness of systematic desensitization (Wilkins, 1971; Yulis et al., 1975).

Both of the above explanations seem plausible for the effects that occur in step four and step five of formal meditation. A third explanation might consider the use of operant punishment, behavioral thought stopping (Wolpe, 1969). In behavioral approaches to thought stopping, whenever the individual realizes the presence of an unwanted aversive thought, he or she covertly yells "Stop!" It is possible that a similar process occurs during meditation, in which using self-instruction the individual stops focusing on thoughts and images and returns to the behavior of breathing.

6.5 Behavioral Programming

THE SECOND of the behavioral self-management strategies is behavioral programming. In behavioral programming, the individual presents him/herself with consequences following the occurrence of a target behavior. These consequences can be either verbal, imaginal, or material self-reward or self-punishment (positive or negative, overt or covert [Mahoney & Thoresen, 1974; Thoresen & Mahoney, 1974]).

Although Zen does not espouse attachment to material possessions (material self-reward), Zen meditation does involve internal processes. Therefore, of particular interest to this discussion is the behavioral literature on covert events, both imaginal and verbal.

It is only within the last ten years that behaviorists have actively begun to pay attention to covert events, finally entering into the "lion's den of private events" (Cautela, 1967, 1971; Mahoney, 1974; Meichenbaum, Note Ten; Ellis, 1962), for several reasons. First, improved scientific instrumentation has made it possible to study some internal processes (e.g., the research on biofeedback [Barber et al., 1971, Shapiro et al., 1973; Stoyva et al., 1972]). Second, animal studies (e.g., Miller, 1969) began to question the traditional distinctions of operant and classical conditioning, especially the interdependence of environmental/ cognitive influence processes and the primary role of "symbolic processes" in behavior change. Third, the clinical experiences of clients and patients have almost invariably involved maladaptive cognitive problems.

As early as 1964, Skinner noted that internal events, even though self-reported and unobservable, are justified in a science of behavior if they delineate functional behavioral relationships. L. Homme (1965), in a seminal article entitled "Control of Coverants, the Operants of the Mind," hypothesized that a behavioral relationship existed between what a person said to himself covertly and his subsequent overt behavior. Several recent studies have attempted to show the relationship between covert events and overt actions. Cautela (1967, 1971) has discussed the use of covert sensitization (covert imagery as punishment) as a technique for modifying maladaptive approach behavior involved in problems such as alcoholism (cf. Ashem & Donner, 1968), inappropriate sexual behavior (Barlow et al., 1969; Davison, 1968a) and obesity. Ferster (1965, 1971) has discussed the use of ultimate aversive consequences in which the individual, say a problem-smoker, imagines an aversive future consequence, rotting lungs, doctors talking over his/her decayed body, every time s/he begins to engage in the maladaptive behavior, lighting a cigarette. The individual thereby learns to modify his/her overt behavior by covertly summoning up aversive future consequences at the onset of his/her present maladaptive activity.

Other studies employing covert responses as examples of behavioral programming have been discussed by Cautela (1967;

1971) and Bandura (1974c). Both authors review studies suggesting that covert desensitization can be used to modify maladaptive avoidance responses, and that covert self-reinforcement, both positive and negative, can be used to modify maladaptive approach or avoidance behavior. Other studies have taken Homme's (1965) coverant control therapy paradigm, based on the Premack principle (Premack, 1965), and successfully applied it to modifying covert thoughts, for instance, increasing positive self-thoughts and decreasing negative self-thoughts (Johnson, 1971; Mahoney, 1971). Further, it has been shown that covertly practicing the behavior, cognitive rehearsal, is a successive approximation of the overt act and increases the likelihood of its successful occurrence (Johnson, 1971).

Based on the research on covert events discussed above, several stress and tension management training packages have been developed (cf. Suinn & Richardson, 1971; Meichenbaum, Note Ten). These training packages have altered the traditional Wolpe paradigm in both theory and practice. As noted earlier, Wolpe believed that relaxation should precede the fear-arousing imagery. In the new paradigm, the fear-arousing situation becomes a discriminative stimulus for relaxation. The two paradigms were compared in a group study involving acrophobics. One group practiced the passive paradigm (relaxation before phobic scene and avoidance of arousal), and one group practiced the active paradigm (fear arousal as a discriminative stimulus for active relaxation and positive imagery). On both self-report and actual performance tests of climbing and looking down from a twelve story building, subjects in the active "stress as a cue to relax" procedure did significantly better (Jacks, Note Eleven.) The latter technique first involves training in deep-muscle relaxation and then teaching the person to discriminate anxiety by imagining the fear-arousing situation and maintaining that situation in imagination. While maintaining the image, the person then practices controlling arousal by means of muscular relaxation, covert self-modeling (self-observation while acting in a competent and successful fashion in the anxiety-arousing situation) and self-instructions to cope with the situation ("relax, I am in control, I can handle the situation," [cf. Goldfried, 1973; Jacks, Note Eleven; Mahoney, 1974; Suinn & Richardson, 1971; Meichenbaum, Note Ten]).

These training procedures involve practices quite different

from both formal and informal meditation. For example, in informal meditation, the individual observes all actions and behaviors throughout the day. In the training package, the individual is instructed to discriminate certain specified "anxiety-arousing" situations, and then to use those situations as discriminative stimuli for engaging in relaxation, covert self-modeling, and self-instruction activities. In informal meditation, although all cues are observed, the individual is instructed to "merely observe, as a witness" and to take no specific action after recognizing any particular cue. In terms of formal meditation, although the beginning meditator may subvocalize such self-instructions as "relax; keep focused on breathing; attention has wandered, better return to breathing again," the goal of meditation is to remove these verbal cues eventually and have an "empty mind," that is, an absence of covert statements and images, step five.

6.6 A Clinical Combination of Zen Meditation and Behavioral Self-Control Techniques

THE PRECEDING discussion has attempted to suggest that there is a common ground between Zen meditation and behavioral self-management techniques. One of the more important clinical questions, however, still remains unexplored: can these techniques complement each other to provide a more effective treatment strategy in combination than either strategy can when practiced alone? To date, there has been almost no research in this area. Therefore, the comments that follow are intended only as plausible hypotheses and must await further research for empirical documentation of their effectiveness.

INFORMAL MEDITATION PLUS
BEHAVIORAL SELF-CONTROL TECHNIQUES:
"CONTINGENT INFORMAL MEDITATION"

Current research suggests that the technique of informal meditation can be converted into a more powerful clinical intervention strategy* by making its performance contingent on certain antecedent cues, and by coupling it with covert self-images, covert self-statements, and focused breathing. In this model, the subject, in addition to observing all events and behaviors occurring throughout the day (informal meditation), also discriminates certain specified cues in the internal and external environment such as tension, anger, anxiety, social events. Once the individual has discriminated those cues, s/he then self-observes in a detached nonevaluative manner, as in informal meditation. However, the individual also focuses on breathing and covertly initiates cues to relax, to feel in control, and imagines acting in a relaxed, competent fashion (cf. Boudreau, 1972; Shapiro, 1976a; Shapiro & Zifferblatt, 1976b).

The research thus far, though suggestive, is cursory, based on case reports. Further replications are necessary to determine the variance of outcome effects attributable to various aspects of the treatment.

FORMAL MEDITATION PLUS BEHAVIORAL SELF-CONTROL TECHNIQUES:

The acquisition of formal meditation behavior might possibly be facilitated by borrowing from certain behavioral self-management techniques. For example, individuals have been given a wrist counter and instructed to punch the counter every time their attention wandered from the task of breathing. The punching of the wrist counter was then made a discriminative stimulus for

---

*It appears that making informal meditation contingent on certain cues and coupling it with covert self-modeling and self-instructions make informal meditation a more powerful clinical strategy for an immediate problem. However, this is in no way meant to suggest that the combination of informal meditation with behavioral self-control strategies makes informal meditation more effective for the goal for which it was originally intended: ongoing awareness of all cues.

Similarly, from a Western perspective, formal Zen meditation is often seen merely as a technique that may be useful when applied to certain clinical problems. However, from an Eastern perspective, Zen meditation is a way of "being" in the world: a total awareness of oneself, of nature, of others. Thus, it is important to note that the technique of formal Zen meditation may be being used for goals other than those for which it was originally intended.

returning attention to the task of breathing. Functionally, a tool used in behavioral self-observation (the wrist counter) took the place of the kwat of the Zen monk (cf. Shapiro & Zifferblatt, 1976a, Van Nuys, 1971). It is possible that biofeedback techniques might also serve to facilitate the acquisition and proper performance of meditation behavior.

Conversely, certain aspects of formal meditation might help complement and facilitate behavioral self-control skills. For example, during formal meditation, the individual learns to unstress (desensitize) himself (step four, Figure 1.2) and to reduce the frequency and duration of covert chatter and images (step five, Figure 1.1). It is hypothesized that this ability to relax and have an empty mind gained during formal meditation will help an individual be more alert and responsive to stress situations occurring at other times, thus facilitating a person's performance of behavioral self-observation of internal and external cues throughout the day (Shapiro, 1978a, 1976; Shapiro & Zifferblatt, 1976a).

Second, formal meditation seems to give practice in noticing when attention wanders from a task. At first, long periods of time usually elapse between the attention wandering and the realization of it. With practice, however, the person may learn to notice it almost as soon as s/he stops focusing on breathing. Similarly, in behavioral self-control strategies, several minutes or longer often pass before the individual realizes that s/he is supposed to have discriminated a cue and subsequently interrupted the maladaptive behavioral chain. For example, the chronic smoker illustrates this lack of awareness (Premack, 1970) as does the heroin addict (Shapiro & Zifferblatt, 1976). The practice of discriminating a stimulus, say wandering attention, developed in meditation may generalize to situations involved in behavioral self-control strategies, such as reaching for a cigarette or the "need" for a fix. As such, the individual practicing meditation may be aided in eventually discriminating the stimulus as soon as it occurs, thereby placing the individual in a much better position to interrupt a maladaptive behavioral sequence.

A third way in which formal meditation might help behavioral self-control strategies involves the cognitive set that meditation can help give to the practitioner. Formal meditation allows the individual an opportunity for fixed reference points in the day during which s/he feels relaxed, calm, and in control. Therefore, when recognizing tension at subsequent points during the day, the individual should be able to say, "I was relaxed, calm and in control this morning," thereby attributing current stress to a specific situation rather than to an "anxious personality trait" (Mischel, 1968), and learning to increase feelings of self-control and self-perception as a responsible individual with the ability to control personal behavior and actions (Lefcourt, 1966; Rotter, 1966, 1969, 1971).

Fourth, although the physiological data are still equivocal (cf. Hirai, 1974) aspects of the technique of formal meditation may make it more powerful than other self-management techniques in certain respects. For example, other self-control techniques, such as autogenic training (Luthe, 1968, 1970), self-hypnosis (Paul, 1969), or relaxation with covert self-statements (Jacobson, 1929, 1971; Meichenbaum, Note Ten), employ certain covert images and self-statements like, "I'm feeling warm; my right arm feels heavy; I am feeling relaxed." In formal Zen meditation, the individual does not say anything to him/herself, nor does s/he attempt to engage in positive covert images or thoughts. This absence of preprogrammed covert thoughts and images seems to allow meditators to observe and become desensitized to "what's on their own mind" (step four, Figure 1.2 Chapter One). Repetition of preprogrammed covert statements and images would seemingly interfere with this process and also would seem to prevent the "mind from becoming empty" as in Figure 1.2, step five. This "emptymind," this absence of verbal behaviors and images, may be important in certain externally oriented situations, such as the counseling setting (Lesh, 1970) and interpersonal relationships (Shapiro, 1978a). The empty mind may also be important for hearing certain internal cues, especially in clinical areas dealing with stress and tension, obesity, tachycardia, migraine, and hypertension.

Finally, because during meditation the individual seems to be able to step back from personal fears, concerns, and worries, and observe them in a detached, relaxed way (Shapiro, 1976, 1978a; Shapiro & Zifferblatt, 1976a, b), it is possible to hypothesize that after meditation the individual should be able to think about the fears and evaluate how s/he wants to act without being overwhelmed or oppressed by them. Within Kanfer's behavioral model of self-management involving self-observation, evaluation, and reinforcement, this type of detached self-observation would

TABLE 6.1 *Meditation and Behavioral Self-Control: Comparison and Contrast*

Topics	*Formal Meditation*	*Behavioral Self-management*	*Informal Meditation*	*Contingent Informal Meditation*
Environmental Planning where intervention strategy occurs	specified setting (e.g., room or in nature); reduced external stimuli to initially help individual focus on object of meditation	*in natural environment where problem behavior occurs; or symbolically in neutral environment*	occurs in natural environment	*same as behavioral self-management*
if stimulus cues are used	stimulus cues (control): e.g. incense; or, in case of concentrative meditation, the object of meditation as stimulus cue	*specified cues in natural environment (programming antecedent or initiating stimuli)* / *self-regulated stimulus exposure*	everything is a stimulus cue for "awareness"	*same as behavioral self-management*
nature of physical posture	or half-lotus, to reduce bodily distractions	*occurs in relaxed posture: e.g., reclining in thick armchair*	posture	posture
if preprogrammed punishments or reinforcers	"KWAT" as preprogrammed punishment for non-alert behavior	*preprogramming of certain punishments or reinforcements*	no preprogrammed punishments or reinforcers	sometimes preprogrammed punishment or reinforcement
Cognitive Variables effects of observation	in formal Zen meditation focusing on behavior of breathing alters the behavior: a stumbling reactive effect (step 1); soon mind wanders, i.e., habituation to task of observing (step 2)	*behavioral self-observation alters behavior observed (generalization one); then there is habituation to task; subject forgets to monitor; when subject stops monitoring, behavior returns to pre-*	goal is that observation have no interference or interruption of daily activities	observation used as a discriminative stimulus to interrupt a maladaptive behavioral sequence *(see also behavioral self-observation)*

Topics	Formal Meditation	Behavioral Self-management	Informal Meditation	Contingent Informal Meditation
what is observed	intially just breathing is focused on (steps 1, 2, 3); eventually openness and receptivity to all stimuli, internal and external (steps 4, 5) occurs	*self-observation phase (generalization two)* *functional analysis: observation of problem behavior, antecedents, and consequences*	all behaviors, actions, and thoughts are observed: global awareness	only specified cues (e.g., anxiety, stress) in internal and external environment are observed
how behavior is observed: self-evaluation and goal setting	thoughts, behavior, breathing, are observed without analysis; no charting, no evaluation, no goal-setting: i.e., "detached" self-observation	*parameters of behavior observed: frequency, latency, duration, intensity; behavior is counted, charted; systematic evaluation is made; and goals are set*	observation without comment and without evaluation	*same as behavioral self-management;* however, also try to maintain detached self-observation at same time
desensitization paradigm; when occurs	relaxation (step 3) precedes feared images (step 4); in formal meditation, a "global" desensitization with no specific cues formal meditation occurs at specific times throughout the day, regardless of antecedent stimuli	*relaxation precedes phobic scene (cf. Wolpe, 1958, 1969) involves subjective hierarchy of disturbing scenes; or, relaxation follows phobic scene (real or symbolically) and is contingent on discriminating certain cues (cf. Goldfried, 1973)*	continuous discrimination of cues in daily environment	relaxation follows phobic scene or certain stress cues

Topics	Formal Meditation	Behavioral Self-management	Informal Meditation	Contingent Informal Meditation
cognitive statements and images; thought stopping	observation without comment (no self-statements); without evaluation (no thinking); covert images are allowed to "flow down the river of consciousness," and are not dwelled on; focus on competing response of breathing helps remove thoughts (step 4)	*covert images and self-instruction used extensively: e.g. covert sensitization (images as punishment); covert rehearsal (images and self-instructions as successive approximation): self-modeling; covert self-reinforcement; covert behavior modification: either alter self-statements, or emit relaxing instructional self-statements; to stop thoughts, covert yelling of word "stop"*	no cognitive statements or images involved in the performance of actions.	use of covert images, self-modeling; and self-instruction: e.g., "I am breath," I am relaxed, in control, I can handle this"
focused attention	in formal Zen meditation, attention focused on breathing (steps 1-4); the KWAT (step 2) helps return the wandering mind to the object of focus; in Raj Yoga (cf. Anandi, Chinna, & Singh, 1961) note the use of internal focusing	*Kanfer and Goldfoot (1966) discuss the use of external focusing as a technique for self-management of pain*	attention focused on the here-and-now action only	in contingent informal breath meditation, attention focused on breathing; in Transcendental Meditation, attention focused on covert sacred syllable
Breathing effects of; type used	breathing from the abdomen; goal is effortless, autonomic breathing plus awareness that breathing; used as a	*"controlled" breathing; voluntary breathing from chest/thoracic area; used in deep muscle relaxation*	relaxed, aware autonomic breathing from abdomen	controlled breathing in contingent informal breath meditation (cf.

Topics	Formal Meditation	Behavioral Self-management	Informal Meditation	Contingent Informal Meditation
	type of relaxation (step 3); an aid in unstressing (step 4) and in thought stopping (step 4)			Shapiro, 1974a); nonfocus on breathing (but rather on sacred sound) in "contingent" Transcendental Meditation (cf. Boudreau, 1972)[16]
Contributions of the Strategies to Each Other	acquisition and proper performance of formal meditation is facilitated by a wrist counter, a device used in behavioral self-observation; naturalistic observation methodology of social learning theory is useful in understanding meditation as a series of behaviors under explicit contingency arrangements	*clear mind gained during step 5 of formal meditation helps facilitate a behavioral functional analysis of internal and external events throughout the rest of the day; practice of discriminating a stimulus (e.g., wandering mind) gaining during formal meditation should help an individual interrupt a maladaptive behavioral chain earlier and more quickly; meditation involves a "detached observation" of concerns, thereby reducing the threat of the concerns and producing optimal conditions for behavior change*	in terms of a clinical intervention stategy, informal is made more powerful by making its performance contingent upon certain internal and external cues, and by coupling it with covert imagery, self-instructions, and focused breathing	This technique is a combination of informal meditation and behavioral self-management strategies; covert imagery, self-instructions, focused breathing, functional analysis all come from the behavioral self-management strategy; however, at the same time the technique involves the use of "detached self-observation", derived from informal meditation

presumably alter the subsequent self-evaluation by reducing the self-evaluative threat, that is, making the problem seem less intense; and by giving the person a sense of strength and control from the firm, centered posture, and relaxed, focused breathing so that s/he need not be subsequently afraid to self-evaluate (Kanfer & Karoly, 1972). Thus, even though during the process of formal meditation there is ideally no thinking or evaluation, subsequent to meditation the individual may be well prepared to think and make decisions. In this way, meditation might help produce "self-observation conditions such that inner feedback for behavior change is optimal" (Goleman, 1971, p. 17). Table 6.1 provides a more detailed descriptive comparison of the different strategies along important dimensions.

6.7 Unanswered Questions: Concluding Remarks

THE FOREGOING discussion leaves several questions unanswered, both with respect to the effectiveness of meditation as a complementary strategy with behavioral self-control skills and also with respect to the exact mechanism by which meditation works. The first set of unanswered questions includes the following: Is formal Zen meditation a necessary part of the intervention? Is it sufficient by itself? Is it the relaxation component of meditation that makes the greatest contribution? As discussed in Chapter Five, is meditation really different from, or more effective than, deep-muscle relaxation (cf. Woolfolk et al., 1976), systematic desensitization, (Kirsh & Henry, 1979) covert imagery, and covert self-statements? Further research is necessary to address these questions and to determine the variance of outcome effects attributable to various aspects of the treatment.

A different set of questions involves the role of breathing in formal Zen meditation. There is a paucity of empirical literature dealing with the effect of breathing. Timmons et al. (1972) have compared different types of breathing in general, and Nakamizo (1974) and Matsumoto (1974) have researched Zen meditation breathing in particular. However, the question is still unanswered as to whether focusing on breathing is more clinically effective than other types of cognitive focusing techniques.

As noted in Chapter One, the Eastern literature is replete with different examples of cognitive focusing techniques (cf. Ornstein, 1971; Shapiro, 1978b). The "objects of focus" can be located in either the external or internal environments. As noted in Chapter One, examples from the external environment include Hindu Yogic focus on a point (trataka), the Taoist focus on the abdomen, early Christian focus on the cross, focusing on a vase (Deikman, 1966), a kasina (disc), a guru or a mandala (a symbol). The meditator can also focus on internal visual images such as a fire in the hearth, the symbol of a guru, sexual mandalas (cf. Mookerjee, 1966; Speigelberg, 1962), the third eye, or the vault of the skull (by Yogins—see Anand, Chinna & Singh, 1961a). The meditator can also focus on words or phrases chanted aloud, such as the Sufi dervish call (cf. Ornstein, 1971) or a mantra (Mishra, 1959). S/he can also concentrate on internally-generated, unspoken sounds such as a bee humming (Mishra, 1959), a prayer, or a sentence like the Zen koan. The meditator can also focus on internal bodily processes, for example, on the heartbeat or on breathing (Datey et al., 1969).

Although different types of meditation can produce different physiological and behavioral indices during meditation (Anand, Chinna, & Singh, 1961a; Kasamatsu & Hirai, 1966) it is not yet clear whether there are in fact any differences after the occurrence of different types of meditation. Although each school of focus seems to make claims and develops rationales for the use of its own particular technique, whether it be Zen's focus on breath (cf. Akishige, 1968; Hirai, 1974) or Transcendental Meditation's focus on an internal mantra (Bloomfield, Cain, & Jaffe, 1975; Kanellakos & Lukas, 1974), there has been almost no research comparing the clinical effectiveness of different types of cognitive focusing (cf. Yamaoka, 1973; Otis, Note Three).

Within the behavioral literature, there has also been an interest in different types of cognitive focusing, including work with delayed gratification (Mischel, Ebbesen, & Zeiss, 1972), the use of different types of imagery in therapy (Singer, 1975), and the use of cognitive focusing on external slides (Kanfer & Goldfoot, 1966) and on music (Yulis et al., 1975). Again, however, systematic comparison of different audiovisual techniques (both overt and covert) has not been undertaken.

What truly seems needed is a convergence of several different fields such as cognitive behavior modification research (Mahoney,

1974, Beck, 1976) imagery research (Singer, 1975), meditation research (cf. Hirai, 1974; Kanellakos & Lukas, 1974; Shapiro & Giber, 1978), behavioral self-observation research (Kazdin, 1974), and biofeedback research (Blanchard & Young, 1974; Schwartz, 1973), to deal with the common problems and issues involved in evaluating the clinical uses of covert processes. With this convergence of academic and clinical scholars, perhaps some of the unanswered questions will begin to be better understood.

This chapter has made an attempt to look at two clinical strategies: Zen meditation and behavioral self-control. Current research has suggested that either technique alone provides potentially effective self-directed attempts to control one's everyday life, thoughts, and feelings. Researchers have found meditation effective in reducing fear (Boudreau, 1972), curbing drug abuse (Benson & Wallace, 1972b; Brautigam, 1971), increasing empathy in counselors (Lesh, 1970), decreasing generalized anxiety (Girodo, 1974), decreasing test anxiety (Linden, 1973), and reducing blood pressure and hypertension (Datey et al., 1969; Wallace & Benson, 1972a). The behavioral self-management literature suggests the effectiveness of social learning strategies applied to a variety of problems, such as reducing weight (Mahoney, Moura, & Wade, 1973; Jeffrey, Note Twelve), curbing smoking (Axelrod, 1973; Premack, 1970), changing negative self-thoughts (Hannum, 1972) reducing fears (Jacks, Note Eleven) and in other clinical areas (cf. Bandura, 1969; Cautela, 1971; Goldfried & Merbaum, 1973; Meichenbaum & Cameron, 1974; Mahoney & Thoresen, 1974; Meichenbaum, Note Ten).

The foregoing research suggests the clinical intervention effectiveness of meditation and behavioral self-control strategies each used alone. Subsequent research should determine whether a combination of the two techniques will, in fact, be more powerful in dealing with applied clinical problems. To this end, pilot studies have applied a treatment package combining Zen meditation and behavioral self-management to such clinical areas as drug abuse (Shapiro & Zifferblatt, 1976a) and stress and tension management (Shapiro, 1978a). Currently, pilot studies are extending these investigations both to rehabilitative programs, such as stress management training (Shapiro, 1980, in press b) and to preventive and educational programs dealing with "positive mental health" (Shapiro, 1978a; Shapiro, 1978b). Although the results of these pilot studies combining behavioral self-control and Zen meditation techniques are tentative and need further replication, the continued exploration of the applied interface between Eastern disciplines and Western psychology promises to be an important and clinically useful area for further investigation.

Chapter Six: Further Reading

MEDITATION AND BEHAVIORAL SELF-CONTROL

Shapiro, D.H. & Zifferblatt, S.M. Zen meditation and behavioral self-control: Similarities, differences, and clinical applications. *American Psychologist,* 1976, *31,* 519-532. (Reprinted in D.H. Shapiro & R.N. Walsh [Eds.], *The science of meditation.* New York: Aldine, 1980).

Shapiro, D.H. *Precision nirvana.* Englewood Cliffs, NJ: Prentice Hall, 1978b.

MEDITATION AND HYPNOSIS

Davidson, J. & Goleman, D. The role of attention in meditation and hypnosis: A psychobiological perspective on transformations of consciousness. *International Journal of Clinical & Experimental Hypnosis,* 1977, *25,* (4), 291-308. (Reprinted in D.H. Shapiro & R.N. Walsh [Eds.], *The science of meditation,* New York: Aldine, 1980.

MEDITATION AND BIOFEEDBACK

Stroebel, C.F. & Glueck, B.C. Passive meditation: Subjective and clinical comparison with biofeedback. In G. Schwartz & D.H. Shapiro [Eds.], *Consciousness and self-regulation,* New York: Plenum, 1977. (Reprinted in D.H. Shapiro & R.N. Walsh [Eds.], *The science of meditation.* New York: Aldine, 1980).

MEDITATION AND OTHER RELAXATION TECHNIQUES

Davidson, R. & Schwartz, G. The psychobiology of relaxation and related states: A multi-process theory. In O. Mostofsky [Ed.], *Psychiatry and mysticism.* Chicago: Nelson Hall, 1976. (Reprinted in D.H. Shapiro & R.N. Walsh [Eds.], *The science of meditation.* New York: Aldine, 1980).

Onda, A. Zen, autogenic training, and hypnotism, *Psychologia,* 1967, *10,* 133-136.

7

Meditation as an Altered State of Consciousness

⁓ THOSE INVOLVED with the psychology of religion (Smith, 1965; Stace, 1960) and those who have studied spontaneous religious experiences (e.g., William James, 1901) note that often during times of meditation there are powerful subjective experiences which individuals claim have radically altered their lives, given them a new sense of meaning and purpose, new values, and a new relationship not only with themselves, but with other people and the world around them. In Eastern traditions some of these are referred to as satori, kensho, samadhi.

These experiences, although of high salience for the individual, are sometimes spoken of as ineffable. Those who experience them have difficulty communicating these experiences to others (Frank, 1977), which presents a dilemma to the researcher who needs some kind of verbal or symbolic representation to help quantify, label, and describe them. Often the task of experimentally validating these experiences has seemed so difficult that some researchers have dismissed the experiences themselves as epiphenomena at best or at worst artificial schizophrenia with complete withdrawal of libidinal interest from the outside world (e.g., Alexander, 1931; GAP Report, 1977). Dismissing the experiences as epiphenomena is based not only on the difficulty of describing the phenomena, but also involves a paradigm clash (as discussed in Section 1.3) between the Western model of physicalistic science and the internal, experiential nature of the altered state phenomena. As Tart has noted (1975), "The philosophy of physicalism is a belief system stating that physical reality exists independent of our perception of it, and is the ultimate reality—physical data are the only data that are ultimately 'real.' Therefore, internal or experiential phenomena, being inherently unreliable and unreal, must be reduced to physiological data to become reliable. If they cannot be so reduced, they are generally ignored" (p. 21, p. 24-25).

The second attitude—that these experiences are like psychotic episodes or schizophrenia—can again be a function of a paradigm clash, overlaying a Western paradigm on an experience within a different context and value system. Just as it may be a mistake to assume *a priori* that all altered state of consciousness (ASC) experiences are unilaterally examples of higher or enlightened consciousness, it may similarly be a mistake to dismiss them *a priori* as delusional. What truly is needed is a precise study of these so-called altered-state phenomena. Again, as Tart noted (1975), "Given the great complexity of spiritual phenomena and discrete altered states of consciousness phenomena and their significance, the need for replication by trained observers to form a data base for future research is of exceptional importance (p. 21)." How might we go about this? First, we need a definition.

7.1 Altered State: Toward a Working Definition; Problems in Studying; Approaches Available

AS A BASIS for our discussion, we will use the general definition of altered states proposed by Tart (1975). He suggested that

> Our ordinary discrete state of consciousness is a *construction* built up in accordance with biological and cultural imperatives for the purpose of dealing with our physical, intrapersonal, and interpersonal environments. A discrete altered state of consciousness is a radically different way of handling information from the physical, intrapersonal, and interpersonal environments, yet the discrete altered state of consciousness may be as arbitrary as our ordinary discrete state of consciousness (p. 24).

Note that this definition is value free. It allows us to study a discrete altered state of consciousness without *a priori* judgment.

At this point, further clarification should be made about my use of the phrase "altered state of consciousness." There are some problems with this phrase which merit comment. First, the problem of defining meditation by its effects needs to be considered. As noted in a previous work (Shapiro & Giber, 1978), we need to distinguish whether meditation as an altered state is conceptualized as an independent variable (causing certain subsequent behavioral changes in a person) or a dependent variable: (i.e. what are the altered-state effects of meditation.) The phrase "meditation as an altered state" does not make that distinction.

Second, the phrase seems to imply a uniform "altered state" unique to meditation. Although there may be certain experiences common to meditation practice (Osis et al., 1973; Kohr, 1977), there are certainly many different types of altered-state experiences which may occur as a result of a specific meditation technique, as well as across different techniques. Further, there are many different methods to attain ASC experiences similar to those which occur in meditation. I have tried to be as precise as possible in discussing these issues throughout the text. As noted earlier (Chapter One, 1.7) the phrase "meditation as an altered state of consciousness" is intended primarily to help researchers differentiate what aspect of meditation they are studying—i.e. its self-regulation qualities, or altered-state qualities.

Given the above definition and discussion, how might we go about studying these altered state phenomena? What are the problems inherent in its undertaking? Tart's comments on this issue are the best to date and are summarized here. The first two problems relate to the nature of the state itself: its ineffability and the problem of state-dependent learning. Another problem is that the person doing the investigation must often be subject, observer, and experimenter.

The first problem, as noted above, is the fact that many of the experiences of an ASC are described as ineffable and therefore beyond conceptualization. Second, there is a problem, seldom mentioned in the literature, of the generalizability of an ASC. We know from research on the state-dependent learning that what is learned in one state, say inebriation (Fischer, 1971), *is not always recalled in the uninebriated state* although it may be *stored* and recallable when once again drunk; learning

therefore does not necessarily generalize to other states of consciousness. Again, as Tart noted, for reasons we know almost
nothing about, the experiences of discrete altered states of consciousness eventually may be transferable to a different state of
consciousness.

> So some people may have a spiritual experience occurring only
> in a particular discrete altered state of consciousness for a
> while, but then find it becomes part of their ordinary discrete
> state of consciousness. We know almost nothing scientifically
> about the degree to which such transfer can take place, the con-
> ditions favoring or hindering it, or the fullness of the transfer.
> (1975, p. 25).

Here we may need to look to the social learning theorist for
the laws of generalization and discrimination training (Bandura,
1977).

Additional problems derive from the need for individuals to
sometimes be subject, observer, and experimenter. Tart suggested that this requires special training in order to develop a
true phenomenology of the spiritual experience. Even such
trained observers need to be cautious of experimenter bias
(Rosenthal, 1962). They need to be aware of the demand characteristics of the training experimental situation (Orne, 1962). Further, Tart noted that the "individual who follows a spiritual path
or tries to reach truth in a discrete altered state of consciousness
may settle for the feeling of certainty rather than pressing on
with his investigations" (1975, p. 48). In other words, the person
may feel that they have an obvious perception of the truth and
therefore not want to question that perception.* In fact, as Tart
noted, the individual may be building fantasy worlds that seem
real to that person, and therefore they create a reality which
they believe to be a truthful *a priori* reality, without questioning
the belief systems they brought to the situation.

In summary, Tart noted that state-specific sciences are possible, though difficult. These state-specific sciences would involve,
in the true scientific tradition, a) observing, b) making public the

---

*It should be noted that this phenomenon is not at all unique to altered-
state-of-consciousness research.

nature of the observation: consensual validation, c) forming logical hypotheses based on the material, d) testability: the looking for testable consequences.

Given these problems, as well as the importance of the phenomena, what approaches might be available to us?

7.2 Subjective Experiences During Meditation

ONE APPROACH to gaining information about subjective experiences during meditation involves only slight variations on the traditional scientific experiment in which the experimenter tries to gather information from the subjects. The first group of these studies to be completed are interesting primarily from a heuristic standpoint.

Maupin (1965) had ordinary subjects focus on breathing for nine sessions. These subjects' meditation experiences were rated on a five-point scale by "blind" judges. Based on their self-report data, described after each session, six of the twenty-eight subjects were rated as high experiencers. A high experiencer was one who reported at least one Type Five experience (concentration and detachment). Ten subjects were rated as having moderate responses to meditation: i.e. no Type Five experience but at least one Type Three or Type Four experience (pleasant body sensations or vivid breathing). Twelve subjects were rated "low response" because they reported nothing more than relaxation (Stage Two) or dizziness (Stage One). Maupin (1965, p. 145) notes that his five-point response scale does not register all observed responses.

> "Subjectively felt benefits similar to those resulting from relaxation therapies were reported by several subjects. Subjects in the high and moderate response group occasionally mentioned the emergence of very specific and vivid effects other than anxiety while they were practicing. These included hallucinoid feelings, muscle tension, sexual excitement, and intense sadness."
> (1965, p. 145)

Lesh (1970) also had subjects practice Zen breath meditation; he adapted Maupin's five-point scale slightly but found essentially the same results.

In a study using external concentration, Deikman (1966) had subjects focus on a blue vase, and he also found strong subjective changes in ordinary subjects' phenomenological perceptions. Every subject noted an alteration in perception of the vase, a shift to a deeper and more intense blue: brighter, more vivid, luminous. Further, subjects noted instability in the vase's shape or size: a loss of the third dimension, a diffusion or loss of perceptual boundaries. One subject noted feelings of merging with the vase, as though "it were almost part of me." Another subject noted complete loss of body feelings (Deikman, 1966).

Kanas and Horowitz (1977) used a content analysis questionnaire devised by Horowitz (1969, 1970) to gain information about subjective experiences during meditation. Subjects were shown a stress film and then asked to estimate the percentage of time spent thinking about the stress film, the experimental task, life issues, fantasies, mantra (where appropriate), other thoughts, and no thoughts, during the ten minutes they meditated or rested.

Kornfield (1979) gathered extensive data from meditators at five two-week and one three-month retreats for intensive insight meditation (Vipassana). Kornfield's data came from reports which the meditators gave their teachers every two or three days and from answers to a series of three questions about 1) sleep/food intake; 2) changes in clarity of perception, concentration, mindfulness; 3) what was currently predominant in meditation experience; any unusual experiences. Although Kornfield's study generated an enormous amount of rich information, the interpretation of these data must be tentative, since the coding instrument was made *post hoc* as a way of sorting the data, rather than prior to the experiment to test the hypotheses. However, this type of heuristic study is necessary initially to give us information about the phenomenology of meditation experience.

These five studies involve having subjects report on their experiences at the completion of the meditation session or in Kornfield's case, at intervals. In Deikman's (1966) and Kornfield's (1979) studies the reports were made directly to the experimenters/teachers, who grouped and reported the data; in the Maupin (1965) and Lesh (1970) studies, raters coded the experiences on a five-part scale, a methodological improvement, *after* sufficient heuristic information has been accumulated via previous studies.

A second group of studies to obtain reports of meditators'

experiences involved having subjects push buttons *during* the meditation session whenever certain thoughts or feelings occurred (Van Nuys, 1973; Banquet, 1973; Kubose, 1976).

Van Nuys had subjects push a button every time they became aware of an intrusive thought. The nature of intrusions reported by subjects in the post-meditation interview included: itches, aches, and other bodily feelings of discomfort; thoughts about the nature and purpose of the experiment; and thoughts about roommates, girl-friends, courses and other current concerns. In addition, many subjects reported such subjective responses as vivid visual experiences, feelings of paranoia, feelings of being "turned on," dreamlike experiences, temporary loss of orientation in time or space, primary-process perceptual distortions (Van Nuys, 1973, p. 67).

Kubose (1976) debriefed meditators after their experience with a questionnaire asking them to divide the thoughts they had into the following categories: a) thoughts about bodily sensations; b) thoughts relating themselves to the present situation; c) thoughts relating themselves to past events; d) thoughts about the future; e) thoughts about ideas and things that did not have a strong time component. His data revealed that subjects in the meditation group categorized most of their thoughts along a present-time dimension, whereas subjects in the control group categorized their thoughts as past and future. As Kubose noted, meditation seemed to minimize the intrusion of distracting thoughts, and relative to a control group, when thoughts did occur, they tended to be categorized as oriented toward the present rather than the past or future.

Banquet (1973) had individuals push buttons to signal thoughts or feelings. He refined the technique of Kubose and had five different buttons for the individuals to push, depending on the category of events during the meditation experience: bodily sensations, involuntary movement, visual images, deep meditation, and transcendence (deepest part of meditation). However, as with any intrusive procedure, there may be difficulties in having a person push a button while in a state of transcendence and attempting to maintain that state.

Finally, two other studies, still within the same scientific tradition of an experimenter trying to gain information from subjects, was undertaken by Osis et al., (1973) and later replicated by Kohr (1977). These studies involved asking meditators to respond to a questionnaire after their sessions, and then performing a factor analysis. Osis et al.'s (1973) research is described in some detail here because it is an interesting application of multivariate statistical analysis to the issue of meditation experience. He gave subjects a premeditation mood questionnaire and a post-meditation questionnaire before and after four different sittings. Both questionnaires were used in the same factor analysis to determine how closely the subjects' meditation and premeditation states were related. Subjects came from a variety of different religious traditions, including Unitarian, Zen, Raja Yoga, Hassidic Judaism, Catholicism. There was an attempt to determine the extent to which meditation experience would cut across different disciplines and different orientations. Osis posited that in most religions the central concept is a belief in a spiritual reality felt to be larger and more valuable than (and often inclusive of) the personal self. The issue of self-selection was mentioned and even maximized; then experimenters tried to select subjects "to whom meditation was a kind of quest for meaning and growth in their lives," (Osis et al., 1973, p. 113). It was found in both the Osis and later the Kohr studies that there was almost no correlation between initial mood and meditation experience, suggesting that meditation did produce a state of consciousness different from the state of consciousness which the person brought to the practice of meditation.

Six factors were replicated in at least three of the meditation experiences: self-transcendence and openness; mood brought to the session (both appeared in all four experiments); intensification and change of consciousness; meaning dimension; forceful exclusion of images; and general success of meditation. Self-transcendence and openness involved the following core items: a feeling of merging with others, unity with the group, oneness with the external. For mood brought to the session the core items were elation, freedom from anxiety, content with self, and greater vitality. The next factor, intensification and change of consciousness, seemed to be the most central and complex. Thirteen core items, half of the items in the post-session questionnaire, are contained in this factor. They include: intensification of consciousness, ways of experiencing change, love and joy, perceptual enrichment, refreshment after session, depth of insight, unity with group, and the feeling that it was a good session. There often seemed to be an organismic arousal during this intensification and change of consciousness. Another factor, the meaning dimension, included core items such as relevant visual images, relevant thoughts, deep insights, alertness, and sense of presence. The next factor, what Osis called "forceful exclusion of images," included negative items. As the authors stated, "The predominant note is one of tension: negative loadings on relaxation, serenity, and affirmation of the external" (Osis et al., 1973, p. 122)." In the fourth experiment, they introduced a negative experience factor. It expresses "the opposites of affirmation and deep acceptance of self and others. It appears to express the feeling that the meditation was interfered with" (p. 130).

In the Kohr experiment (1977), which tried to extend and replicate the Osis experiment, again there was strong bias in the subjects selected: a sampling from members of the Association for Research and Enlightment agreeing to participate in meditation research and answer questionnaires. Some of the refinements that occurred in the questionnaire were breaking the subjects into various subgroups of high and low categories on five variables: anxiety level as measured by the IPAT Anxiety Scale Questionnaire; incidents of perceived personal problems as indicated by the total score on the Mooney Problem Check List, (Mooney & Gordon, 1951); the length of time previously spent engaged in meditation on a fairly regular basis; the amount of previous meditation experience combined with whether a consistent schedule had been maintained in the month prior to the study, and the degree to which the participants adhered to the procedures. (Low anxiety, high anxiety, low problems, high problems, low regular schedule, high regular schedule, low prior experience, high prior experience, low adherence, high adherence.)

The meditators in Kohr's study meditated alone, based on a manual, whereas the subjects in the Osis experiment meditated and discussed their experiences in a small group context. The major factor was intensification and change of consciousness. Kohr found, "This factor conveys the impression of a heightened sense of fullness, deep positive emotion, and intensification of awareness, perceptual change and enhancement, a presence of religious significance and a sense of satisfaction with the session" (1977, p. 200). The authors noted that this factor seemed a blend of the factors of self-transcendence and openness as well as the intensification factor. The "psychological state prior to session" was also a consistent factor, similar to Osis's mood-brought-to-session factor. Importantly, this factor was independent of the other factors except for the tendency for the freedom-from-anxiety item to load with the "negative experience factor" in a majority of the subgroup analysis. This suggests that anxiety can often impair the meditation experience unless one is successful in reducing its effects prior to the session. Kohr noted, "Overall, the cohesiveness of this factor suggests that one's mood and functioning during the day represented a different state of consciousness than the altered state as measured by the post-session questionnaire" (1977, p. 200). The negative experience factor was based on those items added in Osis's fourth experiment plus some additional items. These included sessions characterized by an inability to relax, compounded by the intrusion of unwanted thoughts, some of them anxious residues from the day's experience or anticipations of future events. The mental clarity factor, reflecting retention of awareness and sense of alertness was not observed in the Osis experiment. The physical effects factor—including various physical sensations like an increase in bodily warmth and sensations around the "seven spiritual centers" of Oriental and occult religions—was also weak.

The independence of the psychological-state-prior-to-session factor seems important, in both the Kohr and Osis experiments. As Osis (1973, p. 130) noted, "The items of everyday mood as measured in the pre-meditation questionnaire did not appreciably load on any other factors of the meditation experience and formed a strong common compact factor by themselves. The subjects' free comments support the view that successful meditation leads to altered states of consciousness" (1973, p. 130). Similarly, in the Kohr experiment, the independence of states arises from the fact that "Good sessions frequently occurred regardless of feeling tired or depressed prior to the session. In these sessions there seemed to be an ability to let go of a negative emotion or to move beyond fatigue" (1977, p. 202). The only area where a prior psychological state demonstrated leakage into a meditation period was anxiety associated with having negative experiences. The author noted, "negative experience is not uncommon among individuals who resolve to meditate on a daily basis, especially the novice," a finding already discussed in Chapters One and Two.

As noted, the above studies involve only a slight variation on the traditional scientific experiment in which an experimenter gathers information from subjects. But there is also a different approach to gathering information on the phenomenology of meditation—one in which the subject and experimenter are the same person. The roots of this approach go back to the classical texts, such as the *Adhidhamma* (Goleman, 1972, 1977) and the classical texts of the Mahamudra tradition (Brown, 1977). These texts attempt to develop a scientific phenomenology of meditation, a cartography of the "inner voyage." The scientists are the meditators who use themselves as subjects and through a process of introspective psychology try to chart which experiences and thoughts are helpful in moving toward enlightened experiences, and which are harmful. Their texts provide us with one model derived from long-term experienced meditators. They may or may not be a state-specific science in the sense that we do not know how much the practitioners' own belief systems were looked at carefully as part of the "outcome" success.

The reports in the classical texts give us information from long-term meditators who were presumably not trained in the behavioral sciences. Three studies have been done by behavioral scientists who are also meditators of intermediate, one to several years, experience (Tart, 1971; Walsh, 1977, 1978; Shapiro, Chapter Three). Theoretically, those trained in the behavioral sciences should have more acute and accurate discrimination skills, should be less biased and more willing to admit where the technique of meditation is or is not useful, and should try to communicate those subjective experiences to others in accessible terms. For example, Tart (1971) practiced TM meditation for a year and Walsh (1977, 1978) described his experiences during two years of Vipassana (insight meditation). In a similar vein, Shapiro (Chapter 3) recorded thoughts and images during several meditation sessions, and subsequently analyzed data for number and type of thoughts and cognitions, and percentage of time when there did not appear to be thoughts.

This approach, using behavioral scientists as subject, observer, and experimenter, has several potential pitfalls. However, it does have the advantage of direct experience and reporting by the same person, without the intervening hypotheses and interpretations of another experimenter. At the very least, observing one's own meditation experience should be a rich source of gaining experiential understanding of relevant concepts and of generating hypotheses and refining dependent variables for subsequent research.*

CONCURRENT VALIDITY FOR
SUBJECTIVE EXPERIENCE DURING MEDITATION

Because of the subjective nature of the meditation experience, it is difficult to obtain concurrent validity on subjects' self-report. Maupin (1965) attempted to correlate attention measures (digit span, continuous additions, size estimation) with response to meditation. However Van Nuys (1973) has suggested that these measures were not relevant to the type of attention involved in meditation (see also Galin, 1974). Van Nuys notes that alterations in consciousness occur when attention is relatively fixed and sustained, whereas the tests Maupin used involved tasks that require a constant and rapid shifting of the focus of attention; furthermore, "they invite discursive, analytic thought that is actively restricted in meditation" (Boals, 1978, p. 165).

Van Nuys (1973) developed a simple technique for studying attention during the latter stages of meditation. He had his subjects push a button to report intrusion of "off-task" thoughts that distracted them from the task of meditation. He found that the reports of these intrusions correlated with hypnotizability. Other promising methods of obtaining concurrent validity may be the use of experimenter-controlled buttons to signal physiological values of the meditator to the meditator, requesting a continuing experimenter-subjective report (Herbert & Lehman, 1977), the signal detection format employed in the daydreaming studies of Singer (1975) to obtain reports of occurrence of "task-irrelevant thoughts," and monitoring hemispheric laterality and synchrony to determine brain wave patterns within and between hemispheres during meditation (Davidson, 1976; Galin, 1974).

---

*Whether or not if may be helpful to the meditation practice itself is a different story!—see Chapter Three and the Epilogue.

7.3 Subjective Reports of Changes in Attitudes and Perceptions After Meditation

THE STUDIES reported above have tested short-term, mostly in-state effects of meditation. Other researchers have tried to document perceptual and/or behavioral changes that occur at times other than during meditation. These studies, which look at self-concept and perceived behavior change, have gathered data primarily by use of pencil and paper tests, including Shostrom's Personal Orientation Inventory (Hjelle, 1974; Nidich, Seeman & Dreskin, 1973; Seeman, Nidich & Banta, 1972); the Northridge Development Scale (Ferguson & Gowan, 1977); and the Otis Descriptive Personality List and Otis Physical and Behavioral Inventory (Otis, 1974). All of these studies report that meditators change more than control groups in the direction of positive mental health, positive personality change, and "self-actualization." (Studies that used self-report data, but that focused primarily on anxiety, are not included here.) These changes include such items as self-perceived increase in capacity for intimate contact, increased spontaneity, self-regard, acceptance of aggression, and inner directedness (Table 7.1).

There are, however, several methodological problems with the above studies. First, none of the studies, except Hjelle's (1974), controls for expectations and demand characteristics, and Hjelle's study, as already noted, does not control for commitment (long-term practice). The commitment or motivation of the subjects may be quite important. For example, it appears that five of the original twenty subjects in the experimental condition in Seeman, Nidich and Banta's (1972) study dropped out, a fact that could have biased the experiment in a direction favoring meditation. A second methodological problem of the above studies is that they do not show, aside from paper and pencil test scores, whether the meditating subjects demonstrated behavior change.

In an attempt to learn more about daily changes in behavior, Shapiro (1978a), in addition to pre-tests and post-tests, had subjects self-monitor nine variables daily: feelings of anger, seeing beauty in nature, positive self-thoughts, negative self-thoughts, feelings of anxiety, feelings of creativity. The experimental group

TABLE 7.1 Subjective Changes Following Meditation

Investigator(s)	Focus of Investigation	Ss (N, age, sex, prior experience)	INDEPENDENT VARIABLE — Type and Length of Treatment Training	Frequency of Therapist (t) Contact	DEPENDENT VARIABLE — Subjective Effects (unless otherwise noted)	Follow-up	Type of Design, Quality of Controls, Methodological Problems
Seeman, Nidich and Banta 1972	"Self-Actualization"	Group One: control N=20, 10 male, 10 female. Group Two: meditation N=15, 8 male, 7 female. Prior experience not stated	Standard Transcendental Meditation training. 30–60 min. initial instruction 3 days; verification + further instruction then Ss instructed to meditate 2x daily for 15–20 min	Not stated	Shostrom's Personal Orientation Inventory, 1966 (POI) tested 2 days prior to and 2 months post TM instruction showed meditators moved in positive "self actualizing" direction compared to controls	None reported	Group selection and/or matching procedures not stated. Need behavioral measures of such items as spontaneity, capacity for intimate contact, tolerance for verbal aggression, willingness to self-disclose
Nidich, Seeman and Dreskin 1973	"Self-Actualization"	Group One: N=9 non-meditating controls. Group Two: N=9 meditation	Same as above	Not stated	Shostrom's POI measured pre and post (10 weeks) TM instruction showed meditators moved in direction of "self actualization." Controls showed no significant differences in testing	None reported	Same as above
Stek and Bass 1973	Tested differences between those interested and not interested in meditation in "perceived locus of control" and "personal adjustment"	Group One: N=17 median age 20 yrs, 12 male, 5 female, attended free meditation lectures; paid TM initiation fee. Group Two: N=32 median age 18 yrs, 14 M, 20 F, attended 1 TM lecture. Group Three: N=27 median age 19 yrs, 12 M, 15 F, uninterested in meditation. Group Four: N=30 median age 19 yrs, 18 M, 12 F controls	Tests given pre-meditation training	Not stated	Administration of Rotter's IE Locus of Control Scale (1966) and Shostrom's POI (time competence + internal support) found no significant difference between test scores for all 4 groups and common scores for college students	None reported	Study might indicate that initial group differences between meditators and non-meditators are insignificant; however, group differences may exist in willingness to change, etc.
Hjelle 1974	"Anxiety," "Locus of control" and "Self Actualization"	Group One: N=15, 7 M, 8 F meditating experience = 22.6.3 mo. Group Two: N=21, 11 M, 10 f tested 1 week prior to receiving meditation instruction	Standard TM training	Not stated	Regular meditators (group one) scored significantly lower than beginners on Bending's Anxiety Scale (1956) and Rotter's Internal-External Locus of Control Scale (1966) and significantly higher on 7 of 12 POI scales (Shostrom, 1966)	None reported	Possible demand characteristics in testing; study supports Seeman, Nidich & Banta
Otis 1974	Self concept change, improvement in physical and/or behavioral problems	Group One: (N=30) Transcendental Meditation training for 3 months. All Ss's baseline physiological measurements; pre and post tests. Group Two: (N=15) Passive Controls; took pre and post tests. Group Three: Active Controls: A sitting quietly 15/20 min/2x daily. B "meditative" treatment repeating "I am a witness only," 15–20 min/2x daily	Group One standard TM training for 3 months. All Ss's baseline physiological measurements, for 3 months	Not stated	Psychological tests: Questionnaire on self-concept (Qs, Descriptive Personality List) and checklist on variety of behavioral and physical problems (Qhs, Physical and Behavioral Inventory) found no overall differences between TM and pooled control Ss's. However item analysis revealed TM Ss claimed more specific benefits than passive controls. Interview conducted 3 months post-training indicated that specific benefit claims of active controls and TM Ss's did not differ. Author suggests that simply resting may account for benefits	To 18 months	Treatment conditions not matched for expectation of relief
Udupa et al. 1973	Performance, Intelligence and Memory Quotient(s). Neuroticism. Mental Fatigability and Psychological Health assessed. Plasma Acetylcholine and Serum Cholinesterase monitored	N=12 avg. age 23.0 ± 3.36 yrs. "from a uniform socioeconomic class"	Hatha Yoga exercises (done in group) for 1 hour daily x 6 months. Exercises involved graduated sequence of muscle coordination exercises, postures (asanas), breathing (prāṇāyāma) meditation, etc.	One hour daily x 6 months with trained Yoga instructor	(see Table I below)	None reported	Within subject design: Ss served as own controls

Table I Certain Psychological Changes Induced by the Practice of Yoga

Observations	Test Used	Initial (baseline)	3rd month	6th month	Direction
Performance quotient (PQ)	Alexander's Passalong Test	93.15±12.50	102.6±16.40	108.2±14.70	Increased significantly
Intelligence quotient (IQ)	Koh's Block Design Test	92.17±18.60	100.3±6.40	106.2±16.70	
Memory quotient (MQ)	Wechsler Memory Scale	89.75±9.15	97.3±13.20	100.8±8.60	Increased significantly
Neuroticism index (MPI)	Maudsley Personality Inven.				
N		19.50±8.95	11.40±10.70	9.82±8.40	Decreased
E		27.10±5.60	28.40±6.80	26.54±8.40	
Q		2.66±5.53	1.00±2.19	2.58±5.57	
Mental fatiguability	Digit Cancellation Test				
Time taken		3.52±0.68	3.31±0.90	3.03±0.41	Lowered
Mistake score		5.54±4.69	1.31±1.73	3.64±3.30	
Fatigue index		1.59	0.40	1.20	
Physiological Health Index	Cornell Medical Index				
Physiological complaints		125	83	64	Lowered
Psychological complaints		67	31	30	Lowered

Note: Significant values in decreased complaints or Cornell Medical Index include gastrointestinal, psychoneurological and respiratory complaints (physiological), and anxiety, tension, and inadequacy complaints (psychological).

TABLE 7.1 Subjective Changes Following Meditation (cont'd.)

Investigator(s)	Focus of Investigation	S's (N; age; sex; prior experience)	INDEPENDENT VARIABLE Type and Length of Treatment / Training	Frequency of Therapist (t) Contact	DEPENDENT VARIABLE Subjective Effects (unless otherwise noted)	Follow-up	Type of Design; Quality of Controls; Methodological Problems

Table II. Certain Biochemical Response to the Practice of Yoga

Physiological Data
Mean±S.D. and comparison with initial

Observations	Initial (baseline)	3rd month	6th month
Plasma Acetylcholine in μg/100 ml	181.7±149.3	101.1±34.3 t = 1.825 p < 0.1	58.7±18.05 t = 2.83 p < 0.01
Serum Cholinesterase in pH units/hour	1.17±0.309	0.894±0.313 t = 2.177 p < 0.05	0.95±0.087 t = 2.095 p < 0.05

Note: Both show statistically significant decreases; also found increase in urinary excretion of testosterone and 17-hydroxy corticosteroid; increase in serum proteins and reduction of blood sugar. EEG showed more prominent alpha with less spikes.

Shapiro 1978a | Daily covert behavior and "Global" self-perception. | N=15; college students in class on "Zen Buddhism and Self Management"; no prior meditation experience. | Experimental Group (N=9)
1) 2 weeks behavioral observation on 9 variables
2) weekend Zen experience workshop
3) formal Zen breath meditation practiced 2x daily plus contingent informal breath meditation and continued behavioral observation for 3 weeks.
Control Group (N=6)
1) 5 weeks behavioral observation
2) weekend Zen experience workshop | During intervention phase (weeks 3-5) experimenter had no contact with either group | Data from pre and post testing on Semantic Differential, Rotter's I-E Locus of Control showed no significant group differences but moved in hypothesized (positive) direction Stanford Hypnotic Susceptibility Scale (form C, Group Variant) showed increase in susceptibility for experimental group and decrease for controls

Behavioral Data
Self monitoring of frequency of behaviors with questionnaire (e.g., positive self-statements, negative self-statements; feelings of creativity, feelings of self-control, feeling anxious, becoming angry, noting positive things in nature, relating to only part of a person and not living in the moment) Combined index of behavioral self-observation data showed greater movement in a more favorable (hypothesized) direction for experimental group than controls. | None reported | Modified multiple time series design (c.f. Campbell & Stanley, 1963, pp. 55-57). Positive direction looked at daily change as well as global pre/post. Weakness: need meet co-varying variables with daily self-reported change of feelings.

Lesh 1970 | Counselors measured on empathy and openness to experience | All S's were college students taking counseling courses
Group One: N=16; taught Zen breath meditation.
Group Two: N=12; controls
Group Three: N=11; group "definitely against" meditation exercise. | Group One: Zen breath meditation practiced 30 min./day x 4 weeks. | Meditation instructions given by tape to avoid bias | Pre and Post Treatment Measures:
1) Increased empathy among meditating group on Affective Sensitivity Scale (ASS) responses to videotaped client situation. Both control groups did not show improvement in empathic ability.
2) No correlation found between ASS and blind ratings of subjective response to meditation (Maupin, 1965).
3) Positive correlation found between openness to experience (Experience Inquiry; Fitzgerald, 1966) and response to meditation.
4) Positive correlation between individual scores on openness to experience and ASS.
5) Correlation found between high scores on ASS and "self-actualization" measure (Shostrom's POI). | None reported | Between subjects design; possible selection bias.

Leung 1973 | Counselors measured on empathic ability and ability to respond selectively to clients (e.g., training of "notice authority" statements) | N=57; avg. age 22.75 yrs.; 22 male, 45 female; prior experience not stated.
Group E-1: Deep breathing training first +
Group E-2: External concentration training first + deep breathing training.
Group 3: N=20; controls; given no training. | Training for groups 1 + 2:
7 hrs. training in meditative deep breathing.
7 hrs. training in external concentration on a specific verbal stimuli on tape. Social verbal reinforcement given S's for correct performance of exercises. | Not stated | Criterion Measures:
Group E-1 — Measured S's predictive analytical empathy in response to videotaped sequences of acted client situations (40 min. total). Analytic empathy measurement taken after 10 minute portions of videotape.
Group E-2 — Indicated to E number of "notice authority" statements made by actor "clients" in videotape.
In second part of training the criterion measures were reversed. Both (E) groups showed more accurate analytic empathy and heard more notice authority statements by clients than controls. E-1 showed more predictive ability on self either attitude scale and heard more notice authority statements than E-2. | None reported | Post-test only control group design.

(informal and formal Zen meditation) daily reported data significantly more in a favorable direction: less feelings of anxiety, more feelings of creativity, etc. This longitudinal study was useful because it provided self-report of feelings rather than simply before and after pencil and paper test data of global feeling change. However, it is unclear from the study which parts of the treatment intervention were responsible for what percentage of the variance of the successful outcome. Further, no concurrent covarying overt variables were involved in the study, which still leaves us with the problems of self-reported data.

7.4 Non-Subjective Indices of Attitude and Perceptual Change After Meditation

SEVERAL STUDIES have looked at behavioral indices of attitude and perceptual change.* Some studies† have noted that meditators seemed to have better auditory receptivity and perceptual discrimination than controls, as well as improved reaction times and increased capacity to attend. Meditators, however, were not more adept at learning a novel perceptual-motor skill (Williams, 1978). Linden (1973) and Pelletier (1974), using the Witkin Embedded Figures Test, found differences between meditators and non-meditators in field dependence. The above studies provide useful information about the relationship between meditation and perceptual changes. Two studies that attempt to clinically measure the effects of perceptual changes were done by Lesh (1970) and Leung (1973).

Lesh (1970) found that counselors who had practiced Zen meditation for one-half hour per day for one month had substantially increased accurate empathy, while those in two control

---

*Davidson, Goleman & Schwartz, 1976; Singer, 1975; Pelletier, 1974; Shaw & Kolb, 1977; Brown, Stuart & Blodgett, 1974; Graham, 1971; Pirot, 1973.

---

†Davidson, Goleman & Schwartz, 1976; Shaw & Kolb, 1977; Brown, Stuart & Blodgett, 1974; Graham, 1975; Pirot, 1973; Udupa, Singh & Yadav, 1973; Holt et al., 1978.

TABLE 7.2 Studies on Attention and Perception

Investigator(s)	Clinical Problem	Ss (N, age, sex, prior experience)	INDEPENDENT VARIABLE Type and Length of treatment/Training	Frequency of Therapist (E) Contact	Subjective Effects	DEPENDENT VARIABLE Behavioral, Physiological, Overt, Concurrent Data	Type of Design, Quality of Controls, Methodological Problems
Van Nuys 1973	Meditation, attention and hypnotic susceptibility	N=47, males, prior experience not reported	Task: Concentration on doorstep and flame/breath meditation. Session One: Individual tests of 15 min. focused attention on each object. Session Two: Same	Not reported	Tests given post-task. Session One: Embedded Figures Test. Session Two: Stroop Color Word Test. A's Experience Inquiry. Harvard Scale of Hypnotic Susceptibility, Field Depth of Hypnosis Test. Found correlation between 2 measures of hypnotic susceptibility and number of intrusions reported during meditation	Behavioral: Self-report of intrusions of thought during attention task	None reported	Within subject. Ss served as own controls
Pelletier 1974	Autokinetic perception ("perceptual style")	N=40, avg. age 24.7 yrs., 20 male, 20 female. Group One: Meditators, volunteers from intro TM meeting. Group Two: Sitting controls	Group One: Standard TM instruction. 3 mos. practice. Group Two: Instructed to sit quietly 20 min. each morning (x 3 mos.)	Not reported	Pre and post tests of autokinetic effect shifted towards field indep. On Rod and Frame Test (Cancro & Vuchen Witkin et al.) meditators showed increased accuracy. On Embedded Figures Test (Gardner et al.) meditators showed shorter latency time	None reported	Half of Ss in each group not pretested to control for possible interaction effects of perceptual measures and meditation
Shaw and Kolb 1977	Simple reaction time	Group One: N=9 meditators, one mo. or more experience. Group Two: N=9 non-meditators	1) Learning trials. 2) 100 trials with reaction device. 3) Rest or meditation (20 min.) 4) 100 more trials	Not reported	Report states: "Meditators brighter in mood and more responsive in conversation after meditating"	Behavioral: Meditators had shorter reaction than non-meditators in first test. After resting, meditators improved, non-meditators were slower in reacting	None reported	Test of statistical significance not reported. Matching of groups not reported
Brown, Stuart & Blodgett 1974	1) 2 point threshold determination of skin sensitivity. 2) visual brightness discrimination. 3) simple reaction time. 4) complex reaction time	Group One: N=11, 18-22 yrs. female meditators with experience from "few weeks" to few mos. Group Two: N=11, 18-22 yrs. female non-meditating controls	1) Pre-state performance measurement. 2) Pre-state resting, eyes open) 3 min. 3) Group One: Transcendental Meditation (15 min.) Group Two: resting, eyes closed (15 min.) 4) Post-state resting (eyes open) Note: meditators took 3 min. avg. to open eyes. 5) Post-state performance measures	Not reported	Not reported	Behavioral: Tests given pre and post meditation or sitting for 3 meditators meeting physiological criteria performance improved on all measures. One control also met meditative criteria. Performance of all controls worsened. Physiological: Note heart and respiratory rates, presence of frontal EEG alpha and kappa rhythms used to define "meditation state"—only 3 Ss met this criteria	Small N, short meditation time used (15 min.) and only 1 trial reported. Experimenter anecdotes suggest meditators may have been sleeping
Graham 1975	Frequency and amplitude discrimination of auditory threshold	Study Group: N=8, experience with TM not reported	Condition One: 20 minutes meditation. Condition Two: 20 minutes rest with 3 to 10 days interval between conditions	Not reported	Not reported	Behavioral: Pre and post tests showed greater percentage improvement after meditating (+25 %) than after resting (−37%) in auditory discrimination and +37.0% and −15.1% respectively for frequency discrimination. Meditators seem to evidence lower perceptual thresholds after practice	Ss divided into 2 groups, AB, BA design. Study does not report Ss selection procedures
Pirot 1973	Perceptual auditory discrimination of tones	N=32, 8 in each cell, prior experience not stated	Stimuli: 40 pairs of tones, one 2,000 milliseconds and one 2,225 milliseconds in length (1,000 Hz, 30 dB). Ss had to discriminate longest tone after TM or relaxation	Not reported	Not reported	Behavioral: Meditators performed better post meditation than relaxation, despite the order in which they had meditated. Physiological: CSR, EMG, finger pulse volume and EMG measures to be reported	Four groups with all possible disorders of meditation and relaxation represented. Repeated measures and one-way between groups analysis performed
Davidson, Goleman, and Schwartz 1976	Differences in attentional absorption and trait anxiety	N=58, mean age 20.81 yrs. (S.D. 2.77), 36 male, 23 female	Meditation practice ranged from TM to Zen breath meditation. Group One: (N=11) Controls expressing interest in meditation. Group Two: (N=14) Beginners, one month's meditation exp. or less. Group Three: (N=18) Regular practice of meditation for 1-24 months. Group Four: (N=15) long-term meditators (greater than 24 month's exp.)	Tests given as "take home" among battery of other personality and attitude questionnaires	Ss tested on Shor Personal Experience Questionnaire (PEQ), Tellegen Absorption Scale (TAS), and Spielberger State-Trait Anxiety Inventory (STAI). Reliable increment in PEQ and TAS (e.g. increase in capacity to attend) and reliable decrement in STAI (trait anxiety) observed across groups from controls through long-term meditators.	None reported	Cross-sectional design.

groups did not change. Accurate empathy was measured by an "affective sensitivity" videotape showing a client telling about his/her problem. Subjects were to formulate what they thought the client's problem was. Lesh hypothesized that meditation helped the counselors by giving them an openness to their own inner experiences. The counselor, by knowing what s/he was feeling, was less likely to project those feelings and judgments onto what the client was saying.

In one of the few studies to control for order of teaching different meditation techniques, Leung (1973) taught counselors a deep breathing (internal focus) technique and an external concentration technique. He randomly assigned subjects to treatment groups that reversed the order of teaching the techniques. The criteria for measuring outcome were accurate empathy on a task similar to the one used by Lesh, and also having the subjects count the number of "notice authority" statements made by actor clients on a simulated client situation videotape. Regardless of the order in which the techniques were taught, both groups showed more accurate empathy and heard more notice-authority statements than controls.

7.5 Summary

WHAT CAN WE make of these studies? *First*, it clearly seems important to distinguish between short- and long-term meditation experience. Compared to "Eastern" standards most Western meditators are at a "beginning level" in terms of length of time spent in meditation practice. The classical texts give us a cartography—a context for clarifying different types of long-term meditation experience. *Second*, it seems a useful scientific strategy to have those trained in the behavioral sciences who also meditate be both experimenters, subjects, and observers, although certain conditions must be observed. *Third*, it does seem possible to gain useful and precise information about the phenomenology of the meditation experiences. As Osis et al. noted, "in spite of the almost universal claim that the meditation experience is ineffable, clear dimensionalities emerge" (1973, p. 130). *Fourth*, it appears that even in short-term meditators, relatively strong experiences occur (Deikman, 1966; Maupin, 1965). Further, as the work of Osis and

Kohr suggest, meditation experiences, with the exception of anxiety, were different from the mood brought to the session—evidence for the view of meditation as an altered state of consciousness. *Fifth*, both Osis and Deikman argue that although belief systems may be part of the variance accounting for the effect of the altered state, more than simply belief systems are at work in meditation because "different beliefs of different subjects will on the whole cancel each other out...whereas meditation seems to tap more universal dimensions " (Osis et al., 1973, p. 130). Deikman noted that "hypnotic experiences do not appear to have the ineffable, profoundly uplifting, highly valued quality of the mystic state and are not remembered as such" (1963, p. 340). He noted that there may be strong belief systems, suggestion, and demand characteristics operating but then suggests that the hypothesis of demand characteristics is not consistent with the fact that the highest mystic experiences are similar in their basic content despite wide differences in cultural backgrounds and expectations: a) feeling of incommunicability, b) transcendence of sense modalities, c) absence of specific content, such as images and ideas, and d) feelings of unity with the ultimate. *Sixth*, not all altered states are pleasant and uplifting. For example, in his final experiment, Osis put in questions to tap these negative experiences, and Kohr found a negative experience factor to be a clear dimension. As noted, these negative experiences can also be seen in the earlier reports of Van Nuys, and in an article by French, Schmid and Ingalls (1975) on altered reality testing resulting from too much meditation. Further, a recent article by Otis (in press, 1980) describes the adverse effects of meditation, presumably some of which resulted from experiences during meditation.

Therefore, in conclusion, greater clarity and precision seem necessary in describing altered states. Rather than on the one hand shying away from this area as epiphenomena or dismissing it *a priori* as "psychotic and delusional," or on the other hand calling it "enlightened and higher consciousness," we need to gather more precise information to see when these powerful experiences may in fact be psychotic and when they may be truly enlightened and spritual. Further, with this kind of precise information, in addition to being able to compare meditation with other self-regulation strategies, we also may be able to learn more about meditation as an altered state of consciousness, and thereafter compare it to other altered states such as dreaming (Faber et al., 1978), hypnotic trance, psychosis, sleep, and others.

Chapter 7: Further Reading

OVERVIEW

Tart, C. Science, states of consciousness, and spiritual experiences: The need for state specific sciences. In C. Tart (Ed.), *Transpersonal psychologies.* NY: Harper & Row, 1975.
Tart, C. *States of consciousness,* New York: E.P. Dutton, 1975.

First Approach: Subject and Experimenter Different

Maupin, E.W. Individual differences in response to a Zen meditation exercise. *Journal of Consulting Psychology,* 1965, *29,* 139-145.
Deikman, A.J. Experimental meditation. *Journal of Nervous and Mental Disease,* 1963, *136,* 329-343.
Kohr, E. Dimensionality in the meditation experience: A replication. *Journal of Transpersonal Psychology,* 1977, *9,* (a), 193-203. (Reprinted in D.H. Shapiro & R.N. Walsh [Eds.], *The science of meditation,* New York: Aldine, 1980).

Second Approach: Subject and Experimenter the Same.

Shapiro, D.H., A content analysis of the meditation experience, See Chapter Three.
Tart, C. A psychologist's experience with Transcendental Meditation, *Journal of Transpersonal Psychology,* 1971, *3,* (2), 135-40.
Walsh, R.N. Initial meditation experiences. *Journal of Transpersonal Psychology,* 1977, *9,* (2), 151-92.
Walsh, R.N. Initial meditation experiences. *Journal of Transpersonal Psychology,* 1978, *10,* (1), 1-28. (Reprinted in D.H. Shapiro & R.N. Walsh [Eds], *The science of meditation.* New York: Aldine, 1980).

CLASSICAL TEXTS

Brown, D.P. A model of the levels of concentrative meditation, *International Journal of Clinical & Experimental Hypnosis,* 1977, *25,* 4, 236-273. (Reprinted in D.H. Shapiro & R.N. Walsh [Eds.], *The science of meditation.* New York: Aldine: 1980).

8

Components
of Meditation

8.1 Components, Effects, Mediating Mechanisms: A Distinction

ALTHOUGH THE research discussed in Chapters Five and Seven is relatively conclusive that meditation, broadly conceived, results in powerful subjective experiences and physiological changes, it is not yet clear what variance of the effect is attributable to different components of the technique of meditation. At the simplest level, this chapter tries to answer the question: *What* are the components of meditation which cause the effects? The following chapter, Mediating Mechanisms, tries to answer the questions *why* and *how* do the components cause the effects? Although posing the questions is clear and simple, the answers, unfortunately, are not. Unless we are extremely precise and careful, we can find ourselves in a semantic swamp while discussing effects, components, and mediating mechanisms. This is because certain variables, depending upon the perspective of the observer, may at any given time be either a component, a mediating mechanism, or an effect.

The relaxation literature concretely illustrates some potential difficulties. For example, the relaxation response which Benson

(1975) described and the physiological changes during that response may be the mechanisms mediating the effects of meditation on stress, addictions, and hypertension. Therefore, the relaxation response may be viewed as a mediating mechanism accounting for meditation's effects (Shapiro & Giber, 1978). On the other hand, the relaxation response might be considered a dependent variable, an effect of the components of meditation: attentional training, posture, adherence, etc.

Further, one might argue that decreasing oxygen consumption is the main mediating mechanism and that this decreased oxygen consumption causes a variety of other physiological and subsequent cognitive changes to occur (Watanabe et al., 1972). However, other investigators have looked at oxygen consumption as a dependent variable, an effect of meditation (Pagano, 1978; Fenwick et al., 1977). Thus a given variable may be a component, a mediating mechanism, or an effect, depending *on how it is viewed.*

Therefore, it is critical that a context be formulated and made explicit before proceeding to answer questions about components and mediating mechanisms.

8.2 An Omni-Deterministic Model

THE CONTEXT I will be using in the next two chapters is an omnideterministic model of causality. This model is borrowed from several sources; first, it is indebted to general systems theory, as utilized in structural family therapy (Minuchin, 1974; Minuchin et al., 1978). Each part of the family is thought to influence and interact with the whole, and to focus on any one family member, without acknowledging and dealing with the family context, is seen as anathema to therapeutic success. Second, this model borrows from Skinner (1953, 1966) who outlined a three-form contingency model— functional analysis: antecedents, behavior, consequences. This temporal division previously utilized by Davidson and Goleman (1977) provides an additional helpful structure to our context. Third, Bandura (1978), suggested that our behavior is not solely a function of the environment—a unidirectional view of environment determining behavior; nor is it solely a function of the individual—a unidirectional view of the individual determining environment. Rather there is an interaction effect, a bi-directional model in which each part reciprocally determines the others. By adding an additional variable (cf. Black and Thoresen, Note Thirteen) of the behavior itself (in this case meditation), we have the following interactive model: (Figure 8.1).

E=Environment

P=Person

B=Behavior (meditation)

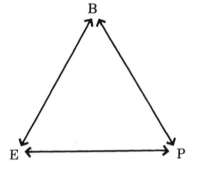

FIGURE 8.1 *An Omni-Determinism Model of Mediating Mechanisms of Meditation*

As an illustration of this model, let us consider the following. High demand characteristics from the external environment influence a person to a stronger belief about the possibilities of meditation, E → P. This belief influences the person's attentional behavior, P → B. The influence of the attentional behavior could in turn cause reduced physical movement, thereby reducing physiological tension. In this way, the behavior should help strengthen the person's attitude and commitment, B → P. Further, if an individual becomes more relaxed, he or she may get more social reinforcement, P → E, so that the individual is affecting the environment. This increased social reinforcement should help the individual continue adherence to the program and the behavior, E → P. And so the cycle continues. Further, the physical environment can have an effect (environmental planning) on the performance of the behavior, E → B, and as we have noted, the actual behavior can determine how the environment is perceived, B → E (cf. Anand, Chinna & Singh, 1961a; Kasamatsu & Hirai, 1966).

In simple terms, we create the environment that creates us. Therefore, I am proposing that we look at the components and mediating mechanisms of meditation as a multi-level process with several different physiological, cognitive, and attentional mechanisms occurring, often simultaneously. In this model it becomes difficult if not impossible to isolate any one most salient component or "one" mediating mechanism in order to determine a "first" cause. Thus, we have what in physics has been referred to as an organismic, omnideterminism, bootstrap theory (cf. Capra, 1976) in which each part effects all others.

I have restricted my discussion of the components of meditation to antecedent, preparatory variables and posture, attention, and breathing. This is a narrowly based definition of the "Components of Meditation." It excludes issues of expectation effects, demand characteristics, non-specific variables, etc. Some researchers rightly label these issues "confounding variables" that therefore should be appropriately discussed with methodological concerns. Some, again rightly, may label them "indirect" components associated with meditation, and therefore appropriately discussed in this chapter. I have chosen to discuss these "confounding variables and indirect components" as mechanisms mediating meditation's effects, and therefore discussed in Chapter Nine. However, as seen in Table 8.1, the "components" of meditation need to be placed within a context.

By breaking meditation into various components, we may be able to a) devise research which can designate the percentage of variance attributable to each component, thereby separating out active from inert variables; b) pinpoint unique aspects of meditation training as opposed to non-specific effects inherent in any self-regulation strategy (e.g., McFall et al., 1971).

8.3 Antecedent or Preparatory Variables

MOST RELIGIOUS traditions have a series of preparations which must be performed before an individual is thought to be ready to begin the spiritual practice of meditation (e.g., Goleman, 1971; Brown, 1977; Deikman, 1980 in press).

TABLE 8.1 *Meditation: An Omni-Determinism Analysis*

A. Antecedents: Variables Preceding Beginning to Meditate

   Psychological Variables
   1. Subject (Client) Variables
      1.1 Expectation Effects
      1.2 Initial Motivation
      1.3 Psychological Profile

   2. Therapist/Training Variables
      2.1 Demand Characteristics
      2.2 Required preparatory rituals (e.g., change of eating habits, lectures)
      2.3 Relationship

   3. Miscellaneous, non-specific variables: Additional placebo effects: e.g., structured training format, being part of a group, sociocultural values of society, etc.
   Physical Variables — Environmental planning — arrangement of the environment to facilitate the desired behavior.

B. Behaviors of Meditation
   Physical Posture
   1. *Movement*
   2. *Stabilized*
      2.1 *Lotus*
      2.2 *Half-Lotus*
      2.3 *Sitting*

   Attentional Focus
   1. *Specific object (e.g., mantra)*
      1.1 *Meaningful*
      1.2 *Meaningless*
   2. *Choiceless awareness*
   Attentional Style
   1. *Active*
   2. *Receptive*

   Regulation of Breathing
   1. *Ignored: "Automatic"*
   2. *Attentive: controlled*
   3. *Attentive: "automatic"*
   Adherence

| Note: the Asterisked (*) items refers to issues discussed in this chapter as components. |

C. Consequences
   Cognitions:
   Social reinforcement: peer pressure, etc.
   Physiological/behavioral/attitudinal changes

These preparations range from the highly structured and complex—changing dietary habits, cultivating feelings of love and compassion, decreasing thoughts of selfishness and greed—to much less complex—preparatory lectures and instructional training. One study (Smith, Note One) has already looked at the relationship between preparation and adherence. The results, discussed more fully in the section on adherence, suggest that the greater the preparation, the greater the adherence.

The primary physical-environmental variable involving antecedent preparation for meditation concerns the room or the place where meditation occurs. There has been no specific research looking at the effect of the actual environmental setting on the effects of meditation. However, environmental planning (stimulus cue) research is quite convincing (Shapiro & Zifferblatt, 1976b; Mahoney & Thoresen, 1974), and common sense as well as anecdotal experience suggest that the actual site in which meditation occurs should influence outcome. For example, a quiet, soundproof room would give one the opportunity to concentrate more effectively than if one were to attempt meditation initially in a more stimulus-demanding environment.

8.4 Posture

WHAT EFFECT DOES physical posture have on successful meditation practice? The Eastern literature believes that bodily self-regulation plays a strong role in determining the subsequent self-regulation of attention. As Ikegami (1973) noted, Zen practice derives very much from the fundamental teachings of the yoga school which suggests we need to "regulate the body in order to obtain peace of mind."

The only series of studies on the role of posture has been carried out by Ikegami (1973), so I report his findings here in some detail. Ikegami began by investigating the relative muscle tension of different postures ranging from lying down to standing. He found that the half-lotus position and the full lotus position and relaxed agura (which is sitting in a full lotus position but without the buttock on a pillow) all showed EMG activity about midway between a standing posture and a supine posture. Ikegami then devised an ingenious experiment in which subjects were asked to sit on a wooden disc which measured fluctuations in body movement. In summary, it was found that:

a) Experience and age of the practitioner had an effect in determining the amount of fluctuation: the more experienced the practitioner, the less that fluctuation occurred.

b) For the experienced meditator, the full lotus posture was the posture that maintained the most balance and best center of gravity.

Ikegami then tried to assess which posture was most stable for naive subjects. He held the attentional component constant by having naive subjects focus on a red digital lamp, and he had these subjects take three different postures, each for thirty minutes. The postures, assigned to the subjects in random order, were *seiza:* a sitting posture with the body weighing on the folded legs, and the buttocks resting on the heels;* *agura:* a cross-legged posture with the buttocks directly on the floor; and half lotus. The least fluctuation occurred in the half lotus and seiza positions.

Ikegami then raised a question regarding the role of attention on the effectiveness of the posture. Subjects were asked to sit in a half-lotus position under two different conditions: condition one involved concentration on a red digital lamp; condition two permitted free eye movement. Concentration on the lamp reduced fluctuation considerably. This study strongly suggests the importance of attentional focus in maintaining firm non-fluctuating posture. Ikegami suggested, however, that these effects may be reciprocally enhancing in that the posture allows one to concentrate better, and the concentration helps maintain a more non-fluctuating physical posture.

These studies raise two interesting and related points. The first question involves which posture is most "balanced and centered." It seems clear from Ikegami's work that the full lotus posture is the "most balanced" for experienced meditators. However, this is not true for naive meditators. Further, anecdotal and personal experiences make it clear that for inexperienced meditators the full lotus posture is more of a hindrance and distraction "to calming the mind" than a help. Further

---

*In the case of the male, the kneecaps are placed apart so the folded legs form the two sides of a triangle.

research should clarify the process and time sequence through which the lotus posture becomes an aid to meditation. The second question deals with the relationship between posture and attentional focus. As noted above, Ikegami first held attentional focus constant and varied posture. Then he held posture constant and varied attentional focus. This latter study showed the importance of attentional focus in posture. We now turn to the attentional literature to see what additional effects the attentional component may have on meditation outcome.

8.5 Attention

WE SAW IN THE previous section that attentional focus on an external object improved the stability of the posture (Ikegami, 1973). Several additional questions need to be addressed concerning the attention variable. For example, is there a relationship between improvement in concentration and clinical improvement? Does attentional absorption increase with practice? What is the type of attention primarily used during meditation—discriminating, analytical; or "holistic," global, intuitive? Are there certain individuals with a better ability to attend? Do they make better meditators? Are there different levels of concentration? Are there differences in the type of concentration involved during "concentrative" versus opening-up (mindfulness) meditation? Does it make any difference whether there is active or passive attention? Does it make any difference whether one stimulus is focused upon or whether a variety of complex stimuli are attended to? Does it make any difference in concentrative meditation whether the stimulus is internal or external?

The literature on meditation and attention has not always been sufficiently precise. Therefore, we need to be careful of our assumptions as we review it. Our definition in Chapter One assumed that attention is a component of meditation, and therefore, is at least in part responsible for its effects. However, others have looked at attention as an effect of meditation (Davidson et al., 1976). Others, as we discuss in Chapter Nine, have viewed it as a mediating mechanism. There have been six studies which look at the relationship between meditation and attention. Let us look at each of these in turn to see what information they might provide about the above questions.

8.5A LENGTH OF
MEDITATION AND
ATTENTIONAL ABSORPTION

Davidson et al., (1976) in a cross sectional design, compared those interested in meditation with those who had practiced meditation for either one month, from one to twenty-four months, or longer than two years. Using the Tellegan Absorption Scale (Tellegan & Atkins, 1974), it was found that more experienced meditators had significantly increased attentional absorption,* and that attentional absorption increased as the length of meditation experience increased. This study about increased ability to attend as one practices meditation is consistent with the physiological literature and the studies by Kasamatsu and Hirai (1966) and Anand et al., (1961a). Longer-term meditators seem to have a better developed ability to voluntarily control attention.

8.5B INCREASED ABILITY
TO ATTEND AND
CLINICAL IMPROVEMENT

Further, it appears that increased ability to attend is positively correlated with clinical improvement (Vahia et al., 1973). Vahia had each of the patients in his study write in their notebooks all thoughts which occurred and disturbed their concentration during their meditation-like practice. Two psychiatrists, who had no knowledge of the patients' improvement, then studied these notebooks several months after the training was over. They noted whether or not there was an improvement or not in concentration during the course of the four-week treatment. A correlation was then made between concentration and clinical improvement which showed that clinical improvement was closely related to improvement in concentration.

---

*It should be noted that absorption is a precise technical term used in classical Eastern texts to describe a specific concentrative state of consciousness which occurs with increasing depth as one attains different jhānas (Goleman, 1972).

8.5C CONCENTRATIVE VERSUS
    OPENING-UP MEDITATION:
    DOES IT MAKE ANY DIFFERENCE
    WHAT THE INDIVIDUAL ATTENDS TO?

It is quite clear from the studies of Kasamatsu and Hirai (1966) and Anand, Chinna and Singh (1961a) that there are pronounced physiological differences between concentrative and opening-up meditation. Whether these differences generalize to the post-meditation period awaits further research.* Further, it appears that during non-meditating time, the Rāja Yogins in Anand, Chinna and Singh's study, and also TM meditators in a study by Wallace (1970), are able to dehabituate to stimuli as well as those who practice opening-up meditation.

Are those who practice opening-up meditation equally able to focus intensely to the exclusion of other stimuli in the environment? Or are different attentional styles being employed in each type of meditation (Pribram & McGinnis, 1975)? How much does one type of learning generalize to the other type? As Brown noted (1977), there is some neurophysiological evidence distinguishing different styles of meditation and the two different modes of awareness—receptive versus active focusing. Two major cortical control mechanisms for the sub-cortical mechanisms involved in selecting and processing information have been reported: a frontal system associated with restrictive processing and a posterior temporal system associated with more wide-ranging information-processing (Pribram, 1971). Brown goes on to note, "The brain may be likened to a camera. It can use either a wide angle lens or a zoom. Or, in cognitive terms, attention can be directed to the more dominant details of the stimulus field or to the entire field" (1977, p. 266). Thus different meditation systems may train different attentional styles.

---

*These post-meditation effects have not yet been documented in Western research literature. However, descriptive information of different post meditation effects on behavior and personality change are available in the classical Eastern texts (see Goleman, 1972, 1977).

8.5D DIFFERENT TYPES OF CONCENTRATIVE
MEDITATION: MANTRA VERSUS NON-MANTRA;
ACTIVE VERSUS PASSIVE FOCUSING

Stroebel and Glueck (1977) suggest that the mantra may be the key variable in the effectiveness of meditation. This was tested in a study by Smith (1976) which looked specifically at the mantra's component role in the effectiveness of meditation. In the first experiment, Smith compared a TM group which focused on a mantra with a PSI group (Periodic Somatic Inactivity) which received similar expectation effects and just sat without any specific instructions to focus on a mantra. In the second experiment, Smith taught two groups what he called "cortically mediated stabilization" (CMS). Specifically, group one (CMS-1) was asked to sit with eyes closed and focus on a mantra—shanti. Group two (CMS-2) was asked to sit with eyes closed and to "engage in thought activity that you intend to be positive . . . fantasy-daydream, story telling, and listening " (Smith, 1976, p. 634). In the first experiment, he found no differences between groups on anxiety scores, symptoms of striate muscle tension, or measures of autonomic arousal. Similarly, in the second experiment, he found no differences between groups on trait anxiety, symptoms of striate muscle tension, and measures of autonomic arousal. The first experiment suggests that it may not be the attentional focusing on a mantra that is the effective component in meditation (cf. West, 1979). The second experiment suggests that focusing on a specific stimulus in a passive manner (mantra) may be equally effective to focusing in an active manner on a variety of stimuli— positive fantasies, thoughts, etc. The second experiment raises a question of whether voluntary regulation of attention may be more important than the nature of the stimuli attended to, whether stimuli are attended to passively or actively.*

An unpublished study by Schwartz, Davidson, and Margolin (Note Six) suggests results somewhat different from Smith's. In this study there were three groups of ten subjects. Group one

---

*There is some question, however, whether Smith's second group was really "anti-meditation" since, as noted in Chapter One, conscious focus of attention is at least part of our definition of meditation. For further discussion of what constitutes a "control" group, see Chapter Ten.

included teachers of Transcendental Meditation who had practiced for at least two years; this group focused in a passive way on an internal mantra. Group two consisted of those trained in a Gurdjieffian form of meditation, involving active voluntary control of attention through a restricted range of somatic and other stimuli. In this study all subjects were required to attend to either a kinesthetic stimulus (sensations in the right hand) or a visual stimulus (photograph of a person). For both groups, during kinesthetic attention, the ratio of occipital to sensory-motor alpha was significantly higher, suggesting activation of the sensory-motor region. During the visual tasks there was relatively greater occipital activation. Further, there was, as predicted, a significantly greater activation of the respective brain regions for the Gurdjieffian meditation group than for the TM group.* The finding of greater cortical specificity in these subjects compared to Transcendental Meditation and control subjects seems consistent with the active versus passive nature of the attentional component in the techniques practiced (Davidson & Goleman, 1977; also Davidson, Schwartz, & Rothman, 1976). Davidson suggested that, "different meditation techniques may lead to the cultivation of different attentional skills which are reflected in a particular patterning of neural processes" (Davidson, Goleman & Schwartz, 1976, p. 238).

How might we account for these seemingly different findings between Smith's study (1976) and Schwartz, Davidson and Margolin's (Note Six)? Or the fact that in Smith's first experiment comparing PSI (just sit) versus focus (TM mantra) there was no difference between groups, whereas in Ikegami's experiment, just-sit versus focus (red light) there were changes?

There are two specific difficulties in comparing the above studies. The first relates to the sensitivity of the dependent variable. As Smith himself noted, when using trait anxiety as a dependent variable, it may be difficult to find changes in periods ranging from eleven weeks to six months, whereas in Schwartz, Davidson and Margolin's study EEG measures were being used. In Ikegami's study, the minute fluctuations, millimeters in physical posture, also provide a more sensitive dependent variable.

---

*Or, as the authors note, the results of the study may merely reflect a subject-selection bias, an increased ability for attentional absorption on the part of the Gurdjieffian group.

A second problem to be addressed is determining what actually happens with the "just-sitting" group. For example, we know that even when individuals are instructed to concentrate on a specific object, the mind often wanders, other thoughts occur. Might the just-sit group also, during their own process of "sitting relaxation" find something to focus on? Maybe they begin to generate positive daydreams, similar to those in Smith's CMS-2 study. Further, just sitting may not be a viable control group because it is in fact a type of Zen Meditation—Shikan-taza (Kapleau, 1967). Also, when "just sitting" is done, and thoughts occur, it may be no different than any other mantra meditation in which thoughts occur, especially if the individual "by chance" picks one thought or object to focus on for the majority of the session. Therefore, the just-sitting group may not be a control group at all, and a debriefing of the just-sitting group may be necessary to determine the degree to which they are consciously directing attention.

8.5E TYPE OF ATTENTION
UTILIZED DURING MEDITATION

In the first study to look specifically at attentional style during meditation,* Maupin (1965) found that attention measures did not predict response to meditation. His measures of attention—digit span, continuous additions, and size estimation—may not have been appropriate measures of type of attention involved. As Van Nuys (1973) suggested, a certain type of attention is necessary for meditation: sustained non-analytic attention, whereas the Strupp and Witkin test involves tasks that necessitate a constant and rapid shifting of attention. Also, such tasks invite discursive, analytical thought. In his study, Van Nuys had subjects focus for fifteen minutes on a candle, and then, after fifteen minutes debriefing, on their breathing. Subjects were asked to push a button noting when they had an intrusion that distracted them from the task at hand. He noted a .91 negative correlation between number of thought intrusions in

---

*The Deikman study (1966) did look at attention (in terms of how well individuals were able to reduce distracting external sounds). However, the prime focus of his study was the phenomenology of meditation.

meditation and hypnotic susceptibility measures. It appears that there was a large variability among subjects, but good hypnotic subjects on the average tended to experience fewer intrusions during meditation than poor ones.*

The Witkin Embedded Figure Test, requiring subjects to be able to pick out a certain form from the context of a distracting stimulus background, is another measure often used to assess attentional change resulting from meditation. At its most concrete level, the test measures field dependence and independence. Results indicate that meditators become signficantly more field independent (Pelletier, 1974; Linden, 1973).

However, the generalizations drawn from this finding and the hypotheses used to justify it may at first appear quite confusing and contradictory. For example, Linden (1973) hypothesized that since the subject's meditation practice trains the individual to focus attention on an object or process (figure) and to resist distracting sources of stimulation (background), meditation might be expected to enhance field independence, which reflects a general disposition to perceive and think in an articulate as opposed to a non-analytic fashion (Witkin et al., 1962). However, Van Nuys' study (1973), in which there was no correlation between the Strupp and Witkin test and the ability to concentrate, accounted for the results by arguing that the Embedded Figures Test is an analytical and discursive test with rapid shifts of attention whereas meditation involves a more pinpointed focus. Therefore different types of attentional training are involved. How can we account for these contradictory findings and theories? Although this issue is dealt with in more detail in the section on mediating mechanisms—discrimination training and hemisphere function—let me suggest here that we might explain these seeming contradictions by noting that although meditation might have a non-analytical focus of attention as a goal, some analysis and discrimination may be necessary to achieve this goal.

---

*Van Nuys assumed that better attenders have fewer intrusions. Might the opposite be the case: the better the attenders, the more they were able to discriminate their attention wandering, and therefore the higher number of intrusions reported?

8.5G ADDITIONAL QUESTIONS ON ATTENTION: IDEAS FOR FUTURE RESEARCH

Many unanswered questions related to attention remain for future research to address. For example, there have not yet been sufficiently well controlled studies to determine whether there are actual differences in clinical outcome depending on whether the focus of attention is internal or external (cf. Leung, 1973), say on breathing or a candle (cf. Van Nuys, 1973). Another important area for future research in the case of concentrative meditation may be to match a person's dominant sensory representational system, be it auditory, kinesthetic or visual with concentrative focus in a non-dominant system (cf. Branstrom, Note Seven). Further research may also wish to investigate the specific cortical training involved in different types of attentional style (cf. Davidson & Goleman, 1977), and to determine whether there is generalization from skill in one mode (non-analytical, single-pointed) to skill in another mode (analytical, discursive). The hypothesized connection between attentional style and hemispheric functioning (Galin, 1974) also awaits documentation. Further, in studies such as Smith's (1976), it would be useful to have a measure of attentional absorption (Tellegen & Atkinson, 1974) or number of intrusions (Van Nuys, 1973; Kubose, 1976) to determine how well the individual is actually concentrating. Future research also needs to look at whether the pinpointed attentional focus on a specific object, say a mantra, is *as effective* in producing successful clinical outcome as discursive thinking about a complex variety of stimuli, say positive daydreaming, fantasy and listening, (cf. Smith, 1976; Goldman, Domitor & Murray, 1979; Boswell et al., 1979). And both need to be compared with opening-up (mindful) meditations.

Another issue raised about the nature of attention in meditation is whether the attentional level is one of drowsiness and lowered arousal, bordering on but not involving sleep (Fenwick et al., 1977) and at the same time, a state of sustained attention (Williams & West, 1975). Is it possible to maintain a combined state of low arousal and high attention—a restful alertness? The work of Hirai (1974), following up on the previous study of Kasamatsu and Hirai (1966), suggests that meditators are able to maintain attentional awareness, a cortical activity, without emotional arousal, a limbic activity, whether the presenting stimulus

is a click, supposedly neutral or a word of high affect, for example their own name. However, an alternative explanation, and
one which may be plausible for concentrative but not opening-up
meditation techniques, is that the clinical success is not due to
calm attentional focus on an object, but rather on cognitive
avoidance. For example, research suggests that a "competing"
focus helps individuals to tolerate pain (Kanfer & Goldfoot, 1966)
or to reduce fears (Yulis et al., 1975). Further research will need
to precisely define the meditation technique and look carefully at
the attentional style involved.

Finally, additional studies, such as Schwartz, Davidson and
Margolin's (Note Six), comparing different techniques with different attentional styles, need to be undertaken. For example,
based on a distinction made by Bagchi (1936) between passive
attention versus "strained" attention, what differences in effects
would we find between the awareness involved in a passive
meditation technique such as TM, compared to a more active,
devotional meditation technique like Bhakti meditation? What
about the difference between focus on a word without meaning
like the TM mantra for Westerners versus focusing on a word
with meaning (cf. Elson, Hauri & Cunis, 1977)? Or the difference
between focus on a self-selected mantra like om versus the spontaneous attentional focus of choiceless awareness?

8.6 Breathing

ONE ADDITIONAL component, which has been largely
ignored in the research literature, *as a component,* is
the role of breathing. Some traditions such as Zen, place a great
deal of importance on breathing. Breath becomes the object of
awareness, and the individual is told to breathe "spontaneously"
and easily. Breath regulation is seen as one of the critical components (e.g., Nakamizo, 1974, Mastumoto, 1974). In Benson's
technique (Benson, 1975), the individual is instructed to count
one on each outbreath. In Transcendental Meditation, breathing
is not directly attended to. In many Yoga traditions, great importance is placed upon voluntary control of breathing, for example, Swan Yoga.

In the one study comparing different types of breathing (Timmons et al., 1972), it was found that diaphragmatic breathing, as

opposed to thoracic, was associated more with EEG alpha. However, the exact role of breathing as a component of meditation awaits further research.

8.7 Summary

THIS CHAPTER has suggested the complexity of component variables, their context, and their interactions, all operating in relationship to the effectiveness of meditation. For example, preparatory behaviors may increase adherence (Smith, Note One), adherence may increase both attentional concentration and posture stability, (Davidson, Goleman & Schwartz, 1977; Ikegami, 1973). If I may take the liberty of an over-generalization about opportunities for research in this area, it seems the type of research that will ultimately be most productive is one which looks at the components listed in Table 8.1, alone, and in various combinations, and determines, through multivariate and multifactorial studies, the specific variance of outcome success due to the various components as well as their interaction with each other.

Chapter Eight: Further Readings

POSTURE

Ikegami, R., Psychological studies of Zen posture. In Y. Akishige *Psychological studies on Zen.* Tokyo, Japan: Kyushu University, Department of Psychology, 1973, 105-135. (Reprinted in D.H. Shapiro & R.N. Walsh [Eds.], *The science of meditation.* New York, Aldine, 1980).

ATTENTION

Pelletier, K. Influence of Transcendental Meditation upon auto-kinetic perception. *Perceptual & Motor Skills,* 1974, *39,* 1031-1034. (Reprinted in D.H. Shapiro & R.N. Walsh, [Eds.], *The science of meditation.* New York: Aldine, 1980).

Davidson, R., Goleman, D. & Schwartz, G. Attentional and affective concomitants of meditation. *Journal of Abnormal Psychology,* 1976, *85,* 235-238. (Reprinted in D.H. Shapiro & R.N. Walsh, [Eds.], *The science of meditation,* New York: Aldine, 1980).

Davidson, R. & Goleman, D. The role of attention in meditation and hypnosis: A psychobiological perspective of transformations of consciousness. *International Journal of Clinical & Experimental Hypnosis,* 1977, *25,* (4), 291-308. (Reprinted in D.H. Shapiro & R.N. Walsh, [Eds.], *The science of meditation.* New York: Aldine, 1980).

Smith, J. Psychotherapeutic effects of Transcendental Meditation with controls for expectation of relief and daily sitting. *Journal of Consulting & Clinical Psychology,* 1976, *44,* 630-637. (Reprinted in D.H. Shapiro & R.N. Walsh, [Eds.], *The science of meditation.* New York: Aldine, 1980).

ENVIRONMENTAL VARIABLES

Shapiro, D.H. & Zifferblatt, S.M. Zen meditation and behavioral self-control: Similarities, differences, clinical applications. *American Psychologist,* 1976, *3,* 519-532. (Reprinted in D.H. Shapiro & R.N. Walsh, [Eds.], *The science of meditation.* New York: Aldine, 1980).

BREATHING

Timmons, B. et al. Abdominal, thoracic respiratory movements and levels of arousal. *Psychonomic Science,* 1972, *27,* 173-175.
Matsumoto, H. A psychological study of the relation between respiratory function and emotion. *Bulletin of the Faculty of Literature of Kyushu University,* 1974, *5,* 167-207.

9

Mediating
Mechanisms

9.1 An Overview

WHY DOES meditation work? Why do the components discussed in Chapter Eight cause the effects discussed in Chapters Five and Seven? Is there any way we can determine whether any one mediating mechanism is significantly salient compared to another?

The list of possible mechanisms mediating meditation's effects is quite lengthy. These explanations as to "why" meditation works include the following: a) a constellation of physiological changes which, taken collectively, constitute a "hypometabolic" state, a relaxation response (Benson, 1975); b) a single physiological change considered to be a primary mediator: oxygen consumption (Watanabe et al., 1972); skeletal muscular relaxation (Davidson, 1976); c) cognitive factors, including the role of self-instruction (Shapiro & Zifferblatt, 1976; Meichenbaum, 1975; Ellis, in press, 1980, Boals, 1978); d) attentional components (Davidson, Goleman & Schwartz, 1976) including global desensitization (Goleman, 1971); the information-processing mechanisms literature (Brown, 1977); sensory deprivation via steady visual fixation and/or repeated auditory stimulation (Piggins & Morgan, 1977); discrimination (Hendricks, 1975);

deautomatization and bimodal consciousness (Deikman, 1971, 1966); sustained nonanalytic attending (Spanos et al., 1978); e) regression in the service of the ego (Maupin, 1965; Lesh, 1970); f) general arousal (Fischer, 1971) and ergotropic/trophotropic shifts (Davidson, 1976); g) sleep (Pagano et al., 1975); h) hemispheric lateralization (Pagano & Frumkin, 1977; Bennett & Trinder, 1977; Galin, 1974); i) interhemispheric synchrony (Haymes, 1977); j) expectation effects (Smith, 1976); k) demand characteristics (Orne, 1962; Malec & Sipprelle, 1977); l) daydreaming (Singer, 1975); m) specific neural activation patterns involving heightened cortical arousal with decreased limbic arousal (Glueck & Stroebel, 1975; Schwartz, 1975; Goleman & Schwartz, 1976); n) habituation, including the ganzfeld experiments (Ornstein, 1971; Anand, Chinna & Singh, 1961a; Banquet, 1973); o) disidentifications from mental content (Walsh, 1977, 1978); p) imagery (Holt, 1964; DiGiusto & Bond, 1979); q) adherence; and r) "non-specific" variables such as structured training format, being part of a group and resultant exposure to other patients practicing the techniques (Galanter & Buckley, 1978), a society's socio-cultural values, the passage of time, and the regulation of lifestyle, including the subject's willingness to adapt to the regimentation of daily sitting.

As noted in Chapter Eight, based on an omni-deterministic model, these variables interact with each other and often occur simultaneously in a multi-level hierarchy. However, because writing and reading require a linear mode, I discuss these mechanisms separately. Further, where an individual has hypothesized a principal or first-cause "underlying" mechanism, this is noted and discussed.

9.2 Physiological Mechanisms

9.2A GENERAL CONSTELLATION OF CHANGES

AS NOTED IN the effects section, Chapter Five, during meditation itself, certain physiological changes have been rather consistently reported. They number *reduced heart rate:* Wallace, 1970; Anand, Chinna & Singh, 1961a; Wegner & Bagchi, 1961; Goyeche, Chihara & Shimizu, 1972; Karambelkar, Vinekar & Bhole, 1968; Das & Gastaut, 1955; Bagchi & Wenger, 1957; *decreased oxygen consumption:* Wallace, Benson & Wilson,

1971; Wallace, 1970; Wenger & Bagchi, 1961; Goyeche, Chihara & Shimizu, 1972; Anand, Chinna & Singh, 1961a; Sugi & Akutsu, 1968; Watanabe, Shapiro & Schwartz, 1972; Allison, 1970; Treichel, Clinch & Cran, 1973; Hirai, 1974; *decreased blood pressure:* Wallace, Benson & Wilson, 1971; Wenger and Bagchi, 1961; Karambelkar, Vinekar & Bhole, 1968; Bagchi and Wenger, 1957; *increased skin resistance:* Wallace, Benson, and Wilson, 1971; Wallace, 1970; Wenger and Bagchi, 1961; Karambelkar, Vinekar and Bhole, 1968; Bagchi and Wenger, 1957; Akishige, 1970; Orme-Johnson, 1973; and *increased regularity and amplitude of alpha activity:* Wallace et al., 1971; Wallace, 1970; Anand, Chinna and Singh, 1961a; Das and Gastaut, 1955; Bagchi and Wenger, 1957; Watanabe, Shapiro and Schwartz, 1972; Hirai, 1974; Akishige, 1970; Kasamatsu and Hirai, 1966; Banquet, 1972; 1973; Williams and West, 1975. It has been hypothesized that these physiological changes during meditation produce a "hypo-metabolic state" (Wallace et al., 1971) or a state of relaxation (Benson, Beary & Carol, 1974). This relaxed state has been considered the central mediating mechanism accounting for meditation's clinical effects, whether for managing stress (e.g., Girodo, 1974), reducing alcohol consumption (Marlatt et al., in press, 1980), decreasing hypertension (Benson et al., 1974a), or aiding psychotherapy (Glueck & Stroebel, 1975; Vahia et al., 1973).

9.2B SPECIFIC PHYSIOLOGICAL VARIABLES

OXYGEN CONSUMPTION:

WATANABE, SHAPIRO and Schwartz (1972) suggested that the reduction of oxygen consumption which occurred in all forms of meditation was the single most important factor in producing the accompanying psycho-physiological changes. Similarly, Kasamatsu and Hirai (1966) and Rao (1968) noted that when air is breathed at high altitudes under reduced pressure, oxygen is lowered and an increase of alpha activity is observed. Certainly there has been a great deal of literature showing that oxygen consumption is reduced during meditation.*

---

*Wallace et al. 1971; Wenger and Bagchi, 1961; Sugi et al. 1968; Allison, 1970; Trichel, 1973; Hirai, 1974; Fenwick et al. 1977.

With regard to respiration, Nakamizo (1968) noted that the ratio of exhalation to inhalation increases during meditation so that the body is literally emptied of air. Timmons et al. (1972) noted a correlation of EEG alpha with increased abdominal, decreased thoracic breathing, a pattern which occurs during meditation.

Certainly, breathing is considered an important variable in most meditation traditions. Both the Zen and Yoga traditions place great emphasis on breathing, counting, observing, or concentrating upon breaths, and in some sects, even hyperventilating. However, at this point, it seems premature to look at oxygen consumption as *the* primary variable inducing subsequent muscular, electro-cortical, and electro-dermal changes. For example, why might not lowered oxygen consumption be merely a function of a lowered arousal level and lowered metabolism?

SKELETAL RELAXATION:

A second variable posited as the primary mediating mechanism is skeletal musculature relaxation (Davidson, 1976). Davidson bases this theory on Gelhorn and Kiely (1972), suggesting the central role of proprioceptive input from the muscles in maintaining ergotropic activation. This ergotropic activation involves a coordinated complex of sympathetic visceral, cerebral, behavioral and skeletal muscle reactions. Curare-like drugs which immobolize skeletal muscles inhibit any responsiveness. Davidson suggested that "a positive feedback loop appears to be operating here in that increased muscle tone produces diffuse ergotropic activation, while the latter induced by other means results in increased muscle tone" (Davidson, 1976). Also, the resulting lower level of muscular activity in meditation may be the cause of the reported decrease in oxygen consumption. He cites as evidence the fact that muscular relaxation has been documented in several studies showing very low electro-myographic activity (Datey et. al., 1969; Das & Gastaut, 1955; Akishige, 1968). In the two studies which have compared oxygen consumption in meditation and Progressive Relaxation, both groups' oxygen consumption decreased (Pagano et al., Note Fourteen; Fee & Girdano, 1978) This finding certainly is not sufficient to justify a primary role for muscular relaxation, but it does suggest it might be one of the mechanisms having a mediating effect.

However, some question exists about the exact connection between muscular relaxation, as first clinically studied by Jacobson (1929), and resultant decrease in autonomic level arousal (cf. Connor, 1974). For example, in the Fee and Girdano (1978) study, muscle tension was significantly reduced with both meditation and EMG biofeedback, but there was a significant decrease in respiration rate only with meditators.

Further, the studies of Ikegami (1973) suggest that the skeletal muscles are maximally relaxed consistent only with the maintenance of the specific posture in which the individual holds him/herself. Ikegami's work showed that the most geometrically stable of the postures, the full lotus, yields the most even distribution of muscular activity and the least random muscle noise. In addition, Glueck and Stoebel (1975) noted that meditation does not seem to be effective for migraine headaches, whereas EMG biofeedback is. Brown (1977) hypothesized, in contrast to the relaxation effects of EMG biofeedback and hypnosis where global muscle tension can be significantly reduced (Green, Green, & Walters, 1970), that realigning and holding fast the meditation posture may not be technically relaxing in the sense of reduced muscle activity. For example, in a study that Davidson cited to support his theory (Datey et al., 1969) breathing exercises were done in a supine posture, not in a sitting or lotus posture.

However, Morse et al. (1977) found meditators did evidence less muscle activity than relaxation or self-hypnosis groups, suggesting that meditation is an effective means of muscle relaxation in the fontalis and temporal regions, and Zaichkowsky and Kamen (1978) found TM and Benson meditation to be as effective as biofeedback in decreasing frontalis muscle tension. Therefore, although it appears that muscular relaxation may be a mediating mechanism, it seems premature at this point to label it as *the* primary mechanism.

9.2C ERGOTROPIC/TROPHOTROPIC STATES

Some additional comments seem appropriate here regarding the trophotropic and ergotropic states. Fischer (1971) and Davidson (1976) describe this theory based on Hess (1938) and, later, Gellhorn and Kiely (1972). The trophotropic state is one of quiescence and relaxation, what Benson (1975) referred to as the relaxation response, and what Wallace et al. (1971) called the hypometabolic state. This state is assumed to involve an integrated hypothalamic response, inhibition of the sympathetic nervous system (Fischer, 1971), and perhaps increased parasympathetic arousal (Benson, 1975) as well as autonomic stability (Orme-Johnson, 1973).

However, some data are at first glance paradoxical or at least unclear. For example, in some studies correlating EEG with subjective experience (Banquet, 1973), generalized fast frequencies of the dominant beta rhythm during states of deep meditation and transcendence were found. A brief report (Das and Gastaut, 1955) reported a similar finding, as did a recent study by Corby et al. (1978). How do we account for this high activation, ergotropic activity in a technique usually intended in Western use* to produce a hypometabolic state of trophotropic activity?

Fischer (1971) tried to explain this by saying that "altered-state experiences" could occur at both ends of an arousal continuum, either at low arousal or at high arousal. Davidson elaborated on this model, suggesting that there was a shift involved from low arousal to high arousal or vice-versa. He based his theory on Gelhorn's model of either an "imbalance resulting from an intense, prolonged trophotropic activation, or the postulated rebound of the ergotropic system, whereby *after cessation* of key excitation, strong ergotropic activation supervenes" (Davidson, 1976, p. 28). This is a finding which may be supported by the work of Schwartz (1973, Note Eight) in which he found higher beta activation after meditation in meditators than in the just-sitting control group.

Davidson (1976) noted that there are certain examples of mystical states of consciousness which occur as a result of intense activity: Sufis' whirling dervish dancing (Naranjo, 1971), and Ishiguro Zen, which includes prolonged shouting and violent abdominal contractions (Akishige, 1968). Davidson suggests that

---

*In Eastern models, meditation is seen as a technique to produce *balance;* via mindfulness, between energy, investigation, rapture, and tranquility, equanimity, concentration (Buddhaghosa, 1976; Kornfield, 1978.)

in these cases the approach to the mystical experience would be ergotropic (E). However, Davidson then suggested, based on work by Sargent (1974), that when people undergo extreme excitation, induced either by psychologic or intense sensory stimuli, a stage is reached in which the subject collapses and extreme changes of mental and physical state supervene, involving altered states of consciousness and greatly heightened suggestibility. Davidson suggested that experiences of altered states of consciousness may be approached from either the E or the T side. For example, a rapid E to T shift is found in orgasm. The opposite switch from T (relative) to E dominance is seen in the transition from slow wave to REM sleep, accompanied by profound alteration in consciousness; and, in sensory deprivation for example, where hallucinogenic activity is correlated with increased E activity.

This model, though provocative as a theory to explain variables mediating meditation's "altered-state" effects, needs further research and specification. In particular, we need to become more precise about our definition of mystical states and ensure we are not lumping quite different types of experience—hallucinogenic, dreamlike, orgastic, meditative—under the same rubric. Further, it seems that the variable of arousal may not be sufficiently precise. For example, Schwartz, Davidson & Goleman (1978) have suggested that there are both somatic and cognitive components to arousal. These somatic components may be further subdivided into autonomic and skeletal (Borkovec, 1976); the cognitive components may be separated into left and right hemisphere arousal. In addition, based on their recent research on advanced meditators showing a simultaneous increase of urinary catecholamines (representing increased sympathetic arousal) and decrease in heart rate reduction (suggesting increased activation of the parasympathetic nervous system), Land, Dehof, Meurer, and Kaufmann (1979) suggest that meditation may cause an increase in both the sympathetic *and* parasympathetic systems. Finally, as Davidson (1976) himself noted, even if these "global" physiological shifts did occur, the cognitive interpretation that one places on them would be an additional mediating variable. We now turn to the literature on cognitions, in order to assess their role as a mediating mechanism of meditation.

9.3 Cognitions

> We are what we think.
> All that we are arises with our thoughts.
> With our thoughts we make the world.
>
> *Buddha (Dhammapada, 1976)*

THOSE OF US who have ever spent more than a few moments closing our eyes and just watching our minds, have some knowledge of the ceaseless and largely uncontrollable flux of thoughts, emotions, and images which continuously but usually only semiconsciously fills and controls our awareness (Walsh, 1977; 1978). Sometimes these take a definite pattern such as purposeful daydreams (Singer, 1975). Sometimes they seem random and incoherent. Within the social learning tradition, several clinicians have suggested the importance of teaching clients how to utilize thoughts (Meichenbaum, 1976; Mahoney, 1974; Ellis, 1962) and images (Cautela, 1967, Ellis, in press 1980; Lazarus, 1978) in precise ways to facilitate desired behavior change. What about the meditation traditions? Certainly, as suggested by the above quote, Buddha recognized the importance of thoughts. What, then, are meditators taught to think and how are they taught to "react" to thoughts?

Meditators are taught that uncontrolled thoughts act as an unrecognized filter which distorts their perception of reality. Thus, uncontrolled thoughts, analysis, and intellect are viewed as hindering a person in his/her search for "true" meaning and reality. Meditators are taught, at least indirectly through modeling, to give themselves cognitions and self-instructions such as, "Do not focus your attention on thoughts, but on the source from which they derive," "You are not your thoughts" (they are epiphenomena), "Watch them, accept them, let them go."

At least in the initial stages of meditation, the meditator continues to have thoughts. However, he or she has now learned a "meta-cognition" to say every time one of these thoughts is discriminated. Therefore, when beginning to meditate, a person may say to him or herself, "I'll never be a good meditator, I'm no good at anything." Once they become aware of that thought, they then may think the meta-cognition, "That's just another thought, let it go" or "thinking, thinking; judging, judging." In essence, the individual is practicing instruction him/herself to stay detached from the thoughts (Shapiro & Zifferblatt, 1976b; Meichenbaum, 1976; Ellis, 1980, in press), either giving "meta-cognitions" as above, or self-instructions relating to returning attention to the task at hand, "keep focused, relax, stay calm," (cf. case study, Chapter Three). The role of these meta-cognitions is insufficiently acknowledged in the Eastern tradition, where it is globally stated that one is to invest less importance in thoughts. Aside from koans, the role of thoughts or self-instructions as a mediating mechanism for reducing thoughts is never explicitly stated.

In addition to thoughts during meditation, there are also thoughts before and after meditation which may mediate outcome. Premeditation thoughts may be thought of in terms of *expectations* and belief systems.

As discussed in Chapter Eight, prior to meditation there are certain preparatory trainings which, whether implicitly or explicitly, set forth a certain vision (i.e. demands) for the student, who is to understand that if these meditation disciplines are correctly practiced, certain positive consequences will follow (Orne, 1962, Franks, 1963). These demands may cause certain expectations for the student. Further, based on self-perception (Bem, 1972) and cognitive dissonance theory (Festinger, 1962), the engaging in preparatory actions such as changing one's eating habits or paying a large initiation fee may cause one to feel that one would never expend so much effort unless the training was significantly valuable.

Further, Shapiro and Giber (1978), discussing research on meditation and the addictions (e.g., Benson and Wallace, 1972), note that there is a strong likelihood that instructions in the initial preparatory training of Transcendental Meditation—stating that drug use adversely affects meditation performance—may have a strong influence on a) the individual's drug taking behavior and/or b) the retrospective self-report of drug usage. Similarly, in the study by Kohr (1977), certain meditators of the Indian tradition noted "vibrations" and warmth at points along their spine, near the "chakras." Might there be a connection between this philosophical system which suggests the importance of the chakras and the actual experiences of the mediator?

In addition, as with biofeedback (Blanchard and Young, 1974) and psychotherapeutic outcomes (Bergin and Garfield, 1971), the individual's belief that a cure is possible may also be an important aspect of the expectation effect. This effect may be intimately related to promotion, in which organizations outline elaborate testimonials of success: in effect, demand characteristics (cf. Smith, 1976; Malec & Sipprelle, 1977). These belief systems (premeditation cognitions) might include the following kinds of self-statements: a) an altered state of consciousness does exist, b) the practice of meditation will help me in attaining that altered state, and c) this altered state and its effects will help me be more the person I would like to be. Also, motivation, cognitions about how much an individual wants to succeed, may to a certain extent determine intention and arousal level, which may in turn mediate variables such as attention. Further, premeditation cognitions may include certain decisions, such as self-contracting, in terms of how long the person wishes to meditate, where, and how often.

Demand characteristics (expectation effects) may influence meditative outcome in two other ways. The first way is the type of "cognitive set" which the meditation disciplines attempt to give to beginning meditators. Specifically, meditation traditions often note that thoughts and images are a hindrance to successful practice. Statements such as, "Be aware of your beliefs," "Do not take ideas too seriously," "Merely focus on focusing," are standard. If an individual believes this message, he or she will likely have a different reaction to thoughts than individuals who, like most in our culture, are at least implicitly instructed to take thoughts seriously.

Second, literature on hypnosis presents evidence that belief in the "magicalness" or "mysticalness" of a technique may contribute to successful outcome, so disrobing meditation of its mystical garb may reduce its effectiveness for those people to whom the mystery is part of the attraction (Katz, Note Two, 1978; Barber & Calverly, 1964). For some individuals the context of religion itself is as important in treatment outcome as the meditation technique itself (Galanter & Buckley, 1978).

EXPECTATION EFFECTS/
DEMAND CHARACTERISTICS

Demand characteristics comprise a relatively confusing issue to separate out from expectation effects. Demand characteristics may be said to come from the external environment—teacher, training organization; expectation effects are the beliefs the subject brings to the practice. We can assess demand characteristics by looking at promotional written statements and verbal and non-verbal cues during the training session. We can assess the subject's expectations by a simple questionnaire. However, there is an obvious interaction between these two and the exact variance and influence of each may be empirically unresolvable (Wilkins, 1978).

One case study (Ikegami, 1973) and one control-group study (Malec and Sipprelle, 1977) have tried to assess the effects of "demand" characteristics on treatment outcome; several other studies with "uniform" demand characteristics across different treatments have tried to create similar expectation effects in subjects (Smith, 1976; Goldman et al. 1979; Boswell & Murray, 1979).

But all these studies assume that presenting uniform demand characteristics automatically controls for expectation effects. A critical mediating variable assessed in only one study is the subjects' belief in the treatment (Kirsch & Henry, 1979). Though experimenters believe their anti-meditation or control-group rationale is credible, subjects may not in fact find it so. Further, Kirsh and Henry (1979), using a credibility questionnaire adapted from Borkovic & Nau (1972), have shown that the subjective estimates of anxiety reduction were augmented by the degree to which subjects perceived the treatment rationale to be credible, thereby suggesting a clear relationship between expectation effects and treatment outcome.

Let us now look at examples of studies that try to assess and/or control for demand characteristics. In Malec and Sipprelle's study (1977) forty students were assigned to one of four groups: a just-sit control group and three meditation groups. The first meditation group was asked to meditate after viewing a videotape demonstrating the Zen exercise "counting breaths" followed by a relaxation outcome. The second group was asked to meditate after viewing a videotape of Zen breath meditation followed by no specific outcome. The third group was asked to meditate after viewing a videotape of Zen counting breaths followed by an arousal outcome. Significant differences appeared between the meditation groups and the control group in terms of respiration rate and frontalis EMG, but there was no significant difference between meditation groups. The authors note that

neither physiological changes nor self-report were related to varying conditions of demand. The authors conclude that although
demand characteristics were varied, no attempt was made to control the subjects' expectation effects and that further investigation should examine the interaction between demand and subject
expectation.

Whereas Malec and Sipprelle called their varying of the effects of the outcome after meditation "demand characteristics,"
Smith (1976) in his study comparing Periodic Somatic Inactivity
(PSI) with TM developed elaborate testimonials about PSI's success rate and bogus research to support the claims in order to
control for "expectation effects." Here again, I would argue that
all that can be said is that uniform demand characteristics,
designed to create expectation of positive outcome, were
presented to subjects. Whether the demand characteristics
created the desired "expectation effect" remains to be assessed.
In Smith's study the control group, practicing PSI, was instructed to "sit quietly" two times a day and was not instructed
to focus on a mantra, as did the TM group. The PSI control
treatment was contrived to match every aspect of TM with the
above exception of the focus on the mantra. It began with two
introductory lectures that outlined what the experimenter considered to be a believable theory explaining why sitting twice a
day would be an effective cure for most psychopathology. In addition to the testimonials and bogus research, subjects were instructed to participate in a fifteen-day fast from illegal drugs,
similar to the TM preparation. Results showed that the TM and
PSI groups did not differ significantly on trait anxiety scores,
symptons of striate muscle tension, or symptoms of autonomic
arousal. However, both TM and PSI post-test means were
significantly lower than the no-treatment control group's means
on all dependent variables. This study, actually comparing the interaction of expectation effects and just-sitting with expectation
effects and just-sitting and concentration on a mantra, suggests
the potentially crucial importance of expectation effects (demand
characteristics) as a contributor to meditation outcome.

Another study supportive of the importance of demand
characteristics was done by Ikegami (1973) with one subject.
Ikegami had the subject sit on a disc that measured the amount
of movement of the meditator as a way of measuring the effect
of previous meditation practice on the amount of fluctuation of

the disc, and found great variability across sessions: increased practice did not seem to produce more stable posture. Two months later the same subject was reinstructed, this time told to "gaze steadily at one point," "to strictly observe the instructed posture," and so on; "these instructions had the purpose of strengthening his mental set for the posture," and led to a significant decrease in the amount of fluctuation and a clear gradient decrease over the eight session trial, an effect perhaps due to additional practice, but quite possibly due to the investigator's demand characteristics.

Finally, there are cognitions which may occur *after* the experience of meditation. One possible significant cognition involves self-statements that an individual might make about his or her ability to relax. An individual, having meditated and having had subjective experiences of feeling calm during meditation, may be more able and more willing to attribute anxiety episodes to situational variables, rather than to a specific anxious personality trait (Mischel, 1968; Shapiro & Zifferblatt, 1976b). This self statement should help a person further reduce the amount of anxiety in his or her life.

A second cognition that may be important is what one says to oneself if there is an experience of "void" or "blankness." Ornstein (1971) reviewed studies involving ganzfeld conditions. An example of these experiments was one in which ping-pong balls, cut in half, were attached to an individual's eyes so that nothing was visible except the inside of the ball. Soon the individual reported the balls disappearing, a period of "blanking out." Simultaneous with the individual's report of the disappearance of the image, a burst of alpha waves was recorded (Cohen, 1957). Ornstein noted that the "period of blanking out" that occurred in the ganzfeld experiment may be similar to the feeling of void or emptiness, or absence of cognition that occurs in many types of meditation.

What is important to our discussion here is how the individual interprets the period of blanking out.* As Ornstein noted, a person in a scientific experiment would describe the experience

---

*Even though the ganzfeld experiments deal only with perceptual habituation (i.e. there still may be thoughts the individual is having), the cognitive system for explaining this perceptual void may be important in determining how the person reacts to it.

of the void very differently from someone who is meditating in a religious or philosophical framework which talks of oneness, of a merging with non-being, or emptiness. In other words, certain of the subjective effects of meditation which occur as a result of prolonged attentional focus, may be due to the subject's cognitions, his/her interpretation of that experience.

For example, Woolfolk (1975) has noted that although samadhi is universally described with terms such as "transcendence" and "bliss" and characterized as a "turning off" of the external world, one Yogin showed cortical excitation in very deep meditation while another clearly evidenced slowing of the EEG. Thus, consistent reports of the phenomenology of meditation may simply reflect similarly shaped verbal sets, rather than regularities along other dimensions (Woolfolk, 1975).*

Davidson has even gone so far as to suggest that an individual's interpretation of the experience of the shift from either ergotropic or trophotropic or vice versa, "depending upon the psychological status of the individual and the circumstances in which he finds himself—may be interpreted as dreaming, hallucinations, psychosis, meditative states, or mystical experiences" (J. Davidson, 1976, p. 43). This assumes, however, that the states in question are quite similar.

A third post-meditation cognitive variable which may account for some of the effects of meditation may be referred to as the William James Box effect (eg., Fadiman & Frager, 1976). William James, during a time of great depression about his inability to resolve the issue of free will versus determinism, made a decision to choose to act as if he lived in a world which allowed freedom of choice. The William James Box actually involves taking matches out of a match box one by one and then putting them back in the box in a continous cycle for five minutes each day. This specific behavior has no particular meaning, but in an existential world where all values are relative, no act has any particular meaning. Meaning comes from the existential decision to choose a certain course of action in one's life. Based on self-perception theory (Bem, 1972), if an individual chooses to

*In this regard, it should be noted that sometimes while S's EEG evidenced alpha production, they reported that their minds were active; other S's reported "blank minds" and yet had high beta EEG activity (Morse et al., 1977). This does call into question the usefulness of the EEG alpha as a measure.

perform an action and then carries it through, he or she may subsequently observe their behavior and label it as willful and highly motivated. Therefore, the very act of meditation (whether or not that behavior has any intrinsic meaning or effect) may in itself be sufficient to allow one to perceive oneself as having increased willpower and motivation.

9.4 Nature of Attentional Process: Active Versus Receptive; Role of Discrimination

DEIKMAN'S WORK on deautomatization (1966) and bimodal consciousness (1971) suggested that mystical experiences occurred because meditation is an attempt to reduce automatic reaction and automatic ways of perceiving the world. Deautomatization or letting go of our cognitive constructs allows us to be more open and receptive to what is around us. Automatic reactions normally have specific intentional focus, causing us to tune out aspects of experience that are not necessary for the goal or do not conform to our expectations (Bruner, 1973). This "active" mode, Deikman noted, is a "state organized to manipulate the environment, a state of striving, oriented toward achieving personal goals that range from nutrition to defense to obtaining social reward...a mode that involves striated muscle systems and sympathetic nervous systems, an EEG showing beta activity and an increase in baseline muscle tension" (Deikman, 1971, p. 481). The receptive mode, Deikman continued, is a state "organized around intake of the environment rather than manipulation. The sensory perceptive system is the dominant agency rather than the muscle system, and parasympathetic systems tend to be most prominent. The EEG tends toward alpha waves and the baseline muscle tension is decreased." Deikman noted that these are two different, functionally specific modes, each with advantages and disadvantages, for specific purposes, and that during meditation there is a shift away from the active mode toward the receptive mode.

Others, such as Washburn (1978), Brown (1977), and Smith (Note Nine) have noted that this "receptive" model of meditation may be accurate for mindfulness meditation, but that in concentrative meditation certain kinds of efforts are necessary. Effort, as well as discrimination, is needed initially to keep the attention on the object of meditation and on fine-honed perceptual differentiation (Linden, 1973). As Washburn noted, it may be a mistake to put all meditation systems under the guise of the receptive mode because in its initial stages concentrative meditation involves many of the aspects of the active mode: a) discrimination of the meditation object and the intent actively to grasp or penetrate it; b) discursive, sequential mental activity, and c) subject object separation.*

Other thinkers (e.g., Welwood, 1977; Smith, Note Nine) have also discussed how the process of discriminating the "figure" from the field is important in meditation. They have both suggested that there is an alternating process which occurs between "convergence," or increasingly focused attention, and "divergence," the focus receding and the background field coming into focus. Welwood referred to this background field as the unconscious. As such, the background forms the context for focal perceptions. During part of the meditative experience, the background becomes the foreground, the field becomes the focus, the unconscious becomes the conscious. Smith viewed this process as cyclical between focus and field, a "natural process which occurs in that most convergence is intrinsically self-limiting and eventually uncovers or triggers a set of divergent processes." Smith noted further that two "traits" may be strengthened by this process—concentration during the convergent phase and acceptance of the field during the divergent phase. To support this he observed that the attentional mechanisms which Davidson and Goleman (1977) discuss are based on the Tellegan Absorption Scale. This scale consists primarily of five factors, based on Tellegan and Atkinson's own factor analytic research: a) reality absorption, b) fantasy absorption, c) dissociation, d) openness to experiences, and e) devotion and trust. Smith (Note Nine) noted that the first three do seem to reflect full, undistracted attention. This would deal primarily with the convergent aspect of his model, and the last two seem to "tap what we have been calling

---

*Washburn (1978) and Brown (1977) note that eventually this kind of active mode is not necessary and "falls aside." However, it may be a mistake not to note it as an important feature in the beginning.

acceptance of experience, as well as concentration: the acceptance aspect of the divergent experience."

Although Smith's model is interesting and supports the importance of the discrimination function, it has certain limitations. Primarily, it deals with beginning meditation steps and makes no distinction between mindfulness and concentrative meditation. Second, it does not seem to state whether this "divergence" will continue indefinitely or if with more practice there will be a greater increase in convergence. Third, it does not discuss the intentional variable, that is, convergence as the result of conscious effort whereas divergence may just happen. As noted in Goleman (1972), Brown (1977), and Washburn (1978) at the most advanced levels of meditation, the discrimination function lessens, subject/object seem to merge, discursive thought diminishes, a feeling of blankness, void, oneness occurs.

We have looked primarily at concentrative meditation in the cognitive analysis above. How does this compare with mindfulness meditation such as the just sitting of Zen (Shikan-taza), the insight meditation (Vipassana) of the Buddha, Krishnamurti's choiceless awareness, and Gurdjieff's self-remembering?

As Washburn noted, mindfulness meditation seems to begin in the receptive mode. However, interestingly, he suggested that the opening-up awareness may end in the same place as concentrative meditation:

> As the intensity threshold of the awareness is lowered, the objects that are received into consciousness become subtler and subtler; and a limit is approached in this way in which they cease being discrete entities, each with a form and nature of its own. In other words, receptivity to experience culminates in the dissolution of differentiated experience and therefore in a transcendence of the receptive function per se. Thus it is said of Buddhist insight meditation that it leads not only to an objectless nirvanic state, but also, beyond this, to a state of cessation (nirodha), which is still a state of awareness, but of no one or no thing (1978, p. 19).

Thus, both concentrative and opening-up meditation seem to end at ultimate states of "non-discrimination." However, particularly in the case of concentrative meditation, discrimination is an important and necessary component in the beginning stages.

The importance of discrimination, especially in the beginning of concentrative meditation, may be one of the reasons why there has not yet been much support for the split-brain theory accounting for meditation's effects (Ornstein, 1972; Davidson, 1976). The basic theory is as follows: The left brain in right-handed people seems to be specialized for verbal, sequential, analytical information processing; the right hemisphere seems to be more specialized for holistic (seeing the entire gestalt), spatial, parallel processing of information (Galin, 1974). Since advanced meditative and mystical experiences are often described as ineffable (Frank, 1977) and since language is "in the left hemisphere" (Sperry, 1969), it was expected that during the "holistic," ineffable experience of meditation, one would see relatively more activation of the right hemisphere (increased beta) and a decrease in activation in the left hemisphere (increased alpha). However, the theory and predictions are not definitively born out (Bennett & Trinder, 1977; Pagano & Franklin, 1977).

This lack of support may be explicable through our discussion on discrimination. If there is a large discrimination function in concentrative meditation, and discrimination of parts is primarily an analytical left-brain function, then in relatively new meditators one would expect ambiguous results (Bennett & Trinder, 1977). Further, this may account for reasons why first-time meditators did not do as well on the Embedded Figure Test (Van Nuys, 1973). Three-week meditators did slightly better (Kubose, 1976) and eighteen-week and three-month meditators did quite well (Linden, 1973; Pelletier, 1974). Discrimination ability may be a function of adherence and practice.

9.5 Information-Processing

BASICALLY, the normal perceptual mode of information processing, based on the work of Bruner (1973) involves a) categorizing based on certain minimally defining perceptual features, b) testing these perceptual hypotheses by scanning the environment, c) confirming and modifying the hypotheses. The phenomenology of concentrative meditation, Brown noted, is "much like perceptual categorizing in reverse; the yogi stops categorizing perceptual objects" (1977, p. 250). Further, as the individual goes into deeper and deeper levels of concentration, as the gaze becomes fixed, there is a reduction in microsaccadic eye movements (Fischer, 1971); as already discussed, the ganzfeld experiments suggest that perceptual images disappear under excessive stimulus constancy. The mechanism for this may be, as Brown noted, analogous to the process of pattern recognition in cognitive psychology, but in reverse. Further, meditation may be reversing the cognitive developmental stages described by Piaget. Piaget assumed certain structural changes—generalization and differentiation, and these are dependent upon constant interaction between the organism and novel stimuli in the environment. As Brown noted, concentrative meditation reverses the fundamental interaction proposition in Piaget's theory:

> The yogi minimizes his interaction with the environment and disrupts this novelty by restricting his concentration to a single object over long periods. An invariant sequence of structural changes and levels of meditation likewise occurs, but in the opposite direction: decreased generalization and de-differentiation of structures (1977, p. 268).

Finally, a similar process may be working on affect construction, that is individuals learn to perceive non-neutral stimuli neutrally. Neurophysiologically, Fischer (1971) described this state as a trophotropic state in which individuals can perceive without high limbic affect (cf. Schwartz, 1975). It may be this quality of finely honed perceptual discrimination without high affective properties that accounts for meditation's effects in reducing fears and phobias.

9.6 Global Desensitization

ANOTHER HYPOTHESIS that attempts to explain meditation's effectiveness in reducing fears and phobias was proposed in a seminal article by Goleman (1971). He described meditation as a type of global desensitization: First, an individual learns to achieve a relaxed state; then, as new thoughts arise, the individuals *learns* to witness the random flow of thoughts from this relaxed state, thereby reciprocally inhibiting the anxiety normally elicited by those thoughts.

Although plausible, this hypothesis leaves many questions unanswered. For example, there is some question as to whether reciprocal inhibition offers the most parsimonious explanation for systematic desensitization. In fact, Jacobs & Wolpin, (1971), Yulis et al. (1975) and Wilkins (1971) suggest that perhaps the important variables are attention shifts and cognitive refocusing (see also Lazarus, 1975). Further, there is no research that supports the hypothesis that the "global desensitization hierarchy is inherently self-regulating" and that "optimal salience is guaranteed" (Goleman, 1971, p. 17). In fact, clinical experience suggests that the original assumptions of Goleman (1971), Otis (1974), and Shapiro and Zifferblatt (1976b) regarding meditation as global desensitization may need more refinement. An individual may not attain a state of sufficient relaxation to deal with unpleasant experiences that arise during meditation. For example, French, Schmid and Ingalls (1975), Carrington and Ephron (1975), and Kanellakos (1974) described complaints from Transcendental Meditators who felt themselves overwhelmed by negative and unpleasant thoughts during meditation. In addition, Otis (1974) noted that Transcendental Meditators who dropped out had more negative self-images before beginning the practice than those who did not drop out. It may be that the meditators who dropped out did so because the unpleasant images that arose during meditation were too unpleasant to deal with. Further, anecdotal accounts of meditators suggest that the thoughts during meditation, rather than being the most important in their life, are often trivial and irrelevant. Based on this latter assumption, Yalom et al. (1977) even used meditators as a control group in a clinical study testing the impact of a weekend group-experience on individual therapy. To document this hypothesis more substantially, future research would have to determine whether the meditator's thoughts are: a) self-paced so that they are never more overwhelming than the individual can deal with; and b) are necessarily concerned with the most important variables in the individual's life.

9.7 Summary: The Technique-Specific and Stage-Specific Nature of Mechanisms

 TO CONCLUDE, reliance on any one exclusive uni-modal mediating mechanism, be it oxygen consumption, skeletal muscular relaxation, general physiological changes, electrocortical activity such as hemispheric laterality or attentional mode does not appear totally satisfactory. What seems necessary is to work toward developing a hierarchic, multi-level, interdependent biopsychological model for mediating mechanisms. This model would require an enormous precision, and would need to be applied to each meditation technique separately, depending both on the effects being measured, as well as the different levels within the technique being experienced. For example, looking only at the variable of attention, there may be differences in attentional style between concentrative and opening-up meditation (Kasamatsu & Hirai; Anand, Chinna & Singh, 1961a); between passive attention and active attention, (Shwartz et al., Note Six); and between different levels within a given technique (Brown, 1977).

Regarding levels of depth of experience, it might be illustrative to look briefly at the five-step model of breath meditation outlined in Chapter One. The initial steps of meditation, described in Chapter One, Figure 1.2, (Step One—reactive effect, Step Two—attention wandering from the task) may be the result of certain mechanisms mediating ordinary awareness. For example, the neurophysiological literature (Pribram, 1971) suggests that the deployment of conscious attention on an automatic activity may interfere with that activity, as we saw in Step One. In Step Two—habituation, attention wandering—the orientation response, or simple distraction, and inability to maintain attentive focus may be operating. Steps Three and Four, as we have noted, involve meditation as a self-regulation strategy. Here the relaxation component of meditation may be important—muscular relaxation, decreased arousal of sympathetic nervous system, etc. (Benson, 1975), as well as counter-conditioning (e.g., Wolpe, 1969; Goleman, 1971). Further, it seems that for Zen breath meditation or concentrative meditation an alternative attentional focus (competing response) may also be responsible for the effects found in stress and tension management, overcoming fears and phobias, reducing blood pressure, and decreasing use of addictive substances. Finally, in Step Five, meditation as an altered state of consciousness, it seems that the relaxation component probably plays a relatively small role. The habituation literature for concentrative meditation, dehabituation literature for mindfulness meditation, and information-processing literature may be more important for understanding some of the phenomenological "enlightenment" experiences of meditation and the findings of increased perceptual clarity. The above comments are made in order to suggest the importance of greater precision in trying to specify mediating mechanisms of meditation—both across meditation techniques and within different levels of a given technique itself.

Chapter Nine: Further Reading: Mediating Mechanisms

PHYSIOLOGICAL

General

Wallace, R.K., Benson, H. & Wilson, A.F. A wakeful hypometabolic state. *American Journal of Physiology,* 1971, *221,* (3), 795-799. (Reprinted in D.H. Shapiro & R.N. Walsh [Eds.], *The science of meditation.* New York: Aldine, 1980).

HEMISPHERIC LATERALITY

Davidson, J. Physiology of meditation and mystical states of consciousness. *Perspectives in Biology & Medicine,* 1976, *32,* 1323-1326. (Reprinted in D.H. Shapiro & R.N. Walsh [Eds.], *The science of meditation.* New York: Aldine, 1980).

Bennet, J. & Trinder, J. Hemispheric laterality and cognitive styles associated with Transcendental Meditation. *Psychophysiology,* 1977, *14,* (3), 293-296. (Reprinted in D.H. Shapiro & R.N. Walsh [Eds.], *The science of meditation.* New York: Aldine, 1980).

Pagano, R. & Frumkin, L.R. The effects of Transcendental Meditation on right hemispheric function. In D.H. Shapiro & R.N. Walsh (Eds.), *The science of meditation.* New York: Aldine, 1980.

ATTENTIONAL—INFORMATION PROCESSING

Davidson, R. & Goleman, D. The role of attention in meditation and hypnosis: A psychobiological perspective on transformations of consciousness. *International Journal of Clinical & Experimental Hypnosis,* 1977, *25,* (4), 291-308. (Reprinted in D.H. Shapiro & R.N. Walsh [Eds.], *The science of meditation.* New York: Aldine, 1980).

Brown, D. A model of the levels of concentrative meditation. *The International Journal of Clinical & Experimental Hypnosis,* 1977, *25,* (4), 236-273. (Reprinted in D.H. Shapiro & R.N.

Walsh [Eds.], *The science of meditation,* New York: Aldine, 1980).

Deikman, A.J. Deautomatization and the mystic experience. *Psychiatry,* 1966, *29,* 324-38.

Deikman, A.J. Biomodal consciousness. *Archives of General Psychiatry,* 1971, *25,* 481-489.

EXPECTATION EFFECTS/
DEMAND CHARACTERISTICS

Smith, J.D. Psychotherapeutic effects of transcendental meditation with controls for expectation of relief and daily sitting. *Journal of Consulting & Clinical Psychology,* 1976, *44,* 630-637. (Reprinted in D.H. Shapiro & R.N. Walsh [Eds.], *The science of meditation,* New York: Aldine, 1980).

Malec, J. & Sipprelle, C. Physiological and subjective effects of Zen meditation and demand characteristics. *Journal of Consulting & Clinical Psychology,* 1977, *44,* 339-340. (Reprinted in D.H. Shapiro & R.N. Walsh [Eds.], *The science of meditation.* New York: Aldine, 1980).

10

Methodological Issues in Meditation Research:
An Applied Clinical Model

10.1 Introduction

MEDITATION, if it is to be considered an empirically effective clinical strategy, needs to be subjected to the same scientific scrutiny as any other psychotherapeutic strategy. Further, it should be apparent from the methodological issues raised throughout the book that many of the research concerns with meditation are similar to those encountered in psychotherapeutic outcome studies. This summary attempts to suggest ways of tightening future research in order to ensure more clinically reliable and valid results.

This summary discussion is guided by the question with which we opened the book and with which we have been concerned throughout, "What effect does the teaching of meditation have on a person who practices, and why?"

In order to answer this question, it has been necessary to look separately at each of the key words in the sentence. In Chapters Five and Seven we reviewed the empirical literature on the *effects* of meditation, both as a self-regulation strategy and as an altered state of consciousness. In Chapter One we noted the importance of the *teaching,* including the therapist's orienta-tion, expectations, belief in the efficacy of the strategy, style of teaching, and relationship variables. In Chapter One and in more detail in Chapter Eight, we discussed the question of what is *meditation,* and what are its components. In Chapter One we explored the issue of the *individual* (or client) who might most benefit from meditation as well as the importance of *practice* or adherence to the technique. Finally, in Chapter Nine, we reviewed difference meditating mechanisms which might help answer the question, *why* does meditation work?

10.2 An Interactive, Omnideterministic Model

WE HAVE DEALT with each of the above issues separately. However, this was only a function of the linear style in which a book is written, and was not intended to imply a lack of interaction between variables. In fact, as suggested in Chapters Eight and Nine, quite the opposite is true. Following general systems theory, I believe in an omni-deterministic model in which each part can and often does interact and effect all other parts. Figure 10.1 presents a general interaction model of therapy in the form of a modified flow chart.

The model is interactive in that therapist and client styles, personalities and belief systems form the basis for not only the relationship, but also such issues as what the clinical concern is, how best to deal with it, whether treatment has been successful, etc. This is not intended to imply a position asserting the client's essential equality of therapeutic knowledge, or to be an abrogation of the therapist's responsibility. However, it is intended to suggest the essential interactive nature of the process and to acknowledge that the client also has a view of the problem, has a certain style and belief system which need to be considered in the teaching process.

The model is represented by a flow chart. For example, when evaluation is made and there is not "treatment success," a reevaluation at all stages may be necessary: is this the most salient concern, the most effective strategy, the best way of teaching this strategy to this particular client? is our relationship facilitating or hindering therapy, and so on?

FIGURE 10.1

An Interactive Systems Theory Model for Utilizing Meditation as a Self-Control Technique in the Management of a Clinical Problem, such as Stress.

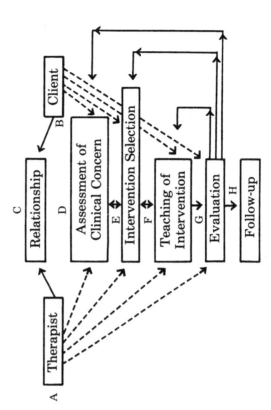

A. The Therapist (Experimenter/trainer)
   —orientation
   —why using strategy
   —what hopes for
   —belief in good/bad aspects of stress (demand characteristics)
   —experience; length of contact

B. The Client (subject pool) (Individual)
   —hopes, expectations, age, sex
   —belief systems, values; freedom response
   —motivation; resistance
   —locus of control/attribution theory
   —response models: e.g., auditory, kinesthetic, visual

C. The Relationship
   —trust, empathy
   —"dynamics" of relationship
   non-technical def. of transference/countertransference voice, etc.

D. Assessment: Nature of the clinical problem (dependent variable)
   —clinical concern
   refinement: e.g., cognitive/somatic anxiety
   Is stress a positive motivator, and to learn to relax is avoidance response; or is person over-stressed and needs to learn how to relax.

E. The Selection of the Clinical Self-Control Strategy (Independent Variable)
   Importance of the theoretical/clinically based rationale between the independent and dependent variables.

F. Method of teaching: How to present strategy
   —Modeling
   —Successive Approximation and Reinforcement
   —Issues of personal responsibility
   —Dealing with adherence and compliance

G. Evaluation e.g., (N=1)

H. Follow up

In this model, I am conceptualizing meditation as a self-regulation strategy and discussing its implications for the clinical problem of stress. I choose this example because it is one which has wide applicability to most clinicians. However, as we have noted throughout the book, I could have as easily labeled the chart, "A Model for Utilizing an Altered State of Consciousness Technique—Meditation—for the Attainment of Spiritual Harmony." Although the terms may be harder to define in the latter example, the model is no less applicable.

In fact, one of the primary weaknesses in meditation studies thus far has been the lack of a clear theoretical rationale linking the independent variable and the selection of the dependent variable. Future research should attempt to clarify precisely the theoretical rationale connecting the independent and dependent variables. This relationship should be the foundation of a proposed research design, not an afterthought; and it should make future researchers decide whether they are conceptualizing meditation as a self-regulation strategy, or as an altered state of consciousness (cf. E in Figure 10.1).

Further, careful consideration should be given to the nature of the independent variable. It is crucial that experimenters report accurately all procedures used. In this way meditation techniques are described behaviorally, and may be compared for clinical efficacy with other cognitive focusing, relaxation, and self-regulatory strategies.

Second, clinician/experimenter orientation and contact should be more precisely described as part of the treatment (A in Figure 10.1). This description should include both length and frequency of contact, and if possible, the actual monitoring of positive verbal and non-verbal statements the experimenter makes to the client. This monitoring of differential reinforcement of client behavior may give experimenters a method of operationalizing one aspect of the concept of demand characteristics (F in Figure 10.1). Demand characteristics are an important part of any therapeutic treatment strategy in a clinical or educational setting. Therefore, rather than reducing demand characteristics by the use of a tape recorder or some mechanical means of training, I would suggest, at least initially, that these demand characteristics be explicitly stated and maximized for clinical success.

Third, experimenters should try to standardize expectation effects. Although the media and cultural milieu cannot be controlled, standard written introductory expectations could be read to all groups participating in the experiment (Barlow, Leitenberg & Agras, 1969; Nidich, Seeman & Dreskin, 1973). In this way, there can be a systematic effort to take subjects' expectations into account as part of the treatment variable (Smith, 1975) (B in Figure 10.1). For example, in certain studies (Smith, 1976; Lesh, 1970), as well as in the introductory and preparatory lectures of TM, the expectation effect is maximized by explicitly stating the benefits of the treatments. In addition, other nonspecific effects, such as a) being in a structured treatment/training framework, or b) the need to reorganize and replan one's life in order to find the time to practice meditation two times a day may also be factors in the therapeutic efficacy of the techniques (McFall & Hammen, 1971). When the technique involves practice at home, the experimenter should make a concerted effort to determine how much the subjects have in fact practiced. This "practice effect" should be reported as part of the intervention (F in Figure 10.1).

Fourth, it may be important to evaluate the quality of the meditation experience. For example, how do we know that the subjects have meditated rather than just sat? How do we know which subjects have learned to focus attention effectively? Vahia et al. (1972, 1973) for example noted that psychoneurotic patients with psychosomatic disorders showed significantly more improvement depending on their differential ability to concentrate. Possible methods for concurrent validity of the meditation experience are suggested by the perceptual studies (Pelletier, 1974), by physiological criteria (Griffith, 1974; Davidson, 1976; Honsberger & Wilson, 1973), and/or rater coding of subjective responses (Maupin, 1965; Deikman, 1966).

Fifth, it may be important to look at the length of treatment. This would also include time per day. Is there an optimal maximum amount of time per day? Can one practice too much (French, Schmid & Ingalls, 1975)? What is the relationship between length of experience and effectiveness (Benson & Wallace, 1972; Shafii, Lavely, & Jaffe, 1975; Otis, 1974). Recent studies, for example, suggest that the effectiveness of meditation as a treatment depends on both steady and prolonged practice of the technique (Lazar et al., 1977, Marcus, 1975).

In summary, future research should also continue to pinpoint answers to the following questions about the independent variable: what are the inert and what are the active variables of the treatment strategy: attention focusing, muscular relaxation, just sitting with eyes closed? What is the role of the demand characteristics? What are the effects of subject's motivation, expectation; therapist's expectation; the structured "non-specific" variables of the research design itself? Insofar as we can begin to specify precisely the above aspects of the independent variable, appropriate research designs may be undertaken, and the answers to the variance of treatment success attributable to various aspects of the independent variable may be determined.

It should be emphasized, however, that from a clinical standpoint, the above questions are of secondary importance. Questions of primary importance include the following: for which clinical populations, under what conditions, for what clinical problems, are what meditation treatments effective?

In order to answer these questions, a few additional comments about subject selection, data gathering and research design are in order. Although standard scientific procedures do not need to be reiterated here, some caveats particular to meditation research may be useful. Regarding subject selection, in addition to subject motivation, expectations, commitment and history of prior meditation, it is important to obtain detailed information about subject's prior clinical history (B in Figure 10.1). For example, Girodo, in his study of anxiety neurosis, found that Yoga treatment was effective only for those with a short prior history (average 14.2 months), and that those with a longer history of illness (average 44.2 months) achieved successful remission of symptoms only with the addition of imaginal flooding (Girodo, 1974). Prior length and severity of illness may also be important in determining the effectiveness of meditation with related problems such as hypertension, insomnia, and asthma.

Subject's prior clinical history may also be important as a means of screening patients to determine their appropriateness for learning meditation. For example, psychotic patients with strong paranoid systems or a poor sense of reality testing may not be appropriate subjects. Further, people experiencing acute anxiety and trauma may be overwhelmed with the emotionally charged material that might present itself during meditation (Patel, 1975). To deal with any "overwhelming" emotional reactions that may develop in their patients, Glueck and Stroebel (1975) had experienced teachers check the patient's meditation process on a daily basis during the first three weeks. They note, as did French et al., (1975) that overt psychotic episodes may be precipitated in individuals with psychiatric disorders who meditate more than the prescribed twenty minutes twice a day. This has been refined by Walsh and Rauch (1979) who note that intensive meditation by individuals with a history of schizophrenia may precipitate psychotic episodes.

Future research should also investigate differences between subjects who begin meditation, and those who do not (Lesh, 1970; Stek & Bass, 1973), as well as differences between those who continue meditation and those who quit. Finally, the relationship between sex of subject and treatment outcome has not, to my knowledge, been explicitly addressed and needs to be.

Regarding data-gathering strategies, future research should attempt to corroborate self-report data with other overt behavior or physiological measures. This should involve the issue of how self-report measures on global paper and pencil tests translate into actual behavior in the patient's life. Clinically oriented studies are also needed to determine whether statistical significance on a pre-post test, for example anxiety, is of clinical significance to the patient (Lykken, 1968).

In addition, future research also needs to pinpoint the nature of the clinical problem as precisely as possible (D in Figure 10.1). For example, Davidson and Schwartz (1976) suggest that there are actually differences between the technique of meditation and other self-regulation techniques, and that it is "the imprecise" measuring of the dependent variable that is lumping the results together. The one study to test this (Schwartz et al., 1978) gave a group of meditators and a group of individuals who exercised an anxiety questionnaire involving both somatic and cognitive components. Subjects who practiced physical exercise reported relatively less somatic and more cognitive anxiety than meditators. Meditators, conversely, reported less cognitive and more somatic anxiety than the exercisers. This study suggests the potential clinical promise of refinement of dependent variables. However, since the study was not a longitudinal design, the results are somewhat difficult to interpret definitively. If further research bears out this hypothesis, however, matching meditation technique to "cognitively anxious" people, exercise to "somatically anxious" people has clear clinical relevance.

Future research may also attempt to combine the independent variable of meditation with other self-regulation strategies (e.g., Woolfolk, 1980 in press; Shapiro, 1978b) to make it a more powerful clinical intervention (Chapter Six). For example, in a well-designed N=1 study, Woolfolk found that formal meditation plus "short" meditations made contingent upon recognizing anger appeared to be more effective than formal meditation alone. Again, these results, though promising, await further replication.

In general, we are developing a literature on subject (client) variables, dependent variables, and their interaction with meditation. This literature should help us choose the intervention best suited to a particular patient and where appropriate, develop refinements and/or combination of treatment interventions.

Future research also needs to be sensitive to the type of research design (G in Figure 10.1). When meditation is conceptualized as a self-regulation strategy for anxiety reduction, stress and tension management, or reduction of fears and phobias as in Chapter Five certain research methodologies are necessary. To support its effectiveness as a treatment of choice, control-group designs involving other self-regulatory strategies need to be employed (Smith, 1975; Goleman & Schwartz, 1976; Woolfolk et al., 1976). These control group designs should address questions of if, how, and to what extent does the state of relaxation during meditation generalize to non-meditating times? Is meditation as effective as other self-regulation techniques such as Progressive Relaxation in the management of stress and tension? or as effective as systematic desensitization in the reduction of fears and phobias? (Kirsch & Henry, 1979). Additional studies may then be necessary to determine relative variance of the different components of meditation as in Chapter Eight: the use of mantra (Smith, 1976); the role of expectations (Smith, 1976; Hjelle, 1974; Malec and Sipprelle, 1978). Other studies will also need to try to determine what may be mediating aspects of meditation's effects: muscular relaxation, just-sitting, reciprocal inhibition, cognitive refocusing, interruption of the threat-arousal-threat spiral and so on, as discussed in Chapter Nine.

These "control" group designs must face the difficult task of determining what, in fact, is a control group. Although investigators have utilized as a control group "just sitting," saying "one," "thinking positive thoughts," each of these, to a greater or lesser extent, may involve "conscious effort to focus attention," which was part of our Chapter One definition of what meditation is! Even the second part of the definition "in a non-analytical manner and an attempt to reduce ruminating thought" implicitly acknowledges that in the initial stages thought does occur, so some overlap would occur with a control group which was to actively generate thoughts. Perhaps a control group doing crossword puzzles or mathematical games which involved continuous active analysis, would be suitable. Although there would be conscious attempts to focus attention in these groups, the awareness would be of a different type, and the implicit instructions for the use of analysis would be the opposite of meditation.

When meditation is conceptualized as an altered state of consciousness (Chapter Seven), a different research methodology may be necessary. As Tart has pointed out, there is a need for detailed mapping of internal states of consciousness. However, since these internal states are subjective phenomena, it may be quite helpful if the subject is also the experimenter. This raises several methodological problems, including experimenter bias and reactive effects of observation (Tart, 1972). For mapping the subjective experiences of altered states, well documented intensive research designs seem necessary.* This is especially true until we have more accurate knowledge about the dependent variables associated with altered states. In addition, we need to continue to search for physiological correlates of these "altered states," such as the promising literature on hemispheric laterality (Davidson, 1976).

Finally, in researching states of consciousness, it is important to decide whether consciousness is viewed as an independent or dependent variable. In other words, is the researcher interested in looking at how meditation techniques produce different states of consciousness (dependent variable), or how altered states of consciousness (independent variable) affects subsequent self-referential attitudes and/or behavior?

---

*Dukes, 1965; Lachenmeyer, 1970; Gottmann, McFall, & Barnett, 1969; Chassan & Bellak, 1966; Mitchell, 1969; Thoresen, 1972; Yates, 1970; Honig, 1966; Sidman, 1960; White, 1972; White, 1971.

10.3 Comments on the
Philosophy of Science

THE ABOVE DISCUSSION on research design suggests an interesting observation: that the philosophy of science necessitates a two-step process. The first step involves forming intuitive hypotheses based on past data, anecdotal reports, and subjective experiences as are most clearly seen in the early clinical studies and with the research on subjective experiences during meditation. These studies are almost exclusively case studies involving within-subject designs. These case studies may cause us to rethink our models and pose questions which challenge our theoretical constructs. They help us gain specific information about the independent variable, possible dependent variables, data gathering strategies, and possible methodological problems.

The second step in the process involves control-group designs to determine treatment variance within the independent variable: expectation effects, nonspecific variables, demand characteristics, etc. Although I believe strongly in the importance of control procedures, I also believe that there are limitations to control group designs in which clinical inferences are based only on statistical significance of group averages as measured by pre- and post-tests. Further, even when control group designs are necessary for pinpointing variance of treatment success, it is important to point out that we can only take this posture because case studies and the testing of intuitive hypotheses were previously undertaken. One cannot have a tight, well controlled research design without a clear dependent variable. The connection between the independent and dependent variable, however, is part of the simultaneous process of theory testing and theory building, and does not spring forth without some prior hypothesis testing.

We may now be at a point in meditation research where, when meditation is conceptualized as a self-regulation strategy, control group designs are useful and even necessary. However, when meditation is conceptualized as an altered state of consciousness, a different methodology may be required. The dependent variables are not as clear, are more delicate, more difficult to ferret out. Therefore, there may still be a need to use well documented intensive designs to gain specific information about the dependent variables, data gathering strategies, and possible methodological problems.

Future researchers need to clarify which dependent variables are being investigated and then determine appropriate methodologies. Both types of methodologies—intensive design and control group designs—can represent scientific inquiry at its best. Both can complement each other and add to our knowledge, so that science truly serves the promotion of human welfare.

10.4 Summary

FUTURE CLINICALLY oriented research needs to include precise descriptions of the independent variable; control for expectation effects and subject motivation; and where clinically appropriate, demand characteristics; exercise care in subject selection and specification of the dependent variable; provide a rationale connecting dependent and independent variables; utilize data-gathering strategies that provide precise information and, where possible, concurrent validity and follow-up data; and finally, emphasize research designs appropriate to the dependent variable investigated.

Because of the excitement and aura of mystery currently surrounding the technique of meditation, there is a tendency to let enthusiasm replace methodology. However, by taking into account the methodological concerns above, it is possible to design clinically oriented research studies that provide relevant information about the efficacy of different types of meditation strategies for specific types of populations with specific concerns. This is the type of research that can truly be of use to fellow researchers, clinicians, and ultimately to patients themselves.

11

Epilogue:
A Personal Essay

I END THIS BOOK with feelings of respect, humility, and acceptance. I have a great and renewed respect for our scientific tradition, and for those researchers who are pushing the frontier of our knowledge by investigating meditation practices. I have a similar respect for those involved in the personal quest on the meditation path. My humility is rooted in the goals I set at the start of the book, a mission of trying to bring these two traditions together. While writing I heard voices criticizing me. The "Western" voices said, "Shapiro is getting soft and anti-scientific; we always knew he was a bit of a flake anyway." The "Eastern" voices said: "Shapiro is corrupting our tradition; he's become too scientific, rigid and analytical; and does not know what he is talking about." I imagine both voices have a certain truth in them. I am not sure I can clearly bridge these two traditions. I feel somewhat humbled at the very idea of it, and, in retrospect, somewhat surprised at the "hubris" that allowed me to try to undertake it.

I have come up against many personal limitations in writing this book, and in my own meditation practice. With regard to the book, I am a clinical psychologist by training and experience. The farther afield I got in pursuing meditation research, the less competent I felt, and the harder I had to try in order to under-

265

stand others' writing. Therefore, the task of pulling together such a large, diverse literature on a theory, research, and clinical level has also been humbling.

This book is subtitled "A Scientific/Personal Exploration." I wanted it, in addition to being a scientific presentation, to reflect my own personal experience: fifteen months study in the Orient, nearly ten years of meditation practice, my attempt to integrate personal, often ineffable experiences with an intellectual, rational, inquiring "mind." This "personal" side is most evident in Chapter Two, in terms of my therapeutic orientation, and in Chapter Three, in the discussion of my meditation experiences. In this epilogue I would like to make explicit some additional issues I have been wrestling with, both in writing this book and in my practice of meditation.

There is a risk in this sharing. Partly it is the vulnerability of openness about my personal feelings. Partly it is the fear that this epilogue may be nothing more than a self-indulgent "true confession." My hope, of course, is that discussion such as this can contribute to a more total understanding of meditation, grounded both in scientific literature and personal experience.

Whether by nature or training, I am a curious, inquiring person. Until ten years ago, my main response to a new situation was, in general, to cope by intellectual means. More often than not that is still the case. Over the past ten years, through flute playing, meditation, poetry writing, and Sumi-e (brush stroke painting), I have worked on cultivating a style different from my rational, intellectual one: a more yielding, non-analytical, delicate mode. However, writing this book in general and the content analysis article in particular (Chapter Three) have made me confront some strong barriers I have to writing about my own meditation experiences. I feared that analyzing that new mode in the service of professional. career could destroy the very thing I was trying to create.

Let me give an example. One morning while meditating on the beach at Laguna, I had a glowing, warm feeling which was, in many ways, overpowering. Images of friends, colleagues, loved ones and enemies came pouring forth. Each person's face had a vivid detail to it. Further, each person's face had a certain pose of delicacy and graciousness. Even when the face of a person whom I did not like appeared, it was in a friendly, kind posture, showing them in their best light. This posture was one which I had in fact seen them in at some point in our relationship. I saw and I experienced an essence of tenderness and gentleness in each person. I could feel and think no evil thoughts; they were transformed into a positive glow.

Now from a scientific standpoint, one could argue quite justifiably that 1) a cognitive reframing, or restructuring was occurring, or 2) a respondent conditioning of negative images paired with a lovely ocean setting was occurring. We could also discuss the role of images and cognitions in shaping behavior.

But this was my peak experience. I did not want this personal experience to be reduced to conform to a scientific model. How to resolve this? On the one hand, I believe that scientific analysis can and should occur regarding altered states. I thought Walter and Harriet Mischel's (1958) experimental analysis of trances was a seminal article. Yet, from a subjective viewpoint, I did not want *my* experience to be reduced to "cognitive restructuring." That is not a rational, but a gut response.

This duality is one I wrestle with frequently. The East says do not research meditation, and do not analyze it. The West says, it is not real unless you can come up with some kind of concrete, valid, replicable study.

That contradiction became particularly acute when, during the September 1977 content-analysis research project, I went to Tassajara, a Zen retreat in Carmel Valley, for a few days. Not only was the above an unresolved issue for me, but there were strong anti-scientific demand characteristics at the monastery. For example, I asked if, when no one else was in the meditation room, I could meditate and conduct my experiment, which involved the use of a tape recorder. I was told absolutely not. Electricity was not allowed in the meditation room—even vacuum clearners were anathema, they cleaned the room by whisk brooms. I felt very scientific, precise, and awkward to be recording and writing down thoughts of meditation. While at Tassajara I gave up my attempt to analyze meditation.

Creative words
    flow down stream
        with the current.

Yet, if we look closely, we can see that the Eastern traditions *do* have elaborate hierarchies and charts of attention and consciousness that must necessarily have been made from the analysis of meditation (see the texts of the Mahāmudra, the *Visuddhimagga*).

Thoughts themselves are not *a priori* wrong. Analysis is not wrong—if it is seen as a tool, a paradigm with which to understand reality. If it is seen as the only tool, then it becomes a blinder separating us from some important and powerful human experiences and ways of interacting with each other (cf. Martin Buber, 1958, 1961). However, by eschewing analysis, I believe we are faced with an equally limiting blinder, an accepting with blind faith all things "esoteric" and mysterious. This can easily lead to dangerous cultism. The issue seems one of balance.

My first experiences of meditation occurred prior to any formal training in psychology in general and psychotherapy in particular. Therefore, I do not have any base-line comparison. It is nearly impossible for me to assess the ways meditation has affected me from a clinical standpoint. In terms of my personal development, I think this has strong advantages. I did not have any preconceived framework in which to place meditation. I had not yet developed good analytical skills with which to analyze why meditation was working or not working, and I had no intention of researching meditation when I first began to learn it.

However, from a research standpoint, there may have been certain disadvantages to this sequence. I may have been more caught up in my belief systems about what meditation might or might not do and less observant about what actually was happening from an experimental standpoint. Meditation may have sharpened my powers of observation, but it may have sharpened a type of observation different from the analytical Western research skills I have since developed. I had a strong reluctance to actually analyze my own meditation experience once I had been trained in Western behavioral sciences. Meditation traditions are clear that analysis, logic and reason get in the way of meditation experience. Therefore, for a long time, I kept the two areas separate: 1) studying the effects of meditation on other individuals, analyzing their experiences and, 2) other than a journal which I have kept daily, doing very little formal analysis of my own meditation experiences. I might add, having completed the content analysis project, that the Eastern traditions are right! Doing this kind of research on meditation does affect the qualitative experience while meditating. I hope, however, that even though short-term meditation experience was more onerous, less enjoyable, eventually it will give us some understanding of meditation that will facilitate other individuals' practice of meditation. A small price to pay for progress?!

Another issue for me relates to my own ego. Meditation traditions are quite clear about the importance of humbleness, honesty, purity and integrity, as important preparatory virtues for facilitating meditation practice. I strongly believe in these virtues and work toward attaining them. Several times during my meditation experiences, I have felt that "inner peace," and, as Mickey Stunkard once jested about his own experience, I too felt, if they gave certificates for enlightenment, I was ready. But my daily existence is filled with ego-oriented events: first and second authorship: annoyance at seeing "my" meditation tape passed over for another's, etc. During my "content-analysis" experiment, I was surprised and not a little disturbed at the number of ego-related competitive thoughts I had. So the vision remains tantalizing; sometimes reached and experienced but lost again; sometimes a self-acceptance, even with the imperfections of the struggle; often not. Again, the goal seems clear; the path difficult.

> Breath soaring
>   a seagull's meditation
>   yielding to the wind.

Another issue for me, and others with similar "goal-orientation," is the problem of approaching meditation in a "Western way"—looking for the end product, rather than at the process. This has two ramifications. First, there are a lot of "shoulds" associated with reaching the goal, and doing so "perfectly." For example, during the initial years of practice, I felt I "should" practice a certain length of time. If I did not, I felt I was failing not only myself but also "The Great Meditation Teacher in the Sky." There is a discipline involved in learning to still one's mind and body; however doing it with a compulsive "I had better succeed" attitude, and trying to compete, if only with myself for "longer times" was not helpful. Rather, as in the case study in Chapter Two, it was just another opportunity for me to be critical about myself. What do I do, for example, when I am trying to meditate for a half hour, and my two and four-year old children come home, rush in, and say "Hi, Daddy." Of course the true Zen master makes them part of his meditation. Sometimes I could, but for me, formal meditation is an important time to clean out, to reduce inputs, and get away from stimulations. I wanted to "finish" and so I would brace as I heard them, try to breathe, hug them, and ask them to give me a few more minutes alone. Then I would continue with meditation, and try to learn to accept "guilty feelings." How discrepant were my visions of whom I wanted to be with how I live each moment, leaving me to wonder if that gap would ever be closed.

Also, once having felt peak experiences, in which I was suffused with a lovely inner peace, I wanted them every time I meditated. Sometimes it would occur so easily. Other times I could try hard, I could try not trying, I could not try, but could not find the "entrance" into that special place. This still remains a frustration to me.

WHAT TASKS ARE LEFT: PERSONALLY/PROFESSIONALLY

How do I integrate a belief in an egoless, cooperative ethic with my individualistic, ambitious style? A belief in graceful, giving simplicity and social commitment with a lifestyle that involves possessions—two homes, two cars, flying at least a thousand miles a week. An inquiring intellectualism with my peaceful inner core experience?

At best I perform these actions sequentially. For me, that is the best compromise I have arrived at. I cannot both be analytical *and* in my peaceful space. It is also hard for me to gear up for a task without being on edge. My sense is I need to try to perfect both styles, and work on integrating them.

I believe the meditation field might benefit from similar advice. We need to 1) become *more visionary* in our attempt for a complete understanding of meditation and its potential for helping us expand our human potential; 2) we need to become *more precise* in our study of that task; and 3) we need to make sure that the two tasks do not lose sight of each other. Otherwise we have vision without grounding; or precision without important substance.

I would like to see each clinician, researcher, and meditation practitioner go more in depth. Our research needs to be more methodologically sophisticated and innovative, as suggested in

Chapters Five, Seven, and Ten. Clinically, we need more in-depth case studies, presenting how in fact meditation might be useful in therapy and health-related fields (Chapters Two and Three). On a practice level, it is hard to understand what you do not know about. We can only teach well what we truly know and understand. Therefore, a greater depth of experiential knowledge is necessary to push the frontiers on a personal level, to share in a precise way the problems, pitfalls, *and* possibilities that we might attain. We also need the theoreticians, with an overview, to give us models. Each of the four parts would require "lifetimes" of work for several individuals. The task for any one individual even to take a beginning, small first step toward accomplishing all four is enormous and, as I noted at the start of this epilogue, teaches humility.

So, the book ends, with respect for two traditions, humility at the size of the task and a recognition of the limitations of our humanness. The challenge remains: to struggle to push the limits of the self, personally, professionally, while remembering to temper the struggle with acceptance.

In peace.
DHS
December, 1979
Laguna Beach, CA.

Appendices

A. Motivation/Expectation/Adherence
    Questionnaire

B. Notes

C. References

Background Note to Motivation, Expectation, Adherence Questionnaire (MEA)

〰〰 MY COLLEAGUES and I are currently involved in a seven-nation study of self-control. One part of this study looks at why people begin to practice different types of self-control techniques, what their motivation is, their hopes, and why they either continue or stop the practice of those techniques.

The MEA is a sub-form of the Shapiro Self-Control Inventory (SSCI) and consists mainly of open-ended questions about an individual's experience with the practice of self-control techniques. Below is a version of the MEA Questionnaire applied to meditation.

*   *   *   *   *   *   *

SSCI (MEA subform):
Meditation

The following questionnaire is being given as part of a seven-nation, cross-cultural study designed to help us gather information about self-control. We appreciate your taking the time to take this survey. Please be as honest and precise as you can, and answer every question. Your responses will be kept confidential.

Thank you for your cooperation.

Please circle the correct answer, or fill in the blank where appropriate.

—Last six digits of social security number ___ ___ ___ ___ ___ ___

1. *Background Information*

1.1 Sex: Male
          Female

1.2 Age: _____

1.3 Level of Education: _____

1.4 Occupation (specify: for example "student", "housewife", "dentist"): _____

1.5 Marital Status: Single ____ Married ____ Separated ____
Divorced ____ Widowed ____

1.6 Race or Ethnic Background: 1. white
2. black
3. oriental
4. Spanish speaking
5. other (specify) _____

1.7 Country of Birth: _____

1.8 Religion: 1. none, atheist or agnostic
2. Protestant
3. Catholic
4. Jewish
5. Buddhist
6. other (specify) _____

1.1. Have you ever meditated before?   Yes   No
If yes, go to question 1.2
If no, go to question 1.1a

1.1a Would you like to learn to meditate?   Yes   No
If yes, please go to question 1.1c.
If no, please go to question 1.1b.

1.1b Could you please put down in a sentence or two some of
the reasons why you don't wish to learn to meditate.
(After answering 1.1b, you are now finished with the
questionnaire: Thank you.)

1.1c Could you please put down in a sentence or two some of
the reasons why you want to learn to meditate.

1.1d What do you believe, in general, to be the qualities of a
truly gifted meditator? (After answering 1.1d you are
now finished with the questionnaire: Thank you.)

1.2 How long have you been meditating?

1.3 Do you meditate formally on a regular basis?   Yes   No
    How long per day?
    How many sittings?

1.4 What type(s) of meditation do you practice?

1.5 Have you practiced other types of meditation in the past?
    If yes, which ones and for how long?

1.6 Why did you stop practicing the other meditation techniques?

1.7 Have you ever stopped meditating for a period of time?
    How long; how often? For what reasons?

1.8 When you don't meditate on a given day, what do you say to
    yourself?

2.1 Why did you begin meditating? Please list as many specific
    reasons as possible.

2.2 What do you believe, in general, to be the personal qualities
    of a truly gifted meditator?

2.3 When you sit down to meditate, what do you think/feel right before the session?

2.4 How do you believe that meditation has influenced your life. Please mention both personal and interpersonal changes.

Positive Influences

Adverse Influences

General Changes

Thank you again for your cooperation in completing this questionnaire.

*   *   *   *   *   *   *

NOTE TO READERS:

If you are interested in filling out the above questionnaire, and would like the results of the study, please send the completed questionnaire, with your name and address to:
Deane H. Shapiro, Jr., Ph.D.
Box 2084, Stanford, CA. 94305

Notes

1. Smith, J. Meditation and preparatory variables. Unpublished manuscript, Roosevelt University 1979.
2. Katz, N.W. & Crawford, C.L. A little trance, and a little skill. Paper presented at the meeting of the Society for Clinical and Experimental Hypnosis, Chapel Hill, NC, October, 1978.
3. Brautigam, E. The effect of transcendental meditation on drug abusers. Unpublished manuscript, City Hospital of Malmo, Sweden 1971.
4. Shapiro, D.H. Cross-cultural study of motivation, expectation, and adherence in meditators. Manuscript in preparation, Laguna Beach, CA.
5. Shapiro, D.H. The Shapiro Self-Control Inventory. (SSCI). Unpublished test. In preparation, Laguna Beach, CA.
6. Schwartz, G., Davidson, R. & Margolin, R. Meditation and the self-regulation of attention. Unpublished manuscript, Harvard University.
7. Branstrom, M. Preferred perceptual mode and biofeedback training. Unpublished doctoral dissertation. Pacific Graduate School of Psychology, 1979.
8. Schwartz, G. Pros and cons of meditation. Paper presented at the annual meeting of the American Psychological Association, Montreal, Canada, 1973.
9. Smith, J. Models of meditation. Unpublished manuscript, Roosevelt University 1979.
10. Meichenbaum, D. Cognitive factors in behavior modification: Modifying what people say to themselves. Paper presented at the meeting of the Association for the Advancement of Behavior Therapy, Washington, D.C., December, 1971.

11. Jacks, R. Systematic desensitization compared with a self-management paradigm. Unpublished doctoral dissertation, Stanford University, 1972.
12. Jeffrey, D.B. Relative efficacy of external control and self-control in the production and maintenance of weight loss. Paper presented at the annual meeting of the American Psychological Association, New Orleans, August, 1974.
13. Black, R. & Thoreson, C. Self-hypnosis: A cognitive social learning perspective. Paper presented at the annual meeting of the American Psychological Association, Toronto, Canada, 1978.
14. Pagano, R., Warrenburg, S., Woods, M., Hlastala, M. Oxygen consumption during transcendental meditation and progressive muscle relaxation. Unpublished manuscript, University of Washington, Seattle, Washington.
15. Shapiro, D. *The psychology of self-control.* Manuscript in preparation, Laguna Beach, CA.

References

Abrams, A.I. & Siegel, L.M. The transcendental meditation program and rehabilitation at Folsom State Prison: A cross validation study. *Criminal Justice and Behavior*, 1975, *5*, (1), 3-20

Akers, T.K., Tucker, D.M., Roth, Randy S., Vidiloff, J.S., Personality correlates of EGG change during meditation. *Psychology Reports*, 1977 *40*, 439-442.

Akishige, Y. (Ed.) Psychological studies on Zen. Kyushu Psychological Studies. *Bulletin of the Faculty of Literature of Kyushu University*, Fukuoka, Japan, 1968, No. 5.

Akishige, Y. (Ed.) *Psychological studies on Zen.* Tokyo: Zen Institute of the Komazawa University, 1970.

Alexander, F. Buddhistic training as an artificial catatonia. *Psychoanalytic Review*, 1931, *18*, 129-45.

Allison, J. Respiratory change during transcendental meditation. *Lancet*, 1970 Ap, *1*, 833-4.

Allport, G. *Becoming*, New Haven, Conn.: Yale University Press, 1955.

American Psychiatric Association. Position statement on meditation. *American Journal of Psychiatry*, 1977 Jun. *134*, (6), 720.

Anand, B., Chinna, G. & Singh, B. Some aspects of electroencephalographic studies in yogis. *Electroencephalography & Clinical Neurophysiology*, 1961a, *13*, 452-6.

Anand, B., Chinna, G. & Singh, B. Studies on Shri Ramananda Yogi during his stay in an air-tight box. *Indian Journal of Medical Research*, 1961b, *49*, 82-9.

Anderson, D. Transcendental meditation as an alternative to heroin abuse in servicemen. *American Journal of Psychiatry,* 1977, *134* (11), 1308-1309.

Ashem, B., & Donner, L. Covert sensitization with alcoholics. *Behavior Research & Therapy,* 1968, *6,* (1), 7-12.

Axelrod, S., Hall, V., Weis, L., & Rohrer, S. Use of self-imposed contingencies to reduce the frequency of smoking behavior. In M. J. Mahoney & C. E. Thoresen (Eds.), *Self-control: Power to the person.* Monterey, Calif.: Brooks/Cole, 1974.

Bagchi, B.K. Mental hygiene and the Hindu doctorine of relaxation. *Mental Hygiene,* 1936, *20,* 424-40.

Bagchi, B.K., & Wenger, M.A. Simultaneous EEG and other recordings during some yogi exercises. *Electroencephalography & Clinical Neurophysiology,* 1957, Suppl. #7, 132-49.

Bandura, A. *Principles of behavior modification,* New York: Holt, Rinehart, Winston, 1969.

Bandura, A. Behavior theory and models of man. *American Psychologist,* 1974a, *29,* (12), 859-69.

Bandura, A. Foreword. In C.E. Thoresen & M.J. Mahoney (Eds.). *Behavioral self-control.* New York: Holt, Rinehart & Winston, 1974. (b)

Bandura, A. Self-reinforcement processes. In M.J. Mahoney & C.E. Thoresen (Eds.), *Self-control: Power to the person.* Monterey, Calif.: Brooks/Cole, 1974. (c)

Bandura, A. Self-efficacy: Toward a unifying theory of behavioral change. *Psychological Review,* 1977 Mar, *84,* (2), 191-215.

Bandura, A. *Social learning theory.* Englewood Cliffs, NJ: Prentice Hall, 1977.

Bandura, A. The self-system in reciprocal determinism. *American Psychologist,* 1978, *33,* (4), 344-58.

Banquet, J.-P. EEG and meditation. *Electroencephalography & Clinical Neurophysiology,* 1973, *33,* 454.

Banquet, J.-P. Spectral analysis of the EEG in meditation. *Electroencephalography & Clinical Neurophysiology,* 1973, *35,* 143-51.

Barber, T.X. and Calverly, D.S. Toward a theory of hypnotic behavior: Effects of suggestibility on defining the situation as hypnosis and defining response to suggestions as easy. *Journal of Abnormal and Social Psychology,* 1964, *68,* 585-592.

Barber, T., DiCara, L.V., Kamiya, J., Miller, N.E., Shapiro, D., & Stoyva, J. (Eds.) *Biofeedback and self-control: An Aldine reader on the regulation of body processes and consciousness.* Chicago, Ill.: Aldine-Atherton, 1971.

Barlow, D.H., Leitenberg, H., & Agras, W.S. Experimental control of sexual deviation through manipulation of the noxious scene in covert sensitization. *Journal of Abnormal Psychology,* 1969, *4,* 597-601.

Beck, A.T., *Cognitive therapy and the emotional disorders.* New York: International University Press, 1976.

Beiman, I.H., Johnson, S.A., Puente, A.E., Majestic, H.W., Graham, L.E. Client characteristics and success in TM. In D.H. Shapiro & R.N. Walsh (Eds.), *The science of meditation.* New York: Aldine, 1980.

Bem, D. Self-perception theory. In L. Berkowitz (Ed.), *Advances in experimental social psychology.* v.6. NY: Academic Press, 1972.

Beneke, W., & Harris, M. Teaching self-control of study behavior. *Behavior Research & Therapy,* 1972, *10,* (1), 35-41.

Bennett, J.E., & Trinder, J. Hemispheric laterality and cognitive style associated with transcendental meditation. *Psychophysiology,* 1977, *14,* 293-296.

Benson, H. *The relaxation response.* New York: William Morrow & Co., 1975.

Benson, H. Yoga for drug abuse. *New England Journal of Medicine,* 1969, *281,* (20), 1133.

Benson, H., & Wallace, R. Decreased blood pressure in hypertensive subjects who practice meditation. *Circulation,* 1972a, Suppl. #2, 516.

Benson, H., & Wallace, R. Decreased drug abuse with transcendental meditation: A study of 1862 subjects. In C.J. Zarafonetis (Ed.), *Drug abuse: Proceedings of the international conference.* Phil: Lea & Febiger, 1972b.

Benson, H., Beary, J.F., & Carol, M.P. The relaxation response. *Psychiatry,* 1974, *37,* 37-46.

Benson, H., Rosner, B.A., Marzetta, B.R., et al. Decreased blood pressure in borderline hypertensive subjects who practiced meditation. *Journal of Chronic Diseases,* 1974a, *27,* 163-9.

Benson, H., Marzetta, B.R., Rosner, B.A., Klemchuck, H.M. Decreased blood pressure in pharmacologically treated hypertensive patients who regularly elicited the relaxation response. *Lancet,* 1974b, (7852), 289-91.

Benson, H. Reply to Muchlman. *New England Journal of Medicine,* 1977, *297,* (9), 513.

Berlyn, D.E. *Conflict, arousal, and curiosity.* New York: McGraw-Hill, 1960.

Bergin, A., & Garfield, S. *Handbook of psychotherapy & behavior change.* New York: J. Wiley, 1971.

Bernard, H. & Efran, J. Eliminating versus reducing smoking using pocket timers. *Behavior Research & Therapy,* 1972 Nov, *10,* (4), 399-401.

Berwick, P. & Oziel, L.J. The use of meditation as a behavioral technique. *Behavior Therapy,* 1973, *4,* 743-5.

Blanchard, E.G., & Young, L.D. Clinical applications of biofeedback training: A review of the evidence. *Archives of General Psychiatry,* 1974, *30,* 573-92.

Bloomfield, H., Cain, M. & Jaffe, R. *TM: Discovering inner energy and overcoming stress.* NY: Delacorte, 1975.

Boals, G. Toward a cognitive reconceptualization of meditation. *Journal of Transpersonal Psychology,* 1978, *10,* (2), 143-182.

Bono, J. An integrated psychological assessment of transcendental meditation. In Shapiro, D.H., & Walsh, R.N. (Eds.). *The science of meditation.* New York: Aldine, in press.

Borkovec, T.D. Physiological and cognitive processes in the regulation of anxiety. In G.E. Schwartz & D. Shapiro (Eds.), *Consciousness and self-regulation:* Advances in research. v.i. New York: Plenum, 1976.

Borkovec, T.D. & Nau, S. Credibility of analogue therapy rationales. *Journal of Behavior Therapy & Experimental Psychiatry, 1972 Dec., 3,* (4), 257-60.

Boss, M. *A psychiatrist discovers India.* London: Oswald Wolff, 1965.

Boswell, P.C. & Murray, G.J. Effects of meditation on psychological and physiological measures of anxiety. *Journal of Consulting and Clinical Psychology,* 1979, *47,* (3), 606-607.

Boudreau, L. Transcendental meditation and yoga as reciprocal inhibitors. *Journal of Behavior Therapy & Experimental Psychiatry, 1972, 3,* 97-8.

Breuer, J. and Freud, S. (1893), *Studies in hysteria. In the standard edition of the complete psychological works of Freud. J. Strachey, (Ed.) Vol. 2. London: Hogarth, 1955.*

Broden, M., Hall, R., & Mitts, B. The effect of self-recording on the classroom behavior of two eighth-grade students. Journal of Applied Behavioral Analysis, 1971, *4,* (3), 191-9.

Brown, D. A model for the levels of concentrative meditation. *International Journal of Clinical & Experimental Hypnosis,* 1977, *25,* 236-73.

Brown, F., Stuart, W., & Blodgett, J. EEG kappa rhythms during transcendental meditation and possible perceptual threshold changes following. In D. Kunellakos (Ed.) *The psychobiology of transcendental meditation.* Menlo Park, CA: W.A. Benjamin, 1974.

Bruner, J.S. *Beyond the information given: Studies in the psychology of knowing.* New York: Norton, 1973.

Buber, M. *Between man and man.* Tr. R. Smith. Lond: Collins, 1961.

Buber, M. *I and thou,* New York: Schribner, 1958.

Buddhashasa, *The path of purification.* Berkeley. Shambhala, 1976.

Cannon, W.B. *The wisdom of the body.* New York: Norton, 1932.

Capra, R. *Tao of physics.* Berkeley, CA: Shambhalla, 1976.

Carrington, P. *Freedom in meditation.* New York: Anchor/Doubleday, 1978.

Carrington, P. & Ephron, H. Meditation as an adjunct to psychotherapy. In S. Arieti & G. Chrzanowski (Eds.), *The world biennial of psychotherapy and psychiatry (III).* New York: J. Wiley, 1975.

Cattell, R.B. *Personality and motivation structure and measurement.* New York: World Book Co., 1957.

Cattell, R.B., Eber, H.W., Tatsuoka, M. *Handbook for the sixteen personality factor questionnaire.* Champaign, IL: Institute for Personality and Ability Testing, 1970.

Cautela, J.R. Covert conditioning. In A. Jacobs & L.G. Jacks (Eds.) *The Psychology of private events: Perspectives on covert response systems.* New York: Academic Press, 1971.

Cautela, J.R. Covert sensitization, *Psychological Record,* 1967, *20,* 459-468.

Cauthen, N. & Prymak, C. Meditation versus relaxation. *Journal of Consulting & Clinical Psychology,* 1977, Jun, *45,* (3), 496-7.

Chassan, J.B. & Bellak, L. An introduction to intensive design in the evaluation of drug efficacy during psychotherapy. In L. Gottschalk & A. Averback (Eds.), *Methods of research in psychotherapy.* NY: Appleton-Century-Crofts, 1966.

Clark, F.V. Transpersonal perspectives in psychotherapy. *Journal of Humanistic Psychology,* 1977 *17,* (2), 69-81.

Coates, T.J. & Thoresen, C.E. What to use instead of sleeping pills. *Journal of the American Medical Association,* 1978, *240,* (21), 2311-2314.

Cohen, W. Spatial and textural characteristics of the ganzfeld, *American Journal of Psychology,* 1957, *70,* 403-410.

Cohen, Y. Inside what's happening: Sociological, psychological, and spiritual perspectives on the contemporary drug scene. *American Journal of Public Health*, 1969, *59*, 2092-7.

Connor, W.H. Effects of brief relaxation training on automatic response to anxiety-evoking stimuli. *Psychophysiology*, 1974, *11*, (5), 591-99.

Conze, E. *Buddhist meditation*, New York: Harper & Row, 1969.

Corby, J.C., Roth, W.T., Zarcone, V.P., Kopell, B.S. Psychophysiological correlates of the practice of Tantric Yoga meditation. *Archives of General Psychiatry*, 1978, *35*, 571-80.

Curtis, W.D. & Wessberg, H.W. A comparison of heart rate, respiration, and galvanic skin response among meditators, relaxers, and controls. *Journal of Altered States of Consciousness*, 1975/6, *2*, 319-24.

Daniels, L. Treatment of psychophysiological disorders and severe anxiety by behavior therapy, hypnosis and transcendental meditation. *American Journal of Clinical Hypnosis*, 1975, *17*, (4), 267-70.

Das, H. & Gastaut, H. Variations de l'activité electrique du cerveau, du couer et des muscles squelettiques an cours de la meditation et de l' extase yogique. *Electroencephalography & Clinical Neurophysiology*, 1955, Suppl. #6, 211-19.

Datey, K., Deshmukh, S.H., Dalvi, C.A. et al. "Shavasan": A Yogic exercise in the management of hypertension. *Angiology*, 1969, *20*, 325-33.

Davidson, J. Physiology of meditation and mystical states of consciousness. *Perspectives in Biology and Medicine*, 1976, *19*, 345-80.

Davidson, R. & Goleman, D. The role of attention in meditation and hypnosis: A psychobiological perspective on transformations of consciousness. *International Journal of Clinical & Experimental Hypnosis*, 1977, *25*, (4), 291-308.

Davidson, R., Goleman, D. & Schwartz, G. Attentional and affective concomitants of meditation: A cross-sectional study. *Journal of Abnormal Psychology*, 1976, *85*, 235-38.

Davidson, R. & Schwartz, G. The psychobiology of relaxation and related states: A multi-process theory. In D.I. Mostofsky (Ed.), *Behavior control and the modification of physiological activity*. New York: Prentice-Hall, 1976.

Davidson, R., Schwartz, G. & Rothman, L. Attentional style under self-regulation of mode specific attention: An electroencephalographic study. *Journal of Abnormal Psychology*, 1976, *85*, 611-21.

Davison, G.C. Counter control and behavior modification. In Hamerlynck, L.A. et al. (Eds.), *Behavior change: Methodology, concepts, practice.* Champaign, IL: Research Press, 1973.

Davison, G.C. Elimination of a sadistic fantasy by a client-controlled counter-conditioning technique: A case study. *Journal of Abnormal Psychology*, 1968(a), *73*, 84-90.

Davison, G.C. Systematic desensitization as a counter-conditioning process. *Journal of Abnormal Psychology*, 1968(b), *73*, 91-99.

Deathridge, G. The clinical use of mindfulness meditation techniques in short-term psychotherapy. *Journal of Transpersonal Psychology*, 1975, *7*, (2), 133-43.

Deikman, A.J. Bimodal consciousness. *Archives of General Psychiatry*, 1971, *25*, 481-9.

Deikman, A.J. Deautomatization and the mystic experience. *Psychiatry*, 1966, *29*, 324-38.

Deikman, A.J. Experimental meditation. *Journal of Nervous and Mental Disease*, 1963, *136*, 329-43.

Deikman, A.J. The state of the art of meditation. In D.H. Shapiro and R.N. Walsh (Eds.) *The Science of Meditation*, New York: Aldine, 1980, in press.

Dhammapada. English. *The Dhammapada.* Tr. Byrom. 1st Ed. New York: Knopf, 1976.

Dicara, L. Learning in the autonomic nervous system. *Scientific American*, 1970, *222*, 30-9.

Dicara, L. & Weiss, J. Effect of heart-rate learning under curare on subsequent non-curarized avoidance learning. *Journal of Comparative & Physiological Psychology*, 1969, *69*, (2), 368-74.

DiGiusto, G.L. & Bond, N.W. Imagery and the autonomic nervous system: Some methodological issues. *Perceptual and Motor Skills*, 1979, *48*, 427-438.

Dillbeck, M. The effect of the transcendental meditation technique on anxiety level. *Journal of Clinical Pyschology.* 1977, *33* (11) 1076-1078.

Dukes, W. N=1. *Psychological Bulletin*, 1965, *4*, (1), 74-9.

Ellis, A. *How to live with a "neurotic."* New York: Crown, 1957. Rev. ed: New York: Crown, 1975.

Ellis, A. *Reason and emotion in psychotherapy.* New York: Lyle Stuart and Citadel Press, 1962.

Ellis, A. The place of meditation in cognitive behavior therapy and rational emotive therapy. In D.H. Shapiro & R.N. Walsh (Eds.) *The science of meditation.* New York: Aldine, 1980, in press.

Elson, B., Hauri, P. & Cunis, D. Physiological changes in yoga meditation. *Psychophysiology,* 1977, *14,* 52-7.

Faber, P.A., Saayman, G.S., Touyz, W. Meditation and archetypal content of nocturnal dreams. *Journal of Analytic Psychology,* 1978, *23,* (1), 1-22.

Fadiman, J. & Fraeger, R. *Personality and personal growth.* New York: Harper and Row, 1976.

Fee, R.A. & Girdano, D.A. The relative effectiveness of three techniques to induce the trophotrophic response. *Biofeedback and Self-Regulation,* 1978, *3,* (2), 145-157.

Fenwick, P.B., Donaldson, S., Gillis, C., et al. Metabolic and EEG changes during transcendental meditation: An explanation. *Biological Psychology,* 1977, *5,* (2), 101-18.

Ferguson, G. *Statistical analysis in psychology and education.* 2nd Ed. New York: McGraw-Hill, 1966.

Ferguson, P.O. & Gowan, J.C. Transcendental meditation: Some preliminary findings. *Journal of Humanistic Psychology,* 1976, *16,* (3), 51-60.

Ferster, C.B. The use of learning principles in clinical practices and training. *Psychological Record,* 1971, *21,* (3), 353-61.

Ferster, C.B. Classification of behavior pathology. In L. Krasner & L.P. Ullman (Eds.), *Research in behavior modification.* New York: Holt, Rinehart & Winston, 1965.

Ferster, C.B. An experimental analysis of clinical phenomenon. *Psychological Record,* 1972, *22,* 1-16.

Ferster, C.B., Nurnburger, J.I., & Levitt, E.B. The control of eating. *Journal of Mathematics,* 1962, *1,* 87-109.

Festinger, L. Cognitive dissonance. *Scientific American,* 1962, *207,* (4), 93-107.

Fischer, R. A cartography of the ecstatic and meditative states. *Science,* 1971, *174,* 897-904.

Frank, Jerome D. Nature and functions of belief systems: Humanism and transcendental religion. *American Psychologist,* 1977, *32,* (7), 555-9.

Franks, J. *Persuasion and healing,* New York: Schocken Books, 1963.

French, A.P. & Tupin, J. Therapeutic application of a simple relaxation method. *American Journal of Psychotherapy,* 1974, *28,* (2),

282-7.

French, A.P., Schmid, A.C. & Ingalls, E. Transcendental meditation, altered reality testing, and behavioral change: A case report. *Journal of Nervous & Mental Disease,* 1975, *161,* 55-8.

Freud, S. *The problem of anxiety.* New York, W.W. Norton, 1936.

Freud, S. *Studies in hysteria,* Collected Papers, New York: Basic Books, 1959.

Freud, S. Dynamics of transferences, (1912) *Standard edition of the complete psychological works of Freud,* J. Strachey, (Ed.) Vol. 2. London: Hogarth, 1955, Vol. 12, 97-98.

Freud, S. Recommendations to physicians practicing psychology, (1912a) *Standard edition of the complete psychological works of Freud,* J. Strachey, (Ed.) Vol. 2. London: Hogarth, 1955, Vol. 12, 109-120.

Fromm, E. Self hypnosis. *Psychotherapy: Theory, Research & Practice,* 1975, *12,* (3), 295-301.

Fromm, E. *Zen Buddhism and psychoanalysis.* NY: Harper & Row, 1960.

Galanter, M. & Buckley, P. Evangelic religion and meditation: Psychotherapeutic effects. *Journal of Nervous and Mental Disease,* 1978, *166,* (10), 685-691.

Galin, D. Implications for psychiatry of left and right cerebral specialization. *Archives of General Psychiatry,* 1974, *31,* 572-83.

"Gallup poll results in upsurge of new religious ideas in U.S.," *San Francisco Chronicle,* Nov. 18, 1976, column 1, p. 17.

Gellhorn, E. & Kiely, W. Mystical states of consciousness. *Journal of Nervous & Mental Disease,* 1972, *154,* 399-405.

Gilbert, G.S. & Parker, J.C., & Claiborn, C.D. Differential mood changes in alcoholics as a function of anxiety management strategies. *Journal of Clinical Psychology.* 1978, *34,* (11), 229-232.

Girodo, M. Yoga meditation and flooding in the treatment of anxiety neurosis. *Journal of Behavior Therapy & Experimental Psychiatry,* 1974, *5,* 157-60.

Glueck, B. & Stroebel, C. Biofeedback and meditation in the treatment of psychiatric illness. *Comprehensive Psychiatry,* 1975, *16,* (4), 303-21.

Goldfried, M. Systematic desensitization as training in self-control. *Journal of Consulting & Clinical Psychology,* 1971, *37,* (2), 228-34.

Goldfried, M. & Merbaum, M. *Behavior change through self-control.* New York: Holt, Rinehart & Winston, 1973.

Goldfried, M.R. Reduction of generalized anxiety through a variant of systematic desentization. In M. R. Goldfried & M. Merbaum (Eds.), *Behavior change through self-control.* New York: Holt, Rinehart & Winston, 1973.

Goldiamond, I. Self-control procedures in personal behavior problems. *Psychological Reports,* 1965, *17,* (3), 851-68.

Goldman, B.L., Domitor, P.J. & Murray, E.J. Effects of Zen meditation on anxiety reduction and perceptual functioning. *Journal of Consulting and Clinical Psychology,* 1979, *47,* (3), 551-56.

Goldstein, J. *Experience of insight: A natural unfolding.* Santa Cruz, CA: Unity Press, 1976.

Goleman, D. The Buddha on meditation and states of consciousness, part II: A typology of meditation techniques. *Journal of Transpersonal Psychology,* 1972, *4,* (2) 151-210.

Goleman, D. Meditation as meta-therapy: Hypotheses toward a proposed fifth state of consciousness. *Journal of Transpersonal Psychology,* 1971, *3,* (1), 1-25.

Goleman, D. The varieties of the meditative experience. New York: E.P. Dutton, 1977.

Goleman, D. & Schwartz, G. Meditation as an intervention in stress reactivity. *Journal of Consulting & Clinical Psychology,* 1976, *44,* 456-66.

Gottmann, J., McFall, R. & Barnett, J. Design and analysis of research using time series. *Psychological Bulletin,* 1969, *72,* 299-306.

Goyeche, J., Chihara, T. & Shimizu, H. Two concentration methods: A preliminary comparison. *Psychologia,* 1972, *15,* 110-111.

Graham, J. Effects of transcendental meditation upon auditory thresholds. In D. Johnson, L. Domash, J. Farrow (Eds.) *Scientific Research on the Transcendental Meditation Program.* Switzerland: MIU Press, 1975, Vol. 1.

Green, E., Green, A. & Walters, E. Voluntary control of internal states: Psychological and physiological. *Journal of Transpersonal Psychology,* 1970, *2,* 1-26.

Greenson, R. *The technique and practice of psychoanalysis,* Vol. 1, New York: International University Press, 1968.

Griffith, F. Meditation research: Its personal and social implications. In J. White (Ed.), *Frontiers of consciousness.* New York: Julian, 1974.

Group for the Advancement of Psychiatry. *Mysticism: Spiritual quest or psychic disorder?* Washington, D.C.: Group for the Advancement of Psychiatry, 1977.

Gundu Rao, H.V., Krishnaswamy, N., Narasimhaiya, R.L. Hoenig, J., Gouindaswamy, M.V. Some experiments on a Yogi in controlled states. *Pratibha, Journal of the All India Institute for Mental Health*, 1958, *1*, 99-106.

Hager, J.L., & Surwit, R.S. Hypertension self-control with a portable feedback unit or meditation-relaxation. *Biofeedback and Self-Regulation*, 1978, *3*, (3), 269-275.

Hannum, J., Thoresen, C.E., & Hubbard, D. A behavioral study of self-esteem with elementary teachers. In M.J. Mahoney & C.E. Thoresen (Eds.), *Self-control: Power to the person*, Monterey, Calif.: Brooks/Cole, 1974.

Hastings, A. & Fadiman, J., & Gordon, J.S. (Eds.), *Holistic medicine*. Rockville, MD: NIMH, in press, 1980.

Haynes, C. Psychophysiology of advanced participants in the transcendental meditation program. In D. Orme-Johnson & J. Farrow (Eds.), *Scientific Research on the TM Program*. v.I. 2nd Ed. Maharishi European Research University Press, 1977.

Heisenberg, W. *Physics and philosophy*. Lond: Allen & Unwin, 1963.

Hendricks, C.G. Meditation as discrimination training. *Journal of Transpersonal Psychology*, 1975, *7*, (2), 144-6.

Herbert, R. & Lehmann, D. Theta bursts: An EEG pattern in normal subjects practicing the transcendental meditation technique. *Electroencephalography & Clinical Neurophysiology*, 1977, *42*, 387-405.

Herrigel, E. *Zen in the art of archery*. NY: McGraw Hill, 1953. (Now entitled *Method of Zen)*

Hess, W. Das Zuischenhim die Regullerung von Lerpzug, Thieme, 1938.

Hesse, H. *Siddhartha*, New York: New Directions Books, 1951.

Hirai, T. *Psychophysiology of Zen*. Tokyo: Igaku Shin Ltd., 1974.

Hirai, T. & Watanabe, Biofeedback and electrodermal self-regulation in a Zen meditator. *Psychophysiology*, 1977, *14*, 103 (abstract).

Hjelle, L.A. Transcendental meditation and psychological health. *Perceptual & Motor Skills*, 1974, *39*, 623-8.

Holt, R.R., Imagery: The return of the ostracized. *American Psychologist*, 1964, *19*, 254-264.

Holt, W.R., Caruso, J.L., & Riley, J.B. Transcendental meditation vs. pseudo-meditation on visual choice reaction time. *Perceptual and Motor Skills*, 1978, *46*, 726.

Homme, L. Control of covenants: The operants of the mind. *Psychological Record*, 1965, *15*, (4), 501-11.

Homme, L.E., & Tosti, D. *Behavior technology: Motivation and contingency management.* San Rafael, Calif.: Individual Learning Systems, 1971.

Honig, K. *Operant behavior: Areas of research and application.* New York: Appleton-Century-Crofts, 1966.

Honsberger, R. & Wilson, A.P. Transcendental meditation in treating asthma. *Respiratory Therapy: Journal of Inhalation Technology*, 1973, *3*, 79-81.

Horowitz, M.J. *Image formation and cognition.* New York: Appleton-Century-Crofts, 1970.

Horowitz, M.J. Psychic trauma: Return of images after a stress film. *Archives of General Psychiatry*, 1969, *20*, 552-559.

Ikegami, R. Psychological study of Zen posture. *Bulletin of the Faculty of Literature of Kyushu University*, 1968, *5*, 105-35.

Jacobs, R.G., Kraemer, H.C. & Agras, W.S. Relaxation therapy in the treatment of hypertension: A Review. *Archives of General Psychiatry*, 1977, *34*, 1417-1427.

Jacobs, A. & Wolpin, M. A second look at systematic desensitization. In A. Jacobs & L.B. Sachs (Eds.), *The psychology of private events.* New York: Academic Press, 1971.

Jacobson, E. The two methods of tension control and certain basic techniques in anxiety tension control. In J. Kamiya, T. Barber, L.V. DiCara, N.E. Miller, D. Shapiro & J. Stoyva (Eds.) *Biofeedback and self-control: An Aldine annual on the regulation of body processes and consciousness.* Chicago, Ill.: Aldine-Atherton, 1971.

Jacobson, E. *Progressive relaxation.* Chicago: University of Chicago Press, 1929.

James. W. *The varieties of religious experience.* New York: Longmans, 1901.

Jevning, R. & O'Halloran, J.P. Metabolic effects of transcendental meditation. In D.H. Shapiro & R.N. Walsh (Eds.), *The science of meditation.* Aldine, New York, 1980, in press.

Jevning, R., Wilson, A. & Smith, W. Plasma amino acids during the transcendental meditation technique: Comparison to sleep. In D. Orme-Johnson & J. Farrow (Eds.), *Scientific research on the transcendental meditation program.* v.I. 2nd Ed. Maharishi European Research University Press, 1977.

Jevning, R., Wilson, A., & Vanderlaan, E. Plasma prolactin and growth hormone during meditation. *Psychosomatic Medicine,* 1978 Jun, *40,* (4), 329-33.

Jevning, R., et al., Alterations in blood flow during transcendental meditation. *Psychophysiology,* 1976, *13,* (2), 168. (Abstr.)

Johnson, S. & White, G. Self-observation as an agent of behavioral change. *Behavior Therapy,* 1971, *2,* (4), 488-97.

Johnson, W.G. Some applications of Homme's coverant control therapy: Two case reports. *Behavior Therapy,* 1971, *2,* 240-248.

Jung, C. (1947) Foreword. In D.T. Suzuki. *Introduction to Zen.* New York: Random House, 1964.

Kanas, N. & Horowitz, M. Reactions of TMers and non-meditators to stress films. *Archives of General Psychiatry,* 1977, *34,* (12), 1431-36.

Kanellakos, D.P., & Lukas, J.D. *The psychobiology of transcendental meditation: A literature review.* Menlo Park, Calif.: Benjamin, 1974.

Kaner, F.H. & Goldfoot, D.A. Self-control and tolerance of noxious stimulation. *Psychological Reports,* 1966, *18,* 79-85.

Kanfer, F.H. & Phillips, J. Behavior therapy: A panacea for all ills or a passing fancy? *Archives of General Psychiatry,* 1966, *15,* (2), 114-28.

Kanfer, F. & Karoly, P. Self-control: A behavioristic excursion into the lion's den. *Behavior Therapy,* 1972, *3,* (3), 389-416.

Kapleau, A. *Three pillars of Zen.* Boston, MA: Beacon Press, 1967.

Karambelkar, P., Vinekar, S. & Bhole, M. Studies on human subjects staying in an air-tight pit. *Indian Journal of Medical Research,* 1968, *56,* 1282-88.

Kasamatsu, A. & Hirai, T. An electroencephalographic study of the Zen meditation (zazen). *Folia Psychiatria et Neurologica Japonica,* 1966, *20,* 315-336.

Kasamatsu, A. & Hirai, T. An electroencephalographic study on the Zen meditation (zazen). *Psychologia,* 1969, *12,* 205-25.

Kasamatsu, A., Okuma, T., Takenaka, S., Koga, E., Ikada, K., Sugiyama, H. The EEG of 'Zen' and 'Yoga' practitioners. *Electroencephaolgraphy & Clinical Neurophysiology,* 1957, Suppl. #9, 51-2.

Kazdin, A.E. Self-monitoring and behavior change. In M.J. Mahoney & C.E. Thoresen (Eds.), *Self-control: Power to the Person.* Monterey, Calif.: Brooks/Cole, 1974.

Kazdin, A.E. Self-monitoring and behavior change. In M.J.

Mahoney & C.E. Thoresen (Eds.), *Self-control: Power to the person.* Monterey, Calif.: Brooks/Cole, 1974.

Keefe, T. Meditation and the psychotherapist. *American Journal of Orthopsychiatry,* 1975, *45,* (3), 484-9.

Kirsch, I. & Henry, I. Self-desensitization and meditation in the reduction of public speaking anxiety. *Journal of Consulting & Clinical Psychology,* 1979, *47,* (3), 536-41.

Kohr, E. Dimensionality in the meditative experience: A replication. *Journal of Transpersonal Psychology,* 1977, *9,* (2), 193-203.

Kolb, D.A., & Boyatzis, R.E. Goal setting and self-directed behavior change. *Human Relations,* 1970, *23,* 439-458.

Kondo, A. Zen in psychotherapy. *Chicago Review,* 1958, *12,* 57-64.

Kornfield, J. Meditation: Aspects of research and practice. *Journal of Transpersonal Psychology,* 1978, *2,* 122-124.

Kornfield, J. Intensive insight meditation: A phenomenological study. *Journal of Transpersonal Psychology,* 1979, *11,* (1), 41-58.

Kretschmer, W. Meditative techniques in psychotherapy. In C. Tart (Ed.), *Altered states of consciousness.* New York: J. Wiley, 1969.

Krishnamurti, J. *Meditation.* Ojai, CA: Krishnamurti Foundation, 1979.

Kubose, S.K. An experimental investigation of psychological aspects of meditation. *Psychologia,* 1976, *19,* (1), 1-10.

Kuhn, T. *The structure of scientific revolutions.* Chicago: University of Chicago Press, 1971.

Lachenmeyer, C.W. Experimentation, a misunderstood methodology in psychological and sociological research. *American Psychologist,* 1970, *15,* 617-24.

Lang, R., Dehof, K., Meurer, K.A. & Kaufman, W. Sympathetic activity and transcendental meditation. *Journal of Neural Transmission,* 1979, *44,* 117-135.

Lao-tzu. *Tao Te Ching.* Tr. G. Feng & J. English. New York: Vintage: 1973.

Lazar, Z. Farwell, L. & Farrow, J. Effects of transcendental meditation program on anxiety, drug abuse, cigarette smoking, and alcohol consumption. In D. Orme-Johnson & J. Farrow (Eds.), *Scientific Research on the Transcendental Meditation program.* v.I. 2nd Ed. Maharishi European Research University Press, 1977.

Lazarus, A.A., *Behavior therapy and beyond.* New York: McGraw-Hill, 1971.

Lazarus, A.A. A cognitively oriented psychologist looks at biofeedback. *American Psychologist*, 1975, *30*, 553-61.

Lazarus, A.A. Psychiatric problems precipitated by transcendental meditation. *Psychological Reports*, 1976, *10*, 39-74.

Lazarus, A.A. In the mind's eye. New York: Rawson Wade, 1978.

Lefcourt, H.M. Internal versus external control of reinforcement: A review. *Psychological Bulletin*, 1966, *65*, 206-220.

Lefcourt, H.M. Belief in personal control. *Journal of Individual Psychology*, 1966, *22*, (2), 185-95.

Lesh, T. Zen meditation and the development of empathy in counselors. *Journal of Humanistic Psychology*, 1970, *10*, (1), 39-74.

LeShan, L. *How to meditate.* New York: Bantam Books, 1975.

Leung, P. Comparative effects of training in external and internal concentration on two counseling behaviors. *Journal of Counseling Psychology*, 1973, *20*, 227-34.

Linden, W. The relationship between the practice of meditation by schoolchildren and their levels of field dependence-independence, test anxiety, and reading achievement. *Journal of Consulting & Clinical Psychology*, 1973, *41*, 139-43.

Luthe, W. Autogenic training: Method, research, and applications in medicine. In C. Tart (Ed.) *Altered states of consciousness.* New York: Wiley, 1968.

Luthe, W. *Autogenic training: Research and theory.* New York: Grune & Stratton, 1970.

Lykken, D. Statistical significance in psychological research. *Psychological Bulletin*, 1968, *70*, (3),151-7.

McFall, R.M. Effects of self-monitoring on normal smoking behavior. *Journal of Consulting & Clinical Psychology*, 1970 Oct, *35*, (2), 135-142.

McFall, R.M. & Hammen, C.L. Motivation, structure, and self-monitoring: The role of nonspecific factors in smoking reduction. *Journal of Consulting & Clinical Psychology*, 1971, *37*, 80-6

McReynolds, W.T., Barnes, A.R., Brooks, S., et al. The role of attention placebo influences in the efficacy of systematic desensitization. *Journal of Consulting & Clinical Psychology*, 1973, *41*, 86-92.

Mahoney, M.H. The self-management of covert behavior. *Behavior Therapy*, 1971, *2*, (4), 575-8.

Mahoney, M.J. *Cognitive behavior modification.* Boston, Mass.: Ballinger, 1974.

Mahoney, M.J. & Thoresen, C.E. *Self-control: Power to the per-*

son. Monterey, CA: Brooks/Cole, 1974.

Mahoney, M.J., Moura, N.G., & Wade, T.C. Relative efficacy of self-reward, self-punishment, and self-monitoring techniques for weight loss. *Journal of Consulting & Clinical Psychology,* 1973, *40,* (3), 404-7.

Malec, J. & Sipprelle, C. Physiological and subjective effects of Zen meditation and demand characteristics. *Journal of Consulting & Clinical Psychology.* 1977, *44,* 339-340.

Marcus, J.B. Transcendental meditation: Consciousness expansion as a rehabilitation technique. *Journal of Psychedelic Drugs,* 1975, *7,* (2), 169-79.

Marlatt, G., Pagano, R., Rose, R., Margues, J.K. Effect of meditation and relaxation training upon alcohol use in male social drinkers. In D.H. Shapiro & R.N. Walsh (Eds.), *The science of meditation.* New York: Aldine, 1980, in press.

Maslow, A. *Toward a psychology of being.* New York: Van Nostrand, 1968.

Matsumato, H. A psychological study of the relation between respiratory function and emotion. *Bulletin of the Faculty of Literature of Kyushu University,* 1974, *5,* 167-207.

Maupin, E. Individual differences in response to a Zen meditation exercise. *Journal of Consulting Psychology,* 1965, *29,* 139-45.

Maupin, E. Meditation. In H. Otto & J. Mann (Eds.), *Ways of growth.* New York: Viking, 1968.

Meichenbaum, D. Cognitive factors in biofeedback therapy, *Biofeedback and Self-Regulation,* 1976, *1* (2), 201-216.

Meichenbaum, Donald. *Cognitive behavior modification: An integrative approach.* New York: Plenum, 1977.

Meichenbaum, D. & Cameron, R. The clinical potential of modifying what clients say to themselves. In M.J. Mahoney & C.E. Thoresen. *Self-control: Power to the person.* Monterey, CA: Brooks/Cole, 1974.

Michaels, R., Huber, M. & McCann, D. Evaluation of transcendental meditation as a method of reducing stress. *Science,* 1976, *192,* (4245), 1242-4.

Miller, N. Learning of visceral and glandular responses. *Science,* 1969, *163,* (3866), 434-445.

Minuchin, S. *Families and family therapy.* Cambridge, MA: Harvard University Press, 1974.

Minuchin, S., Rosman, B.L, & Barker, L.: *Psychosomatic*

families: Anorexia nervosa in context. Cambridge, MA: Harvard University Press, 1978.

Mischel, W. *Personality and assessment.* New York: J. Wiley, 1968.

Mischel, W. & Mischel, F. Psychological aspects of spirit possession. *American Anthropologist,* 1958, *60,* 249-60.

Mischel, W., Ebbesen, E., & Raskoff-Zeiss, A. Cognitive and attentional mechanisms in delay of gratification. *Journal of Personality & Social Psychology,* 1972 Feb, *21,* (2), 204-18.

Mishra, R. *Fundamentals of Yoga.* New York: Julian, 1959.

Mitchell, K. Repeated measures and the evaluation of change in the individual client during counseling. *Journal of Counseling Psychology,* 1969, *16,* 522-7.

Mookerjee, A. *Tantra art.* New York: Ravi Kumar, 1966.

Mooney, R.L. & Gordon, L. *Mooney problems check list.* New York: Psychological Corp, 1951.

Morse, D.R., Martin, S. Furst, M.L. & Dubin, L.L. A physiological and subjective evaluation of meditation, hypnosis, and relaxation. *Psychosomatic Medicine,* 1977, *39,* 304-24.

Muchlman, M. Transcendental meditation. *New England Journal of Medicine.* 1977, *297* (9), 513.

Nakamizo, S. Psychophysiological studies on respiratory patterns. *Bulletin of the Faculty of Literature of Kyushu University,* 1974, *5,* 135-67.

Naranjo, C. Meditation: Its spirit and techniques. In C. Naranjo & R. Ornstein. *On the psychology of meditation,* New York: Viking, 1971.

Naranjo, C. & Ornstein, R. *On the psychology of meditation.* New York: Viking, 1971.

Nidich, S., Seeman, W. & Dreskin, T. Influence of transcendental meditation on a measure of self-actualization: A replication. *Journal of Counseling Psychology,* 1973, *20,* 565-6.

Onda, A. Zen, autogenic training, and hypnotism. *Psychologia,* 1967, *10,* 133-136.

Onda, A. Autogenic training and Zen. In W. Luthe (Ed.), *Autogenic Training.* New York: Grune & Stratton, 1965.

Orme-Johnson, D.W. Autonomic stability and transcendental meditation, *Psychosomatic Medicine,* 1973, *35,* (4), 341-9.

Orne, M.T. On the social psychology of the psychological experiment: With particular reference to demand characteristics and their implications. *American Psychologist*, 1962, *17*, (10), 776-83.

Ornstein, R. *The psychology of consciousness*. San Francisco; W.H. Freeman Co., 1972.

Ornstein, R. The techniques of meditation and their implications for modern psychology. In C. Naranjo & R. Ornstein. *On the psychology of meditation*. New York: Viking, 1971.

Osis, K., Bokert, E., Carlson, M.L. Dimensions of the meditative experience. *Journal of Transpersonal Psychology*, 1973, *5*, (1), 109-135.

Otis, L.S. If well-integrated but anxious, try TM. *Psychology Today*, 1974, *7*, 45-46.

Otis, L.S. Adverse effects of meditation. In Shapiro, D.H. and Walsh, R.N. (Eds.), *The science of meditation*. New York: Aldine, 1980, in press.

Pagano, R. & Frumkin, L. Effect of TM in right hemispheric functioning. *Biofeedback & Self-Regulation*, 1977, *2*, 407-15.

Parker, J.C., Gilbert, A.S., Thoreson, R.W. Reduction of autonomic arousal in alcoholics. *Journal of Consulting and Clinical Psychology*, 1978, *46* (5), 879-886.

Patel, C. Yoga and biofeedback in the management of hypertension. *Lancet*, 1973, 2, 1053-55.

Patel, C. Randomized control trial of Yoga and biofeedback in management of hypertension. *Lancet*. 1975a. *11*, 93-4.

Patel, C. Twelve-month follow-up of Yoga and biofeedback in the management of hypertension. *Lancet*, 1975b, *1*, 62-5.

Paul, G. Physiological effects of relaxation training and hypnotic suggestion. *Journal of Abnormal Psychology*, 1969, *74*, 425-37.

Pelletier, K. Influence of TM upon autokinetic perception. *Perceptual & Motor Skills*, 1974, *39*, 1031-34.

Pelletier, K. & Peper, E. The chutzpah factor in altered states of consciousness. *Journal of Humanistic Psychology*, 1977, *17*, (1), 63-73.

Piggins, D. & Morgan, D. Note upon steady visual fixation and repeated auditory stimulation in meditation and the laboratory. *Perceptual and Motor Skills*, 1977, *44*, 357-358.

Pirot, M. TM and perceptual auditory discrimination. Unpublished manuscript (Univ. of Victoria), 1973.

Polanyi, M. *Personal knowledge*. Chicago: Univ. of Chicago Press, 1958.

Pollack, A.A., Weber, M.A., Case, D.B., Laragh, J.H. Limitations of transcendental meditation in the treatment of essential hypertension. *Lancet,* 1977, *8,* 71-73.

Pomerleau, O.F. Behavioral medicine. *American Psychologist,* 1979, *34,* 654-663.

Premack, D. Reinforcement theory. In D. Levine (Ed.), *Nebraska Symposium on Motivation* (Vol. 13). Lincoln: University of Nebraska Press, 1965.

Premack, D. Mechanisms of self-control. In W. Hunt (Ed.), *Learning and mechanisms of control in smoking.* Chicago, Ill.: Aldine, 1970.

Pribram, K. *Languages of the brain: Experimental paradoxes and principles in neuropsychology.* Englewood Cliffs, NJ: Prentice-Hall, 1971.

Pribram, K. & McGuiness, D. Arousal, activation, and effort in the control of attention. *Psychological Review,* 1975, *82,* 116-49.

Rahula, W. *What the Buddha taught.* New York: Grove Press, 1959.

Random House dictionary of the English language, J. Stein & L. Urdang. (Eds.) Unabridged. New York: Random House, 1973.

Rao, S. Oxygen consumption during Yoga-type breathing at altitudes of 520m and 5800m. *Indian Journal of Medical Research,* 1968, *56,* 701-5.

Rogers, C. *Client centered therapy.* Boston: Houghton Mifflin, 1951.

Rogers, C. *On becoming a person.* Boston: Houghton Mifflin, 1961.

Rogers, C.R. Necessary and sufficient conditions for therapeutic personality change. *Journal of Consulting Psychology,* 1957, *21,* (2) 95-103.

Rosenthal, R., Persinger, G. & Fode, K. Experimenter bias, anxiety and social desirability. *Perceptual & Motor Skills,* 1962, *15,* (1), 73-4.

Rotter, J.B. External control and internal control. *Psychology Today,* 1971, *5,* (1), 37-42, 58-9.

Rotter, J.B. Generalized expectancies for internal versus external control of reinforcement. *Psychological Monographs,* 1966, *80,* (1), (Whole #609).

Rotter, J.B. Internal-external control scale. In J. Robinson & P. Shaver (Eds.), *Measures of social psychological attitudes.* Ann

Arbor: University of Michigan Press, 1969.

Sargent, W. *The mind possessed: The physiology of possession, mysticism, and faith healing.* Phil: J.B. Lippincott, 1974.

Schacter, S. & Singer, J. Cognitive, social, and physiological determinants of emotional state. *Psychological Review.* 1962, *69*, (5), 379-99.

Schuster, R. Empathy and mindfulness. *Journal of Humanistic Psychology,* 1979, *19*, (1), 71-7.

Schwartz, G., & Weiss, S. What is behavioral medicine? *Psychosomatic Medicine,* 1977, *36*, 377-381.

Schwartz, G.E. Biofeedback as therapy: Some theoretical and practical issues. *American Psychologist,* 1973, *28*, 666-673.

Schwartz, G. Biofeedback, self-regulation, and the patterning of physiological processes. *American Scientist,* 1975, *63*, 314-25.

Schwartz, G., Davidson, R. & Goleman, D. Patterning of cognitive and somatic processes in the self-regulation of anxiety: Effects of meditation versus exercise. *Psychosomatic Medicine,* 1978, *40*, 321-8.

Seeman, W., Nidich, S. & Banta, T. Influence of TM on a measure of self-actualization. *Journal of Counseling Psychology,* 1972, *19*, (3), 184-7.

Selye, H. *The stress of life.* New York: McGraw-Hill, 1956.

Shafii, M. Silence in the service of ego: Psychoanalytic study of meditation. *International Journal of Psychoanalysis,* 1973, *54*, (4), 431-43.

Shafii, M., Lavely, R. & Jaffe, R. Meditation and marijuana. *American Journal of Psychiatry.* 1974, *131*, 60-3.

Shafii, M., Lavely, R. & Jaffe, R. Meditation and the prevention of alcohol abuse. *American Journal of Psychiatry,* 1975, *132*, 942-45.

Shapiro, D., Tursky, B., & Schwartz, G. Differentiation of heart rate and systolic blood pressure in man by operant conditioning. *Psychosomatic Medicine,* 1970, *32*, (4), 417-23.

Shapiro, D. & Tursky, B., Schwartz, G.E., & Shnidman, S.R. Smoking on cue: A behavioral approach to smoking reduction. *Journal of Health and Social Behavior,* 1971, *12*, 108-113.

Shapiro, D., Barber, T., DiCara, L.V., Kamiya, J., Miller, N.E. & Stoyva, J. (Eds.) *Biofeedback and self-control: An Aldine annual on the regulation of body processes and consciousness.* Chicago, Ill.: Aldine, 1973.

Shapiro, D.H. A combined personal self-management and environmental consultation strategy. In J.P. Krumboltz and C.E. Thoreson (Eds.) Counseling methods. New York: Holt, Rinehart & Winston, 1976.

Shapiro, D.H. Zen meditation and behavioral self-management applied to a case of generalized anxiety. *Psychologia.* 1976, *19*, (3), 134-8.

Shapiro, D.H. Behavioral and attitudinal changes resulting from a Zen experience workshop in Zen meditation. *Journal of Humanistic Psychology*, 1978a, *18* (3), 21-9.

Shapiro, D.H. *Precision nirvana.* Englewood Cliffs, NJ: Prentice-Hall, 1978b.

Shapiro, D.H. Instructions for a training package combining Zen meditation and behavioral self-management strategies. *Psychologia.* 1978, *21* (2), 70-76.

Shapiro, D.H. Meditation and holistic medicine. In A. Hastings, J. Fadiman, J. Gordon (Eds.) *Holistic medicine.* Rockville, MD: NIMH, 1980a, in press.

Shapiro, D.H. Meditation and stress management: Use of a self-regulation strategy in anxiety reduction. In D. Logan (Ed.) *A comprehensive approach to the treatment of anxiety.* New York: Springer, in press.

Shapiro, D.H. & Giber, D. Meditation and psychotherapeutic effects. *Archives of General Psychiatry*, 1978, *35*, 294-302.

Shapiro, D.H. & Walsh, R.N. (Eds.) *The science of meditation.* Aldine: New York, 1980 in press.

Shapiro, D.H. & Zifferblatt, S.M. An applied clinical combination of Zen meditation and behavioral self-management techniques: Reducing methadone dosage in drug addiction. *Behavior Therapy*, 1976a, *7*, 694-5.

Shapiro, D.H. & Zifferblatt, S.M. Zen meditation and behavioral self-control: Similarities, differences and clinical applications. *American Psychologist*, 1976b, *31*, 519-32.

Shapiro, J. & Shapiro, D.H. The psychology of responsibility. *New England Journal of Medicine*, 1979, *301* (4), 211-212.

Shaw, R. & Kolb, D. Improved reaction time following TM. In D. Orme-Johnson & J. Farrow (Eds.), *Scientific research on the transcendental meditation program.* V.I. 2nd Ed. Maharishi European Research University Pr., 1977.

Sidman, M. *Tactics of scientific research.* New York: Basic Books Inc., 1960.

Singer, J.L. Navigating the stream of consciousness: Research in daydreaming and related inner experience. *American Psychologist,* 1975, *30,* 727-38.

Singer, J.L. *Imagery and daydream methods in psychotherapy and behavior modification.* New York: Academic Press, 1974.

Skinner, B.F. What is the experimental analysis of behavior? *Journal of the Experimental Analysis of Behavior,* 1966, *9* (3), 213-18.

Skinner, B.F. Behaviorism at fifty. In T.W. Wann (Ed.), *Behaviorism and phenomenology.* Chicago, Ill.: University of Chicago Press, 1964.

Skinner, B.F. *Science and human behavior.* New York: Mac-Millan, 1953.

Smith, H. *The religions of man.* New York: Harper, 1965.

Smith, J. Meditation and psychotherapy: A review of the literature, *Psychological Bulletin,* 1975, *32,* (4), 553-64.

Smith, J. Personality correlates of continuation and outcome in meditation and erect sitting control treatments. *Journal of Consulting & Clinical Psychology,* 1978, *46,* (2), 272-9.

Smith, J. Psychotherapeutic effects of TM with controls for expectations of relief and daily sitting. *Journal of Consulting & Clinical Psychology,* 1976, *44,* (4), 630-7.

Solomon, G.G., & Bumpus, A.K. The running meditation response: An adjunct to psychotherapy. *American Journal of Psychotherapy,* 1978, *32* (4), 583-592.

Spanos, P.H., Rivers, S.M., & Gottlieb, J. Hypnotic responsivity, meditation, and laterality of eye movements. *Journal of Abnormal Psychology,* 1978, *87,* (5), 566-569.

Sperry, R. A revised concept of consciousness. *Psychological Review,* 1969, *76,* 532-6.

Spiegelberg, F. *Spiritual practices of India.* New York: Citadel, 1962.

Stace, W.T. *Mysticism & philosophy.* 1st. Ed. Phil: Lippincott, 1960.

Stek, R. & Bass, B. Personal adjustment and perceived locus of control among students interested in meditation. *Psychological Reports,* 1973, *32,* 1019-22.

Stone, R. & DeLeo, J. Psychotherapeutic control of hypertension. *The New England Journal of Medicine,* 1976, *294,* (2), 80-4.

Stoyva, J., Barber, T., DiCara, L.V., Kamiya, J., Miller, N.E., & Shapiro, D.H., (Eds.). *Biofeedback and self-control: An Aldine annual on the regulation of body processes and consciousness.*

Chicago, Ill.: Aldine-Atherton, 1972.

Stroebel, C. & Glueck, B. Passive meditation: Subjective and clinical comparison with biofeedback. In G. Schwartz & D. Shapiro (Eds.), *Consciousness and self-regulation.* New York: Plenum, 1977.

Stuart, R.B. Behavioral control of overeating. *Behavior Research & Therapy,* 1967, *5,* (4), 357-65.

Stunkard, A. New therapies for the eating disorders: Behavior modification of obesity and anorexia nervosa. *Archives of General Psychiatry,* 1972, 26, 391-398.

Stunkard, A. Interpersonal aspects of an Oriental religion. *Psychiatry,* 1951, *14,* 419-31.

Sugi, Y. & Akutsu, K. Studies on respiration and energy metabolism during sitting in Zazen. *Research Journal Physical Education,* 1968, *12,* (3), 190-206.

Suinn, R. & Richardson, F. Anxiety management training: A nonspecific behavior therapy program for anxiety control. *Behavior Therapy,* 1971, *2,* (4), 498-510.

Surwit, R.S., Shapiro, D., Good, M.I. Comparison of cardio-vascular biofeedback, neuromuscular feedback, and meditation in the treatment of borderline hypertension. *Journal of Consulting and Clinical Psychology,* 1978, *46* (2), 252-263.

Suzuki, D.T. Lectures in Zen Buddhism. In E. Fromm (Ed.), *Zen Buddhism and psychoanalysis.* New York: Harper-Colophon 1960.

Suzuki, D.T. Manual of Zen Buddhism. Lond: Rider, 1956.

Tart, C. (Ed.) *Altered states of consciousness.* New York: J. Wiley, 1969.

Tart, C. A psychologist's experience with T.M. *Journal of Transpersonal Psychology,* 1971, *3,* (2), 135-40.

Tart, C. States of consciousness and state-specific sciences. *Science,* 1972, *186,* 1203-10.

Tart, C. *Transpersonal psychologies.* New York: Harper & Row, 1975.

Tellegen, A. & Atkinson, G. Openness to absorbing and self-altering experiences . . .*Journal of Abnormal Psychology,* 1974, *83,* (3), 268-77.

Thomas, D. & Abbas, K.A. Comparison of transcendental meditation and progressive relaxation in reducing anxiety. *British Medical Journal,* 1978, *2,* (6154), 1749.

Thoresen, C.E. & Mahoney, J.J. *Behavioral self-control.* New

York: Holt, Rinehart & Winston, 1974.

Thoresen, C. The intensive design: An intimate approach to counseling research. Paper presented at annual meeting of American Educational Research Association, 1972.

Timmons, B., Salamy, J., Kamiya, J., & Girton, D. Abdominal, thoracic respiratory movements and levels of arousal. *Psychonomic Science,* 1972, *27,* 173-175.

Travis, T., Kondo, C. & Knott, J. Subjective aspects of alpha enhancement. *British Journal of Psychiatry,* 1975, *127,* 122-6.

Travis, T., Kondo, C. & Knott, J. Heart rate, muscle tension, and alpha production of transcendental meditation and relaxation controls. *Biofeedback & self-regulation.* 1976, *1,* (4), 387-94.

Treichel, M., Clinch, N. & Cran, M. The metabolic effects of transcendental meditation. *The Physiologist,* 1973, *16,* 472. (Abstr.).

Truax, C.B. & Carkuff, R.R. *Toward effective counseling and psychotherapy.* Aldine: New York, 1967.

Tulpule, T. Yogic exercises in the management of ischaemic heart disease. *Indian Heart Journal,* 1971, *23,* 259-64.

Udupa, K.N., Singh, R.H. & Yadav, R.A. Certain studies on psychological and biochemical responses to the practice of Hatha Yoga in young normal volunteers. *Indian Journal of Medical Research,* 1973, *61,* 237-44.

Vahia, H.S., Doengaji, D.R., Jeste, D.V. et al. A deconditioning therapy based upon concepts of Patañjali. *International Journal of Social Psychiatry,* 1972, *18,* (1), 61-66.

Vahia, H.S., Doengaji, D.R., Jeste, D.V. et al. Psychophysiologic therapy based on the concepts of Patañjali. *American Journal of Psychotherapy,* 1973, *27,* 557-65.

VanNuys, D. Meditation, attention, and hypnotic susceptibility: A correlational study. *International Journal of Clinical & Experimental Hypnosis,* 1973, *21,* 59-69.·

VanNuys, D. A novel technique for studying attention during meditation. *Journal of Transpersonal Psychology,* 1971, *3,* (2), 125-34.

Wallace, R. The physiological effects of transcendental meditation. *Science,* 1970, *167,* 1751-4.

Wallace, R., Benson, H. & Wilson, A. A wakeful hypometabolic physiologic state. *American Journal of Physiology,* 1971, *221,* (3), 795-99.

Walrath, L. & Hamilton, D. Autonomic correlates of meditation and hypnosis. *American Journal of Clinical Hypnosis,* 1975, *17,* (3), 190-7.

Walsh, R. Initial meditative experiences: Part I. *Journal of Transpersonal Psychology,* 1977, *9,* (2), 151-92.

Walsh, R. Initial meditative experiences: Part II. *Journal of Transpersonal Psychology,* 1978, *10,* (1), 1-28.

Walsh, R. Behavioral sciences and the consciousness disciplines. *American Journal of Psychiatry,* in press.

Walsh, R. & Rauche, L. The precipitation of acute psychoses by intensive meditation in individuals with a history of schizophrenia. *American Journal of Psychiatry,* 1979, *138* (8), 1085-6.

Walsh, R. & Vaughan, F. *Beyond ego: Readings in transpersonal psychology.* Los Angeles: J.B. Traecher, in press.

Walsh, R. & Shapiro, D.H. (Eds.). *Beyond health and normality: Explorations of extreme psychological well-being.* New York: Van Nostrand, 1980, in press.

Washburn, M. Observations relevant to a unified theory of meditation. *Journal of Transpersonal Psychology,* 1978, *10,* (1), 45-66.

Watanabe, T., Shapiro, D. & Schwartz, G. Meditation as an anoxic state: A critical review and theory. *Psychophysiologia,* 1972, *9,* 279.

Watts, A. The sound of rain. *Playboy,* April 1972, 220.

Watts, A. *Psychotherapy east and west.* New York: Ballantine Books, 1961.

Weide, T. Varieties of transpersonal therapy. *Journal of Transpersonal Psychology,* 1973, *5,* (1), 7-14.

Weinpahl, P. *Matter of Zen.* New York: University Press, 1964.

Welwood, J. Meditation and the unconscious. *Journal of Transpersonal Psychology,* 1977, *9,* (1), 1-26.

Wenger, M. & Bagchi, B. Studies of autonomic functions in practitioners of Yoga in India. *Behavioral Science,* 1961, *6,* 312-23.

West, M.A. Physiological effects of meditation: A longitudinal study. *British Journal of Social and Clinical Psychology,* 1979, *18,* 219-226.

White, O. *A manual for the calculation and use of the median slope: A technique of progress estimation and prediction in the single case.* Working paper 16, University of Oregon, Eugene, 1972.

White, O. *The split middle: A quickie method of trend estima-tion.* Working paper 1, University of Oregon, Eugene, 1971.

Wilbur, K. *Spectrum of consciousness.* Wheaton, IL: Theosophical Publishing House, 1977.

Wilkins, W. Desensitization: Social and cognitive factors underlying the effectiveness of Wolpe's procedure. *Psychological Bulletin,* 1971, *76,* 311-317.

Wilkins, W. Expectancy effect vs. demand characteristics. *Behavior Therapy,* 1978, *9,* (3), 363-7.

Williams, L.R.T. Transcendental meditation and mirror tracing skills. *Perceptual and Motor Skills,* 1978, *46,* 371-378.

Williams, P. & West, M. EEG responses to photic stimulation in persons experienced at meditation. *Electroencephalography & Clinical Neurophysiology,* 1975, *39* (5), 519-22.

Witkin, H.A., Dyk, R.B., Fattuson, H.F., Goodenough, D.R., Kerp, S.A. *Psychological differentiation.* New York: Wiley, 1962.

Woolfolk, R. Psychophysiological correlates of meditation. *Archives of General Psychiatry,* 1975, *32,* (10), 1326-33.

Woolfolk, R. Self-control, meditation and the treatment of chronic anger. In Shapiro D.H. & Walsh, R.N. *The science of meditation.* Aldine: New York, 1980, in press.

Woolfolk, R., Carr-Kaffeshan, L., McNulty, T.F. Meditation training as a treatment for insomnia. *Behavior Therapy,* 1976, *7,* (3), 359-65.

Woolfolk, R. and Franks, C. Meditation and behavior therapy. In Shapiro, D.H. & Walsh, R.N. *The science of meditation,* New York: Aldine, 1980 in press.

Wolpe, J. *Psychotherapy by reciprocal inhibition.* Stanford, CA: Stanford University Press, 1958.

Wolpe, J. *The practice of behavior therapy.* New York: Pergamon Press, 1969.

Yalom, I., Bend, D., Bloch, S., Zimmerman, E., Friedman, L. The impact of a weekend group experience on individual therapy. *Archives of General Psychiatry,* 1977, *34,* 399-415.

Yamaoka, T. Psychological study of mental self-control. *Bulletin of the Faculty of Literature of Kyushu University,* 1974, *5,* 225-271.

Yamaoka, T. Psychological study of self control. In Y. Akishige (Ed.), *Psychological studies on Zen.* Tokyo: Zen Inst. of Komazawa University, 1973.

Yates, A. The experimental investigation of the single case. *Behavior Therapy.* New York: John Wiley & Sons, 1970.

Younger, J., Adrianne, W. & Berger, R. Sleep during transcendental meditation. *Perceptual & Motor Skills*, 1975, *40*, 953-4.

Yulis, S., Brahm, G., Charnes, G., Jacard, L.M., Piccta, E., & Retman, F. The extinction of phobic behavior as a function of attention shifts. *Behavior Research & Therapy*, 1975, *13*, 173-76.

Zaichkowsky, L.D. & Kamen, R. Biofeedback and meditation: Effects on muscle tension and locus of control. *Perceptual and Motor Skills*, 1978, *46*, 955-958.

Zifferblatt, S.M. & Hendricks, C.G. Applied behavioral analysis of societal problems. *American Psychologist*, 1974, *29*, (10), 750-61.

Zuroff, D. & Schwartz, J. Effects of TM and muscle relaxation on trait anxiety, maladjustment, locus of control, and drug use. *Journal of Consulting & Clinical Psychology*, 1978, *46*, (2), 264-71.

Author Index

Akishige, Y., 123, 150, 183, 231, 232, 234
Alcers, 31
Alexander, F., 6, 187
Allison, J., 150, 231
Allport, G., 16
Anand, B., 3, 13, 15, 16, 31, 33, 150, 183, 212, 217, 218, 230, 231, 249
Anderson, D., 141
Ashem, B., 172

Bagchi, B.K., 150, 224, 230, 231
Bandura, A., 4, 33, 40, 165, 166, 171, 184, 190, 210
Banquet, J.-P., 87, 150, 193, 230, 231, 234
Barber, T.X., 26, 57, 172, 238
Barlow, D.H., 172, 257
Beck, A.T., 184
Beiman, I.H., 30, 31, 33, 65, 156, 159
Bem, D., 237, 242
Beneke, W., 169
Bennett, J.E., 230, 246
Benson, H., 4, 12, 14, 20, 37, 141, 142, 143, 150, 151, 184, 209, 224, 229, 231, 233, 234, 237, 249
Bergin, A., 237

Berlyne, D.E., 38
Bernard, H., 169
Berwick, P., 2, 30, 135
Black, R., 211
Blanchard, E.G., 184, 237
Bloomfield, H., 183
Boals, G., 198
Bono, J., 2, 30, 33
Borkovec, T.D., 235, 239
Boss, M., 3
Boswell, P.C., 151, 156, 223, 239
Boudreau, L., 135, 139, 175, 184
Braushom, M., 66, 223
Brautigam, E., 141, 142, 143, 184
Breuer, J., 39, 82
Broden, M., 167
Brown, D.P., 20, 86, 95, 197, 212, 218, 233, 243, 244, 245, 249
Brown, F., 202
Bruner, J.S., 243, 246
Buber, M., 268

Cannon, W.B., 140
Capra, R., 212
Carrington, P., 2, 14, 45, 46, 47, 67, 248
Cattell, R.B., 30
Cautela, J.R., 128, 166, 172, 184, 236

Cauthen, N., 36, 86, 151, 152, 154
Chassen, J.B., 261
Clark, F.V., 3
Coates, T.J., 64
Cohen, W., 241
Cohen, Y., 142
Connor, W.H., 233
Conze, E., 14
Corby, J.C., 13, 87, 234
Curtis, W.D., 86, 151, 154, 160

Daniels, L., 135
Das, H., 13, 150, 230, 231, 232, 234
Datey, F., 143, 184, 232, 233
Davidson, J., 13, 25, 134, 154, 232, 233, 235, 246, 257, 261
Davidson, G.C., 58, 171, 172
Davidson, R., 12, 34, 36, 48, 66, 160, 163, 164, 198, 202, 210, 216, 217, 220, 223, 225, 229, 244, 259
Deathridge, G., 139
Deikman, A.J., 14, 16, 20, 87, 166 192, 204, 205, 212, 221, 230, 243, 257
Dillbeck, M., 135, 139
Dukes, W., 261

Ellis, A., 85, 172, 229, 236, 237
Elson, B., 154, 224

Faber, P.A., 205
Fadiman, J., 242
Fee, R.A., 232, 233
Fenwick, P.B., 153, 210, 231
Ferguson, P.C., 2, 139, 199
Ferster, C.B., 166, 169, 172
Festinger, L., 237
Fischer, R., 13, 189, 230, 233, 234, 247
Frank, J.D., 34, 187, 246
Franks, J., 6, 237
French, A.P., 2, 47, 48, 135, 205, 257, 259
Freud, S., 4, 38, 39, 43, 44, 45, 82
Fromm, E., 3, 15

Galanter, M., 230, 238

Galin, D., 165, 198, 223, 230, 246
Gellhorn, E., 232, 233
Giber, D., 134
Gilbert, G.S., 159
Girodo, E., 135, 139, 258
Glueck, B.C., 4, 19, 34, 37, 38, 69, 139, 140, 153, 158, 159, 163, 230, 231, 233, 258
Goldfried, M., 165, 173, 184
Goldiamond, I., 166
Goldman, B.L., 27, 36, 156, 239
Goldstein, J., 95
Goleman, D., 2, 3, 15, 20, 24, 41, 67, 86, 135, 139, 154, 171, 182, 197, 212, 217, 218, 223, 229, 230, 245, 247, 248, 249, 260
Gottmann, J., 261
Goyeche, J., 150, 230, 231
Graham. J., 202
Green, E., 233
Greenson, R., 39, 43, 45
Griffith, F., 257
Group for Advancement of Psychiatry Report 1977, 6
Gundu Rao, H.V., 3

Hager, J.L., 156
Hannum, J., 184
Hastings, A., 2
Heisenberg, W., 6
Hendricks, C.G., 229
Herbert, R., 198
Herrigel, E., 14, 24
Hess, W., 233
Hesse, H., 44
Hirai, T., 12, 13, 150, 164, 165, 177, 183, 184, 223, 231
Hjelle, L.A., 2, 135, 139, 199, 260
Homme, L.E., 85, 128, 166, 167, 172, 173
Honig, K., 261
Honsberger, R., 135, 257
Horowitz, M.J., 192
Huber, 85

Ikegami, R., 36, 214, 215, 216, 220, 225, 233, 239, 240

Jacks, R., 173, 184
Jacobs, A., 248
Jacobs, R.G., 143
Jacobson, E., 128, 166, 170, 177
James, W., 187
Jevning, R., 154
Johnson, S., 167
Johnson, W.G., 173
Jung, C., 3

Kanellakos, D.P., 183, 184
Kanas, N., 32, 34, 36, 87, 154, 192
Kanfer, F.H., 166, 167, 177, 182,
    183, 224
Kantor, R., 33
Kapleau, A., 123, 164, 221
Karambelkar, P., 150, 230, 231
Kasamatsu, A., 3, 15, 18, 36, 150,
    166, 183, 212, 217, 218, 223,
    231, 249
Katz, N.W., 26, 238
Kazdin, A.E., 128, 166, 167, 184
Keefe, T., 2, 45, 46
Kirsch, I., 156, 157, 159, 182, 239,
    260
Kolb, D.A., 167
Kohr, E., 2, 20, 87, 88, 189, 193,
    195, 196, 205, 237
Kondo, A., 139
Kornfield, J., 87, 192, 234
Kretschmer, W., 15
Kubose, S.K., 27, 87, 193, 223,
    246
Kuhn, T., 4, 5

Lachenmeyer, C.W., 261
Lang, 235
Lao-tsu, 6
Lazar, Z., 139, 141, 142, 257
Lazarus, A.A., 2, 40, 47, 48, 79,
    236, 248
Lefcourt, H.M., 177
Lesh, T., 2, 31, 46, 87, 177, 184,
    191, 192, 202, 204, 230, 257,
    259
Leung, P., 46, 202, 204, 223

Linden, W., 135, 139, 184, 202,
    222, 244, 246
Lykken, D., 259

McFall, R.M., 167, 212, 257
McReynolds, W.T., 42, 46
Mahoney, M.H., 85, 128, 165, 167,
    169, 171, 172, 173, 183, 184,
    214, 236
Malec, J., 26, 230, 238, 239, 240,
    260
Marcus, J.B., 141, 257
Marlatt, G.A., 19, 37, 86, 156, 231
Maslow, A., 4, 41
Matsumoto, H., 182, 224
Maupin, E., 20, 27, 30, 31, 33, 87,
    164, 191, 192, 198, 204, 221,
    230, 257
Meichenbaum, D., 15, 85, 120,
    128, 166, 172, 173, 177, 184,
    229, 236, 237
Michaels, R., 153
Miller, N., 3, 172
Minuchin, S., 210
Mischel, W., 35, 183, 241, 267
Mitchell, K., 261
Mookerjee, A., 183
Mooney, R.L., 195
Morse, D.R., 36, 86, 151, 152, 153,
    154, 159, 160, 233, 242
Muchlmaner, M., 151

Nakamizo, S., 182, 224, 232
Naranjo, C., 13, 15
Nidich, S., 2, 27, 199, 257

Onda, A., 164
Orme-Johnson, D.W., 150, 151,
    231, 234
Orne, M.T., 42, 88, 190, 230, 237
Ornstein, R., 3, 230, 241, 246
Osis, K., 2, 6, 20, 87, 88, 189, 193,
    194, 195, 196, 204, 205
Otis, L.S., 29, 32, 34, 47, 135, 183,
    199, 248, 257

Pagano, R., 153, 154, 210, 230,
    246
Parker, J.C., 156

Patel, C., 143, 258
Paul, G., 15, 177
Pelletier, K., 33, 34, 202, 222, 246
Piaget, J.,247
Piggins, D., 229
Pirot, M., 202
Polanyi, M., 5
Pollack, A.A., 143
Pomerleau, O.F., 41
Premack, D., 173, 176
Pribram, K., 13, 218, 249

Rahula, W., 19, 128, 166
Rao, S., 231
Rodgers, C.R., 40, 43, 58, 82
Rosenthal, R., 88, 190
Rotter, J.B., 29, 31, 177

Sargent, W., 235
Schuster, R., 2, 45, 46
Schwartz, G.E., 2, 35, 41, 65, 219,
    220, 224, 230, 234, 235, 247
Seeman, W., 2, 27, 199
Selye, H., 140
Shafii, M., 2, 141, 142, 257
Shapiro, D., 3, 146, 169, 172
Shapiro, D.H. , 1, 2, 3, 16, 19, 22,
    23, 25, 35, 48, 65, 81, 85, 90,
    128, 129, 133, 134, 135, 141,
    142, 143, 150, 154, 164, 175,
    176, 177, 183, 184, 189, 199,
    210, 214, 229, 237, 241, 248,
    260
Shaw, R., 202
Sidman, M., 261
Singer, J.L., 15, 183, 184, 198,
    202, 230, 236
Skinner, B.F., 40, 172, 210
Smith, H., 187
Smith, J.C., 26, 29, 30, 31, 33, 37,
    38, 65, 66, 134, 135, 139, 150
    157, 160, 214, 219, 220, 223,
    230, 238, 239, 240, 243, 244,
    245, 257, 260
Solomon, G.G., 164
Spanos, P.H., 230
Sperry, R., 246
Spiegelberg, F., 166, 183
Stace, W.T., 187

Stek, R., 29, 259
Stone, R., 143
Stoyva, J., 172
Stroebel, C.F., 2, 28, 36, 47, 48,
    219
Stuart, R.B., 169
Stunkard, A., 169
Sugi, Y., 150, 231
Suinn, R., 173
Surwit, R.S., 157
Suzuki, D.T., 3, 5, 6, 165

Tart, C., 3, 5, 15, 85, 87, 88, 160,
    188, 190, 197, 261
Tellegan, A., 217, 223, 244
Thomas, P., 156
Thoresen, C.E., 166, 169, 171, 261
Timmons, B., 126, 182, 224, 232
Travis, T., 86, 152, 154
Treichel, M., 150, 231
Truax, C.B., 43, 58
Tulpule, T., 135

Udupa, K.N., 1, 202

Vahia, H.S., 1, 2, 33, 82, 135, 139,
    140, 158, 159, 217, 231, 257
Van Nuys, D., 47, 87, 124, 176,
    193, 198, 221, 223, 246

Wallace, R., 13, 20, 150, 151, 152,
    153, 184, 230, 231, 234
Walrath, L., 151, 154
Walsh, R., 3, 4, 33, 47, 49, 87, 88,
    134, 197, 230, 236, 259
Washburn, M., 244, 245
Watanabe, T., 12, 150, 210, 229,
    231
Watts, A., 43, 168
Weide, T., 3
Weinpahl, P., 128, 164
Welwood, J., 244
Wenger, M., 3, 150, 230, 231
West, M.A., 219
White, O., 261
Wilbur, K., 5
Wilkins, W., 171, 239, 248
Williams, L.R.T., 202
Williams, P., 150, 223, 231

Witkin, H.A., 222
Wolpe, J., 40, 82, 128, 129,
    170, 171, 173, 249
Woolfolk, R., 2, 34, 64, 134,
    135, 139, 159, 163, 182, 242,
    260

Yalom, I., 48, 248

Yamaoka, T., 183
Yates, A., 261
Young, J., 154
Yulis, S., 171, 183, 224, 248

Zaichkowsky, L.D., 233
Zifferblatt, S.M., 165

Subject Index

Abhidamna, 20, 86
addiction, 2, 8, 10, 134, 141, 142, 210, 257
affectothymia, 31
alcohol abuse, 142, 231
alcoholism, 140, 172
  and anxiety, 156
Altered State of Conciousness (ASC) 3, 6, 8, 10, 24-27, 31, 47, 85, 120, 126, 187-205, 235, 238, 249, 254, 256, 261, 262
  definition, 188
  and inebriation, 189, 190
  and manic depression, 190
  as schizophrenia, 188
amphetamines, 142
anaerobic state, 12
anger, 128, 130, 175, 260
animal studies, 172
anxiety, 2, 7, 23, 30, 31, 34, 47, 65, 66, 70, 73, 78, 123, 129, 130, 139, 156, 159, 184, 258, 260
arousal, 219, 233, 235
assertiveness training, 48, 80, 84
attention focus, 9, 216-224
Autia, 30
autogenic training, 37, 140, 164, 177

awareness, 128, 165, 166
  (see also Altered States of Conciousness)

basal skin resistance, 154, 231
behavioral changes, 85
behavioral medicine, 2, 39, 40, 41
behavioral programming, 171, 172, 173
belief system, 42, 254
Bendig Anxiety Scale, 139
Benson's Method Relaxation Response, 156
Bhagavad Gita, 126
biofeedback, 37, 48, 66, 120, 140, 143, 156, 159, 172, 176
blood plasma, 153
blood pressure, 26, 134, 143, 231
body Sensations, 109, 110
body control, 3, 120
boredom, 47
brain hemispheres, 235, 249
  (see also split brain research)
brainwaves, 121, 123
  (see also EEG)
breathing, 12, 20-23, 72, 88, 89, 94, 98, 121-130, 135, 183, 204, 224, 225, 232
  and thought intrusion, 88, 97, 98, 99, 100, 101, 102, 103,

112, 117, 123, 124
breath meditation, 67, 81, 90, 93, 120, 123, 128, 143
bronchial asthma, 135, 258
Buddha, 50
Buddhaghosa, 86
Buddhism, 14

Catholicism, 59
chanting, 109, 183
clinical orientation, 56
cognitive focusing, 183, 261
companionship, 78, 79, 82
conscience, 139
Control procedures, 134, 142, 260, 262
cortically mediated stabilization (CMS), 219
counting, 67, 71, 72, 89, 94, 116, 117, 123, 124, 130, 232
cults, 58, 121

data gathering, 94, 134, 135, 192-197, 258, 262, 263
in Altered State of Conciousness Study, 191
in drug use studies, 142
demand characteristics, 87, 88, 237-243, 256, 258
in Altered State of Conciousness Study, 190, 205
in drug use studies, 142
depression, 1, 47, 48
diet, 60
dream analysis, 59
dreaming, 205, 242
dropouts, 28, 29, 34, 35, 36, 248
drowsiness, 46
drug use, 140-142, 184, 237
(see also addiction)

Eastern philosophy, 3, 50
Ego, 38, 40, 41, 42
Electroencephalograph (EEG) activity, 17, 32, 87, 134, 152, 153, 154, 220, 225, 232, 234
Alpha activity, 17, 18, 31, 123, 150, 231, 241, 243, 246
Beta activity, 243, 246

Electromyogram (EMG), 152, 153, 214
and migraine headaches, 233
Embedded Figure Test, 264
employment, 60, 81
Ergotropic State, 233, 234, 235, 242
Existentialism, 3
expectation effects, 87, 256, 257, 258
experimenter bias, 88, 113, 114, 190,

face tension, 68
Fear Survey Schedule, 31
fears, 1, 64, 78, 135, 173, 175, 177, 247, 260
Fitzgerald Experience Inquiry, 31
fixed concentration, 18
follow-up, 134, 143, 263
formal meditation, 90, 124, 126, 127, 128, 130, 170, 174, 175, 176, 177, 270
Frau Elizabeth Von R., 44
Freudian psychoanalysis, 38
frontalis EMG, 239
frontalis muscle tension, 233

galvanic skin response (GSR), 151, 152, 153

hashish, 142
habit, 133
hallucinations, 121, 242
Hatha Yoga, 13
(see yoga)
heart attack, 135
heart beat, 69, 129, 183
heart rate, 121, 134, 139, 150, 230
Heroin addicts, 23, 176
holistic medicine, 2, 38, 40
humanistic psychology, 38, 39, 40
humanistic psychotherapy, 2
hyperactive children, 48
hypertension, 8, 10, 134, 143, 156, 177, 184, 210, 231, 258
hypertensives, 48
hyperventilation, 232
hypnotic subjects, 222

hypnotic trance, 205

ideal self, 2
informal meditation, 83, 91, 124,
    128, 129, 130
India, 3
insomnia, 58, 59, 64, 65, 69, 72,
    84, 139, 258
Internal-External Locus of Control
    Scale, 31
Interruption of Sequence and
    Competing Response, 129

Japanese martial arts, 121
Jhānas, 20

Kensho, 24
Koan, 15, 16, 67

Lazarus' Inner circle, 79
loneliness, 69
lotus positions, 18, 122, 123, 214,
    215, 233
lowered awareness, 115
LSD, 142

Mahamudra, 86, 95, 268
maladaptive behavior, 129
Malnak vs. Yogi, 121
Mandalas, 66, 183
Mantras, 17, 18, 66, 67, 219
marijuana, 141, 142
Maupin's five point scale, 191
meditation,
    adherence, 7, 9, 35-38, 66, 89,
        90, 91, 127, 214, 225, 257
    adverse effects, 2, 10, 32, 33, 47-
        51
    Benson meditation, 233
    Bhakti, 224
    Christian, 15, 16, 183
    components, 209-225, 254
    and concentration, 217
    concentrative meditation, 15,
        46, 48, 50, 67, 143, 183, 204,
        245, 246, 249
    contraindications, 47, 64
    definition, 12-15
    Gurdjiefian, 220, 245

instructions, 120, 122-25
mirror meditation, 90
mindful meditation, 15, 17, 50,
    67, 90, 115, 127, 218, 244,
    245, 249
negative experiences, 47, 48, 49,
    50
neurophysological difference be-
    tween styles, 218
and physiological changes, 150,
    218, 249
position or posture, (see also
    Lotus position) 122, 124,
    214-216, 225, 283
practice, 35-38, 66, 68, 72, 89,
    91, 125, 130, 254, 257
prior experience, 7, 9, 164
process, 123
psychoanalytic theory, 39
resistance to, 10, 44, 45
setting, 93, 116, 122, 124, 169,
    170, 211, 212, 214
teaching, 1, 7, 8, 10, 38-51, 66,
    220, 254
techniques, 10-15, 42, 66
trancendent qualities, 7, 47
visionary experiences, 7
levels, 8, 10
metabolic changes, 153
migraine headaches, 48, 177, 233
Minnesota Multiple Personality
Index (MMPI), 32, 140
muscle tension, 219
myocardial infarct, 135

neurosis, 1, 140
Nirvana, 24

obesity, 169, 177
Opiates, 142
orgasm, 235
Oxygen Consumption, 134, 150,
    210, 229, 230, 248

Patañjali graded exercises, 139,
    140
Periodic Somatic Inactivity, (PSI)
    219, 220, 240
Personal Orientation Inventory

(POI), 27, 29
phasic skin conductance, 139
phobias, 1, 23, 82, 135, 247
phosphorous imbalance, 60
physiological responses, 134, 151,
    152, 153, 230, 248
praxernia, 30
psychedelic drugs, 121
psychiatric patients, 28, 47, 139,
    140, 257
psychoanalysis, 3, 45
psychoneuroses, 140
psychosomatic complaints, 1, 140
Psychotics, 47, 258, 259
Psychotherapy, 30, 139, 231, 237
Psychotic breaks, 33

Rāja - Yogins, 15, 16, 17, 18, 31,
    218
Rapid Eye Movement (REM)
    sleep, 235
Raynaud's Disease, 48
relaxation, 12, 26, 27, 37, 48, 64,
    66, 81, 116, 121, 130, 143,
    173, 209, 229
    and systematic desensitization,
        17, 170, 171, 248
relaxation technique, 65, 128, 143
religion, 5, 42, 122, 238, 242
religious orientation, 56
repressed material, 2, 39
respiration, 152, 239
    (see also breathing)
retrospective content analysis, 87
retrospective self-reports, 141
    (see also self-reports)
role playing, 79, 84
resistance, 10, 44
Rotter Internal/External Locus of
    Control Scale, 29, 31
Rorschach test, 31, 50, 140
running, 164

Samadhi, 24, 242
Sammurai warriors, 121
Satori, 24
schizophrenic, 33, 140
schizothymia, 30

self concept, 30, 45
self control, 133
self-criticism, 30, 49, 50, 60, 63,
    65
self-hypnosis, 57, 177
self-instruction, 70, 81, 128, 229
self-management, 167, 168, 169,
    175
self-observation, 166, 167, 168,
    182
self-regulation, 2, 4, 8, 10, 25, 26,
    35, 41, 57, 60, 70, 71, 83, 85,
    86, 117, 120, 122, 133, 134,
    249, 253, 256, 260
self reports, 88, 135, 172, 198,
    202, 259
    in altered State of Conciousness
        Studies, 198
    in drug use study, 142, 237
    in meditation study, 88
self-statements, 109, 110, 113
sexual behavior, 172
shyness, 59, 60, 65
skeletal muscular relaxation, 229,
    232, 248
skin response, 134
    (see also basal skin resistance)
sleep, 61, 62, 72, 73,
    (see also in insomnia)
sleepiness, 22
sleep onset, 139
smoking, 172, 176, 184
social interaction, 62, 69, 84
Speigelberger's State-Trait Anxi-
    ety Inventory, (STAI), 31, 37,
    139
split brain research, 165, 246
    (see also brain hemispheres)
Stimulus Control, 169
stress, 1, 10, 26, 57, 59, 60, 63, 66,
    81, 128, 134, 135, 139, 177,
    210, 256
    pharmacological treatment, 41
stress management, 8, 57, 184
stress reduction, 139
study skills, 169
Subjects, 27, 28, 197, 220, 254,
    258, 259
    belief system, 89, 91

journal entries, 92, 93, 113, 116
meditation experience, 134
Subject background, 89, 90
Subject motivation, 89, 91, 141,
258
in drug use studies, 142
Subject profile, 28-35, 58-63, 114-
115
subject selection, 134, 258
sample bias in drug use experiment, 141
in Self-Regulation Comparisons
Study, 151-152
substance abuse, 1
(see addictions)
Subi whirling dervish, 13, 183, 234
Sullivanian Interpersonal Theory,
3

Tai Chi, 13
Taoism, 15, 16, 183
taped instruction, 68, 71, 93, 119,
120
target behavior (TB), 128
Tassajara, 267
Taylor's Manifest Anxiety Scale,
135, 140
Tellegan Absorption Scale, 217,
244
Tennessee Psychosis Scale, 30, 34
Tennessee Self Concept Scale
(TSCS), 30
Tennessee Self-Criticism Scale, 30
tension, 128, 129, 135, 173, 175,
177
Test Anxiety Scale for Children,
139
therapists, 45, 46, 119
therapist contact, 134
therapy duration, 58
third eye, 16
thought coding, 89, 95, 106, 107,
108, 109, 110, 111, 112

Thought Coding Instrument, 96,
113, 117
thought intrusion, 87-97, 104-106,
108, 114, 221, 236
thought stopping, 128, 129, 171
Trancendental Meditation (TM), 4,
13, 18, 27, 29, 30, 31, 33, 36,
87, 119, 121, 134, 140, 159,
183, 197, 218, 219, 220, 224,
233, 240, 257
and Alpha rhythm, 152
and drug use, 141
transference, 43, 45
Transpersonal meditation, 41
transpersonal psychology, 39
transpersonal psychotherapy, 3
trophotropic state, 233, 234, 242,
248,
(see also relaxation response)

Urinalysis, 142

Valium, 59, 61, 72, 73, 78, 81
Vipassana, 13, 14, 18, 95, 117, 245
Visuddhimagga, 86

walking meditation, 126
weight reduction, 184
withdrawal symptoms, 143
Witkin Embedded Figure Test,
222
wrist counter, 124, 130, 135, 176

Yoga, 4, 13, 120, 134, 140, 258
Yoga Masters, 120
Yogin Cakra, 15

Zen, 13, 14, 18, 20, 28, 90, 93, 127,
129, 168, 171, 221, 245
Zen breath meditaion (zazen), 120
164, 232, 239
Zen Masters, 15, 22, 43, 120, 123

Milton Keynes UK
Ingram Content Group UK Ltd.
UKHW040013071024
449327UK00011B/214